DATE DUE

Management of Persons with Chronic Neurologic Illness

Management of Persons with Chronic Neurologic Illness

Mark N. Ozer, M.D.

Professor, Department of Neurology, Georgetown University School of Medicine, Washington; Director, Program for Clinical Excellence, National Rehabilitation Hospital, Washington

Foreword by
Kenneth M. Viste, Jr., M.D.

Clinical Professor of Neurology, University of Wisconsin Medical School, Madison; Medical Director, Physical Rehabilitation Unit, Mercy Medical Center, Oshkosh; Medical Director, Physical Rehabilitation Unit, St. Agnes Hospital, Fond du Lac

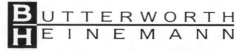

BUTTERWORTH HEINEMANN

Boston • Oxford • Auckland • Johannesburg • Melbourne • New Delhi

Every effort has been made to ensure that the drug dosage schedules within this text are accurate and conform to standards accepted at time of publication. However, as treatment recommendations vary in the light of continuing research and clinical experience, the reader is advised to verify drug dosage schedules herein with information found on product information sheets. This is especially true in cases of new or infrequently used drugs.

Recognizing the importance of preserving what has been written, Butterworth–Heinemann prints its books on acid-free paper whenever possible.

 Butterworth–Heinemann supports the efforts of American Forests and the Global ReLeaf program in its campaign for the betterment of trees, forests, and our environment.

Library of Congress Cataloging-in-Publication Data
Ozer, Mark N.
  Management of persons with chronic neurologic illness / Mark N. Ozer ; foreword by
Kenneth M. Viste, Jr.
       p. ; cm.
  Includes bibliographical references and index.
  ISBN 0-7506-7005-3 (alk. paper)
    1. Nervous system--Diseases. 2. Chronic diseases. 3. Nervous
system--Diseases--Patients--Rehabilitation. I. Title.
    [DNLM: 1. Central Nervous System Diseases--diagnosis. 2. Central Nervous System
Diseases--rehabilitation. 3. Chronic Disease--rehabilitation. WL 300 O99m 2000]
  RC346 .O99 2000
  616.8--dc21
                                                                99-053895

British Library Cataloguing-in-Publication Data
A catalogue record for this book is available from the British Library.

The publisher offers special discounts on bulk orders of this book.
For information, please contact:
Manager of Special Sales
Butterworth–Heinemann
225 Wildwood Avenue
Woburn, MA 01801-2041
Tel: 781-904-2500
Fax: 781-904-2620

For information on all B-H medical publications available, contact our World Wide Web home page at:
http://www.bh.com

10 9 8 7 6 5 4 3 2 1

Printed in the United States of America

To Sam and Max

Contents

Contributing Authors

Pamela H. Ballard, M.D.
Assistant Director, Spinal Cord Injury Program, Department of Medical Affairs, National Rehabilitation Hospital, Washington

Allan L. Bernstein, M.D.
Associate Professor of Clinical Neurology, University of California, Davis, School of Medicine, Davis; Chief of Neurology, Kaiser-Permanente Medical Center, Santa Rosa

Robert D. Gerwin, M.D.
Assistant Professor of Neurology, Johns Hopkins University School of Medicine, Baltimore; Active Staff, Department of Medicine, Washington Adventist Hospital, Takoma Park, Maryland

Robert J. Gumnit, M.D.
Clinical Professor of Neurology, Neurosurgery, and Pharmacy, University of Minnesota Medical School—Minneapolis; President, MINCEP Epilepsy Care, Minneapolis

Lauren B. Krupp, M.D.
Associate Professor of Neurology and Co-Director of the Comprehensive Multiple Sclerosis Care Center, State University of New York at Stony Brook School of Medicine Health Sciences Center

Andrew D. McCarthy, M.D.
Medical Director, Brain Injury Program, National Rehabilitation Hospital, Washington

Susan M. Miller, M.D.
Assistant Professor of Neurology, George Washington University School of Medicine and Columbian College School of Arts and Sciences, Washington; Director of Residency Training Program and Assistant Medical Director, National Rehabilitation Hospital, Washington

Kenneth J. Ottenbacher, Ph.D.
Professor and Vice Dean, School of Allied Health Sciences, University of Texas Medical School at Galveston

Mark N. Ozer, M.D.
Professor, Department of Neurology, Georgetown University School of Medicine, Washington; Director, Program for Clinical Excellence, National Rehabilitation Hospital, Washington

Jonathan H. Pincus, M.D.
Professor of Neurology and Chairman Emeritus, Georgetown University School of Medicine, Washington; Attending, Department of Neurology, Georgetown University Hospital, Washington

Foreword

Persons with chronic disease represent an increasingly large component of our population. People can now live long lives with their diseases, and, thus, the goal for physicians should be to "add life to the person's years." The management of persons with chronic neurologic disease should reduce the amount of "illness" or disruption of life the person experiences as a result of the neurologic disease. Major opportunities exist to improve the quality of medical care. The days of making a diagnosis without concern for the ongoing life of the person experiencing the disease have passed.

This book provides a blueprint for such ongoing continuity and enhancement of care. It emphasizes the principles of quality medical care and illustrates their application to a variety of neurologic illnesses. The concept of *principal care* must be brought to these complex illnesses. The themes include not only continuity of care but also comprehensive care—dealing with the disease, the person, and the setting in which the person lives. Comprehensive care provides a needed addition to the character of the management of illness through its emphasis on expanding and enhancing the role of the patient and family as the primary participants in the planning and evaluation of treatment. Their involvement in the review and revision of disease management can make medical care more responsive to the need to control costs while making treatment more responsive to the needs of the patients and families involved. It is gratifying that it is possible to meet the requirements of one by emphasizing the other.

I recommend this book to physicians of every specialty who come into contact with persons with chronic neurologic problems to help them meet the demands for quality and compassion—the twin goals guiding the future of American medical care.

Kenneth M. Viste, Jr.

Preface

The management of persons with chronic neurologic illness requires change in the character of patient care from that of neurologic disease. For example, diagnostic issues based on anatomic localization are less prominent. In general, the need for anatomic diagnosis was based on a focus on treatment of neurologic disease. Although breakthroughs in the management of the disease process have occurred, such as in Parkinson's disease and, more recently, in stroke, major efforts continue to be focused on the management of the person with functional limitations or illness that can interfere with the ongoing life of the person with neurologic disease. Knowledge of the natural history of the disease process remains important; however, it is also important to assess the environment in which the person with the disease functions. The character of patient care must focus on the ongoing management of the ways in which one's life is affected. The goal is to "add life to years"—that is, to reduce the degree of disability.

Because the goals are different, the methods must also differ. Health care can be considered an ongoing planning and review process. The product of such interactions is a treatment plan that is subject to ongoing review and revision. The methods by which this can be done generally require an ongoing rather than episodic form of care. In addition to continuity, it is necessary to consider that the needs of persons with disability cannot be met by medical treatment alone or by the patient alone. The problems affect the ability of the person to function within the family and the larger community. A need exists for a more comprehensive approach that may require a team of professionals to deal with the problem.

The question has been asked as to the "added value" that accrues by such ongoing interaction over time and in the context of more complex systems. Disabled persons consume a relatively large portion of health resources. Changes must be made to reduce the costs and the utilization of such care. In addition to continuity of care and comprehensive care, a need exists for greater sharing in management. Attention must be paid in particular to the relationship between the patient and/or family and the health professional(s). The professional must reconcile him- or herself to this new goal of *care* rather than *cure*. The professional also should consider that he or she gains by enabling the patient to contribute to the management rather than taking on the full responsibility of management. One shift can be toward more conjoint or collaborative care. The person with chronic illness and/or the caregiver can be empowered to develop management skills with the result being a greater degree of self-management. The interaction between the health professionals and the primary participants is a more consultative one with this new focus on education.

Because the person with disabilities is now a member of the planning/treatment team, a need and an opportunity exist for that person to help define his or her problems in the context of his or her own life and to identify meaningful goals. The opportunity also exists to clarify the methods by which one can improve results. In these various ways, by the ideas contributed and through the very process of making such contributions, the likelihood is greater that the person with chronic illness will commit energy to accomplishing the plans that are made. Enhancing the degree of participation in the development and ongoing review of one's health plan can lead to a greater degree of participation in the implementation of those plans with improved results.

This shift in focus can be illustrated in a range of chronic disease processes affecting the nervous system. Each will vary in terms of its character. Some are progressive, others are less so but are intermittent in their effects, and others have a sudden onset with long-lasting residual impairment. Diseases may also differ in terms of the parts of the nervous system affected. One must be cognizant not only of the disease process but also of the people in whom the diseases occur. For example, the frequency of spinal cord injury and head injury in young men has major implications for the type of disability and the appropriate treatment plans. The distribution of stroke over a wide range of adults, including those of working age as well as the more elderly, has different implications. It is the interaction between the disease and the person affected that is illustrated in each of the several chapters. The underlying principles of patient care remain the same.

The book is divided into two sections. The first section deals with principles, the second with the application of those principles to the various disease areas. The three chapters in the first section form the guidelines for the structure of the chapters in the Applications section. In the first section, for example, there is a generic approach to the "Nature of the Problem" in management of chronic neurologic illness, a generic approach to the "Character of the Solution," and a generic approach to the "Measurement of Effectiveness." These same three aspects are repeated throughout each of the chapters in the second section. Each of the specific entities discussed in the second section was selected because of its significance as a major cause of disability and health care service use. I recommend reading the first three chapters before beginning any of the chapters in the second section.

The format in each of the chapters in the Applications section illustrates the overall planning process that is generally carried out in the individual case. The first step in dealing with an individual with a disease entity is to define the problem. The next step is to carry out a planning process that exemplifies the principles of continuity and comprehensiveness while also collaborating with the patient and/or family. This must be joined with an ongoing evaluation of effectiveness intrinsic to the clinical efforts. A description of the various evaluation measures used with specific problems is presented, along with a critical assessment of each. Some are more generic and widely used, whereas others are more specific to a particular disease entity.

In some instances, the chapters in the Applications section describe protocols developed to exemplify these attributes. When protocols are not available, case reports are used to illustrate the application of these principles. Selected references are provided as a basis for further reading without attempting to be exhaustive of the available literature.

The order of the chapters in the second section reflects the application of principles of neurologic rehabilitation practice. The first three chapters deal with stroke, spinal cord injury, and head injury, with focus on the preparation of the client for continuing care in community life. These are the prototypical problems associated with in-patient training to deal with the effects of sudden impairment. The subsequent chapters illustrate the application of rehabilitation principles to the management of chronic neurologic illness. Chapters 7–9 deal with progressive illness associated with neuromuscular diseases, demyelinating disease, and Parkinson's disease. These all require ongoing modification of treatment plans in response to the character of the disease process. Chapters 10–12 describe the application to generally less progressive but still disabling disease processes such as seizures, chronic pain, and headache.

This book is designed to be used by practicing physicians who would have occasion to treat persons with chronic neurologic illness. This can include, in some instances, the internist or gerontologist or specialists such as neurologists or physiatrists who are also interested in providing primary or principal care to persons with these illnesses. This book can be particularly useful for physicians training in these fields or others interested in re-examining their practice styles. All physicians, regardless of specialty, may consider the implications of this approach to systems such as cardiac, pulmonary, and rheumatic, which now form the ever-larger part of overall medical practice.

Mark N. Ozer

Acknowledgments

This book represents the efforts over many years to bring the principles of patient care to the management of persons with a wide range of neurologic illnesses. It is impossible to mention all the various influences over my entire career that have brought me to bring about this synthesis. My work with children and their families in their ongoing efforts to cope with the difficulties of developmental disorders provided the opportunity at the Children's Hospital National Medical Center in Washington, to develop what was a truly interdisciplinary approach to this set of problems. It became increasingly clear that the results of treatment were not only in the hands of professional staff regardless of their specialty. The energy and skill needed were ultimately from those who were most directly involved with the problems. In this case, they were the parents and the teachers in the school and the child. The role of the professional must be to enhance the energy and skill of these primary participants.

After developing a model of community-based treatment with focus on the primary participants, I then applied these principles to persons with spinal cord injury in the Veterans Administration and more specifically at the McGuire Medical Center in Richmond, Virginia, where systems for care were available over the lifetime of persons with impairment caused by spinal cord injury. Further application with persons with stroke permitted the integration of these approaches within a receptive clinical setting with physiatric colleagues at the National Rehabilitation Hospital in Washington.

My aim in this book is to widen the scope of application to the full range of neurologic illness. The opportunity to do this is the result of encouragement from a number of neurologists, as well as physiatrists who have welcomed this concept of management over the life of the person. Particular credit must go to Dr. Roger Rosenberg and Dr. Kenneth M. Viste, Jr., from the American Academy of Neurology who provided support at crucial times. The residents in training within the Department of Neurology at the Washington Veterans Medical Center and the Georgetown University School of Medicine program provided a critical but important audience.

I particularly appreciate the support I have received over the past few years from the staff and administration of the National Rehabilitation Hospital. The entire staff of the Stroke Recovery Program and the physicians who have been my colleagues there, Dr. Fatemah Milani and Dr. Brendan Conroy, have provided a living laboratory for the implementation of this model. I also have been encouraged by the further efforts of the staff to implement this model over the range of illnesses cared for in several programs at the National Rehabilitation Hospital as reflected in the various chapters of this book written by colleagues there. The actual production of the book has been possible only because of its support over the past several years from Dr. John Toerge, who serves as Medical Director, and Mr. Edward Eckenhoff, whose vision in founding the hospital still directs its work.

Part I
Principles

Chapter 1
Nature of the Problem

Mark N. Ozer

Extent of the Problem

Prevalence of Disabilities

The most recent United States census (1990) provides estimates of disability. *Disability* is defined as any limitation in outside mobility (difficulty in going outside the home alone) or self-care (difficulty in caring for personal needs, such as bathing, dressing, or getting around inside the home). In addition, there is an estimate of *work disability*, which is defined as inability to perform work that results from a physical, mental, or other health condition of 6 months' duration or longer. Categories are *nonsevere*, defined as limitation in the type or amount of work a person can perform, with *severe* defined as the inability to perform work of any type.

In 1990, 13 million persons older than 16 years of age had some mobility or self-care disability. The overall incidence of mobility disability was 43 in 1,000, with 22 in 1,000 in the working-aged population (ages 16–64 years) and 155 in 1,000 in those older than 65 years. For self-care, the overall incidence was 48 in 1,000, with 34 in 1,000 in the younger group and 120 in 1,000 in those older than 65 years. In general, 6 million of those older than 65 years had one or the other disability, and 30% (approximately 1.8 million) had both.[1] Thus, a substantial proportion of persons in the United States have mobility or self-care disabilities. Although the incidence is higher in the elderly, the total prevalence is high even for those in the working-aged population, with some 7 million in that group. The

overall incidence of self-care disability is higher than for mobility. It is noteworthy, however, that mobility problems are particularly important in the older age group, with approximately 25% greater incidence than self-care disability. The elderly group with both types of disability is considered to be particularly needy.

In 1990, approximately 13 million persons of those aged 16–64 years had a work disability. Slightly more than one-half had a severe work disability, indicating inability to perform work of any type.[2] It appears from the data presented that approximately twice as many persons in the working-aged group have problems in work than have the other, perhaps more serious, measures of disability. Cost of such work disability has been estimated as approximately $110 billion per year in direct and indirect medical costs and lost wages. The total effect of disability on work is underestimated by virtue of the definition of greater than 6 months' duration. Ongoing intermittent work disability is not reported.

In general, increases in disability of various kinds over the years have coincided with the reduction in age-specific mortality in the United States. It can be expected that the total numbers of disabled persons, as well as the incidence of disability, will continue to increase as the population continues to age. It is anticipated that, using the Census Bureau "middle mortality" projections, the numbers of persons older than 65 years will rise to 52 million by 2020.[3]

More in-depth studies were carried out in the 1991–1992 Survey of Income and Program Participation (SIPP). This is an ongoing nationally representative survey of the noninstitutionalized U.S. population focused on economic status, income transfers, and service programs. It defines disability as "limitation in a functional activity or in a socially defined role or task," which is broader than the definition used by the Census Bureau, described previously. An overall rate of severe disability, defined as "inability to perform a functional activity or role," is estimated to occur in approximately 10%.[4] In the working-aged population, the rate for blacks was 20% greater than for the total population. The figure for whites was approximately 25% lower than the average. The import of this study is its recognition that disability is related to some degree to economic status and educational level.

A parallel rise has occurred in the numbers who require personal assistance as a measure of rather severe disability.[5] In a study carried out in 1991–1992 by SIPP, it was found that approximately 7 million adults (15 years or older) have difficulty in carrying out activities of daily living (ADL), such as bathing, dressing, using the toilet, or transferring from bed to chair.[5] The largest number (2.7 million) need help with bathing, with lesser numbers (2 million each) needing assistance with dressing and transferring. The primary source of help is family members (82%), with spouses providing the largest percentage (38%), daughters next (20%), and other relatives (including sons) providing 20%. Approximately 9% have paid attendant care. Providing personal assistance for the disabled individual, whether paid or unpaid, creates an important burden.

Major efforts need to be expended to reduce the degree of disability, with its attendant overall costs as well as burden on the population. One of the national health objectives for the year 2000 has been to increase the span of healthy life for persons in the United States and to reduce the proportion of persons who experience disability from chronic conditions to a maximum of 8% (from a baseline of 9.4% in 1988). The impact of this degree of disability extends beyond work lost and the requirement for personal assistance to costs attributed to the health system.

Impact on the Health System

Estimates of the relationship between disability and health status are difficult to interpret due to varying definitions. Several different data sets are collected periodically, which serve as a basis for various reports. The National Health Interview Survey (NHIS) is one, done most recently in 1992. Another is the National Medical Expenditures Survey (NMES), done most recently in 1987 and updated to 1990.

Thus far in our discussion, we have been referring to disabilities. The underlying impairments are measured as disturbances from normal health. They include deficits in senses such as hearing and vision, absence of limbs, and paralysis. These impairments are coded in accordance with a scheme developed by the National Center for Health Statistics and used in the NHIS. The underlying diseases and injuries that may cause the impairments are coded differently in accordance with the *International Classification of Disease* (*ICD-9*). Thus, a person who had a limb amputated secondary to diabetes would have the absent limb coded as an impairment and the underlying disease of diabetes coded separately.

The relationship between disabling conditions and health status is a complex one. The most recent data come from the 1992 NHIS. *Disability* is defined rather broadly as limitation in usual activities. For example, for adults, the definition relates to one who cannot work or do housework or is limited in the amount or kind of work, housework, or other activities. Approximately 38 million Americans were so identified. Slightly more than one-third have two or more disabling conditions. In particular, those with multiple disabling conditions have poorer health and use more medical services.[6] Those who have multiple disabling conditions are more frequently elderly. However, the absolute number (7 million) is greater in the working-aged population, particularly in the older working-aged group (ages 45–64 years). Those older than 65 years number 6 million. Both the older working-aged group and those aged 65–74 years have an average of 3 months per year of restricted activity and nearly 6 weeks spent in bed. After age 75 years, activity is restricted for almost 4 months per year. Illness in terms of restrictions in activity is a major component of the experience of disabled persons.

These statistics translate into increased use of the health system by persons with disability. Physician visits are comparable throughout the various age cohorts with some increase after age 75 years. Individuals with disabilities average 14 physician visits per year. Those with two or more disabling conditions have almost two times as many visits as those with only one such condition (19 versus 11). Hospital discharges also increase in those older than 75 years. The frequency of hospitalizations steadily rises with age and number of conditions. For example, those older than 75 years with multiple disabling conditions have nearly 50 hospital discharges per year per 100 persons. It is clear that persons with disabilities have increased use of the health system. Both inpatient and outpatient use increases concomitant with the rise in degree of disability.

The NMES estimated medical costs for persons with chronic health conditions or impairments. These were updated to 1993. Americans with disabilities spend four times as much on average as their nondisabled counterparts. Composing 17% of the population, they account for 47% of medical expenditures.[7] Not only do they use services more frequently, they do so with proportionately greater cost. They are apparently sicker, representing 38% of those hospitalized but 57% of hospital expenditures. Similarly, persons with disabilities represent 19% of those who visit physicians but 42% of physician expenditures. Similar ratios exist in relation to prescription drugs (20% of persons account for 50% of costs). People with disabilities account for a disproportionately large share of expenditures for every age and gender group. For example, in the older working-aged group, they account for twice the average health costs.

The total effects on health care of chronic conditions are far greater than encompassed within the category of persons with disability.[8] The majority of persons with chronic conditions are neither disabled nor elderly. Using data from the 1987 NMES, linkage was possible of disability days, health care use, and expenditure data in relation to the conditions of the person. Unlike the studies described previously (SIPP, NHIS), the NMES does not limit itself to persons with activity limitations. Using the *ICD* code, a condition was considered chronic if classified as an impairment or as a disease that was not self-limited but created persistent and recurring health consequences that lasted for years. Costs were calculated up to 1990, including both direct costs and indirect costs of wages lost.

Using these criteria, 90 million Americans were identified with chronic conditions. One may recall that the number of persons with activity limitation due to chronic conditions was far less (32 million), with approximately 9 million unable to carry on their major activity as appropriate for their age. Rates of chronic conditions were highest in the elderly, 88% of whom had at least one such problem. However, more than one-third of young adults (18–44 years) and two-thirds of middle-aged adults (45–64 years) has at least one chronic condition. Working-aged adults (18–64 years) accounted for 60% of all noninstitutionalized persons with chronic conditions. Having more than one chronic condition, defined here as comorbidity, adds to the burden. More than one-fourth of young adults, one-half of middle-aged adults, and 69% of the elderly had more than one condition to manage.

The costs of health services and supplies in 1990 for these persons (including nursing home costs) totaled $425 billion. They represented 80% of hospital days, with an average length of stay (LOS) 80% greater than others. Similarly, 83% of prescription drugs, 66% of physician visits, and 55% of emergency department visits were made by persons with chronic conditions. Morbidity costs in 1990 as a result of work loss days amounted to $73 billion. Mortality due to premature death also represents a tremendous burden to society. Mortality combined with morbidity totaled $234 billion as indirect costs. Uncounted are the nonmonetary costs for these persons, who, not necessarily disabled, lead normal lives. They do so, however, with the threat of recurrent exacerbations, higher health care costs, more days lost from work than others, and the risk of long-term limitations and disabilities as well as excessive out-of-pocket costs for health care. Uncounted also are the caregiver costs. With the large number of persons involved, nearly every family in the United States may well be affected, providing some sort of unpaid support. With increasing numbers of elderly persons, it is estimated that by 2030 the number of persons with chronic conditions will rise to 148 million, with a concomitant rise in costs.

Despite the magnitude of the problem, the U.S. health care system is still largely based on the construct of acute illness and often fails to meet the needs of persons with chronic conditions. Growth in services designed to maintain health and independent living, particularly for persons with nonfatal chronic conditions, remains subordinate to advances in episodic health care. It is clearly necessary to transform our health care delivery system so that it better meets the needs of those who live with chronic conditions.

Chronic Neurologic Conditions

The contribution to this problem made by neurologic conditions is difficult to determine from the various data sets that are available. The most recent and most complete data come from the NHIS, derived in 1992.[9] A sample set of 50,000 households containing 128,000 noninstitutionalized persons are interviewed and the estimates extrapolated to the entire population. During the interview, if limitation in one's major activity is present, the chronic health condition that may be related is determined. Limitation in one's major activity for the nonelderly consists of working at a job and keeping house. There is also assessment in those with limitation and in the elderly of the need for help with basic personal needs (ADL), such as bathing and dressing, as well as with more complex needs, such as household chores, shopping, or getting around in general. One cannot assume that difficulty in one area necessarily applies to another. For example, some have limitation in basic ADL but are nevertheless able to carry on without limitation in work. A condition is considered chronic if it has lasted at least 3 months or is on a list of conditions that are considered chronic. Such conditions are subdivided into "impairments" and "health disorders." Neurologic impairments derived from the scheme of NHIS include deficits of body structure or function, such as vision, hearing, and sensation, or of speech and paralysis. The health disorders category is derived from *ICD-9* and includes diseases of the nervous system as one of its components.

Under the category of impairments, estimates of prevalence related to the neurologic system are as follows: problems of vision present in approximately 1 million, speech impairments in 500,000, quadriplegia in 50,000, paraplegia in 60,000, hemiplegia in 100,000, and plegia of one of the upper extremities in an additional 50,000. Paresis or partial paralysis is listed separately with hemiparesis and partial paralysis of one limb or another in approximately 450,000, with 50,000 additional

persons with paraparesis. Therefore, the numbers projected for impairments suggestive of spinal cord injury (SCI) are in the range of 160,000–200,000. The number of those with impairments suggestive of stroke or brain injury is approximately 1 million. Estimates based on *ICD* codes suggest that Alzheimer's disease (AD) affects 150,000; Parkinson's disease (PD) affects approximately 200,000; multiple sclerosis (MS), 225,000; amyotrophic lateral sclerosis (ALS), 100,000; epilepsy, 600,000; and migraine, approximately 400,000. Peripheral nerve disorders affect 600,000 persons and include nerve roots and plexus disorders, Bell's palsy, and a number of other conditions of lesser frequency.[10]

Overall, diseases of the nervous system are chronic and high in their primacy. The latter signifies that they are considered a major cause of the limitation, thus serving as a rough measure of severity. Tetraplegia, for example, has particularly serious consequences as evidenced by the degree to which it is attributed primacy and to which respondents are proxies for the person with the condition. MS and AD are also high in primacy. The actual figures for prevalence of the various neurologic conditions must be considered to be approximate. For example, other studies on the prevalence and incidence of stroke provide far higher figures. As the result of a sampling, they are subject to error. Also excluded are persons institutionalized in nursing homes who may suffer from some of these same conditions. These figures merely serve to illustrate the magnitude of the problem.

Each of the chapters in the second section of this book deals with the extent of the problem in terms of the data more specific to the condition being discussed.

In recognition of the severity and extent of the problem of chronic neurologic conditions, interest in the development of services appropriate for their care has increased. It is unclear how widely accepted will be the concept of principal care physicians dealing with the ongoing care of persons with chronic conditions. These are physicians with specialty training in neurology, physiatry, internal medicine, or gerontology who will provide what is otherwise considered to be primary care for persons with chronic conditions.

The principles of primary care are first contact, continuous, comprehensive, and coordinated care.[11] The proposed character of "principal care" is for one physician to take overall responsibility for all the daily aspects of care with the skills of the specialist and the approach of the generalist.

For those who have undergone a period of rehabilitation, such as after SCI, traumatic brain injury (TBI), or stroke, the outcomes sought include (1) averting unnecessary rehospitalization, (2) offering access to timely primary care, and (3) responding to new health needs as persons with disabilities become older.[12] Rehabilitationists, whether physiatrists, neurologists, or other specialists, can also provide ongoing care for those who ordinarily receive rehabilitation services. Another complementary source of staff would be neurologists interested in providing primary care for persons with chronic neurologic conditions, such as demyelinating disease, tumors, movement disorders, motor system diseases, epilepsy, and primary neuromuscular diseases. Shorter term neurologic involvement of a consultative nature is suggested as appropriate for cerebrovascular disease, dementia, headache, and sleep disorders.[13]

It is for health professionals interested in providing such ongoing care and physicians trained in physiatry, neurology, or other medical specialties that this book has been designed.

International Classification of Impairments, Disabilities, and Handicaps

The World Health Organization (WHO) model developed to describe rehabilitation has long been widely used to clarify the various aspects of treatment in the management of persons with chronic neurologic illness.[14] The *International Classification of Impairments, Disabilities, and Handicaps (ICIDH)* describes four levels on which analysis can be performed: pathology or disease, impairment, disability, and handicap.[15] Recent modifications of this basic scheme, presently in draft form, recognize the impact of environmental aspects in the degree to which persons with disability are able to participate in their wider social roles.[16] The more neutral term *participation* will replace *handicap*. Another change in terminology suggested in this new model is to use *activities* to replace the term *disabilities*.

Other more complex models have been proposed to describe the "disablement process" for planning for prevention and other population-based research.[17] The main pathway in the disablement process is as follows: Pathology (presence of disease) leads to impairments (anatomic and structural abnormalities), which in turn can lead to functional limitations (restrictions in basic physical and mental actions), which can then lead to disability (difficulty in performing activities of daily life).

A model has been proposed by the Institute of Medicine that focuses on the opportunities for reversibility of the various categories.[18] It also substitutes *functional limitations* as the descriptor of the effects of the impairments on the life of the person and reserves the term *disabilities* for the effects on the social role, thus eliminating the problematic term *handicaps*.

In general, all these formulations distinguish among phenomena that pertain to tissues or organs, those that relate to people, and those that pertain to people in interaction with their environments. The basic *ICIDH* model is used here, with recognition of newer emphasis on both the concept of potential for reversibility between these categories and the multifactorial nature of the disabling process. Particularly important is recognition of the interaction between the person with impairments and the environmental aspects that interfere with function or, if modified, that could facilitate function.[19]

Nature of the Disease

Pathology refers to the damage or abnormal processes that occur within an organ or organ system inside the body. The level of the disease is the traditional focus of medical care leading to diagnosis. One can further identify the etiology, anatomy, biochemistry, or genetics of the disorder. Prognosis can also be addressed in relation to the disease level of analysis.

The natural history of the disease process is the fundamental background on which the management of the person must depend. The character of the disease, whether diffuse or focal and whether progressive or relatively static, and the site(s) within the nervous system where the disease process manifests itself are important variables. For example, TBI, SCI, and stroke are all sudden and relatively devastating in their onset. Stroke differs in that it is a reflection of an underlying progressive disease process involving the vascular system and is therefore subject to recurrence. Demyelinating disease is also frequently progressive and subject to recurrence. Movement disorders such as PD are progressive, as are the various genetically based motor system diseases. Seizure disorders are by their very nature intermittent, as is headache. Neither of these is necessarily progressive but may become unremitting. Chronic pain is by definition unremitting.

The significance to the person of the progressive nature of the disease process includes the need for ongoing treatment to deal with changes over time. The implication of an apparently inexorable course must have enormous impact on the person and his or her ability to deal with the consequences of the disease. What is generally a progressive disease may permit a greater degree of reversibility in practice than is at first apparent or predicted. For example, in the case of stroke, clear opportunities exist to modify the course of progression from initial ischemia to the stage of infarction with the use of thrombolytic agents. The course may also potentially be modified between the presence of infarction and subsequent impairment of function by judicious use of drugs.

The degree to which recurrence is likely and the unpredictability of this recurrence are important variables in relation to headache and seizure disorders even if they are not necessarily progressive. For example, this principle is recognized in assessing the burden that a seizure disorder places on the person. The percentage of "impairment of the whole person" is determined not only by the frequency of the seizures.[20] The degree of impairment for purposes of disability evaluation is quite low (0–14%) in those persons with paroxysmal disorders when unpredictability of occurrence is associated with predictability of characteristics. It appears that a consistent pattern of prodromal symptoms can lessen the degree to which the person's life is adversely affected. In these conditions, one could have enough warning to seek safety and avoid injury if a seizure does occur. The unpredictability of time when seizures occur can lead to disruption in one's life despite the predictability of prodromal symptoms if the frequency becomes greater.

In a similar way, one of the major issues in the management of demyelinating disease is its degree of unpredictability of recurrence as well as its likelihood of progression. To the extent that a person with demyelinating disease becomes better able to identify the early signals of recurrence, that aspect ceases to be as crucial. At times, the likelihood of recurrence and its severity can become somewhat less when early intervention is possible. In a similar way, for those with chronic recurrent headache, awareness of the early signs of recurrence can limit its frequency and severity by judicious use of medication. One of the objectives of ongoing management is to develop for the person with the chronic condition the ability to define some of the possible precipitating factors so that they can be controlled.

The fact that treatment is readily available in the case of PD despite its progressive nature can reduce the impact of its progression. For the person with genetically based motor system disease, the decision to bear children and the impact of the knowledge of the genetic aspects have major implications. For example, one man with motor system disease spoke about his mother not telling him about the family disease until he had experienced it in adulthood after having married and sired children. Her guilt about having a family history had deprived him of the ability to make an informed decision about his own family plans. Similarly, many persons with seizure disorder were not able to speak about it because of its supposedly genetic aspect and its perception as a stain on the family. One such person describes the secrecy she was enjoined to maintain about her seizures as its most devastating quality.

The anatomic sites and their degree of distribution have significant impact on the kinds of impairments they cause. The divisions of the nervous system are broadly defined as the cerebrum (anterior and middle fossa), brain stem, and cerebellum (posterior fossa); spinal cord; peripheral nerves; neuromyal junction; and muscles. Diseases of the brain overall such as TBI may be diffuse, such as with diffuse axonal injury, or more focal, as with gunshot wounds. Stroke is classically focal, involving one side, but is frequently multifocal and bilateral and within the cerebrum and brain stem, or both. Distribution of stroke can be in the deep structures of the cerebrum or in the cortical areas. Headaches and seizures are considered to be cerebral in origin. PD is a disease of the deep structures of the brain. Demyelinating disease is by definition multifocal, with possible involvement of the cerebrum, brain stem, spinal cord, or a combination thereof. SCI can affect different levels of the spinal cord with appropriate consequences. The basic distinction is between injury affecting upper cervical cord with subsequent difficulties with breathing, lower cervical cord with involvement of all four extremities, midthoracic cord with problems in control of blood pressure as well as paraplegia, and lumbosacral cord with different patterns of impairment of bladder, bowel, and sexual function. The motor system diseases variously affect the spinal cord, nerves, and muscles with their significant impact by definition on the motor system.

Equally important in management are the age and sex of the persons who are likely to incur the disease. The major distinction is between those of working and child-bearing and -rearing age and those who are older. Seizure disorders, headache, chronic pain, genetically based motor diseases, TBI, and SCI are primarily diseases of the younger age cohort. Stroke and PD are primarily, albeit not exclusively, diseases that appear in the older age group. Age can also be a factor in the ability to recover from the effects of injury of whatever etiology when the onset is acute. The elderly are also more likely to have concomitant medical problems such as cardiac disease and arthritis that may affect their ability to carry out alternative approaches to deal with problems in mobility. TBI and SCI are primarily diseases of younger men, and MS is mainly a disease of younger women. These gender differences are coupled with differences in social roles and intrapersonal and interpersonal characteristics.

Nature of the Impairments

Impairments are the direct consequences of the underlying pathology. These are described as symptoms or signs such as one would assess in the course of the medical/neurologic examination. The *ICIDH* definition of impairment is "any loss or abnormality of psychological, physiological, or anatomical structure or function."[15] Normal medical practice uses impairments to deduce the underlying pathology or disease process. The aim is to reduce the degree of impairment with the use of medication or other techniques.

Examples of common neurologic findings at the level of impairment are weakness of a limb, sensory loss, and pain. Impairments affect actions, which in themselves have no meaning but are a result of the mode of examination. For example, weakness of elbow flexion can be tested. However, the action of the elbow must be considered as a component in the more total activity of the arm in carrying out tasks such as feeding oneself, dressing, and writing one's name on a check.

It is important to remember that not all pathology causes impairment: witness the presence of silent brain infarction. Conversely, not all impairments can be attributed to pathology: witness the lack of findings in many instances in persons with seizures or headaches. The anatomic sites determine the impairments. The "total burden" of impairment has importance. For example, in assessing the burden for rating purposes, the degree of overall impairment increases as a result of the multiplicity of the systems involved.[20]

Cerebral disease is specific in bringing about major impairments in language, mental status, and integrative functions as well as emotional behavioral disturbances. Difficulties in attention, learning, and memory can have particular significance. Behavioral disturbances and emotional problems as well as cognitive impairments can affect the training of the person to participate in his or her management as well as the ability to carry out the use of the compensatory strategies that would be necessary. Cerebral disease is also specific in causing general impairment of consciousness or episodic impairments of consciousness such as with seizure disorders. Major effects can be caused by visual field defects due to involvement of the visual system. Motor and sensory system impairments can occur anywhere in the nervous system with the pattern depending on the site. Brain stem impairments are specific for dysfunction of the cranial nerves, which can manifest itself as diplopia and disturbances in hearing and balance as well as swallowing and dysarthria. Spinal cord involvement leads to impairments of both motor and sensory systems as well as bowel, bladder, and sexual function.

Ultimately, the significance of the impairments depends on their functional consequences. Crucial to the reduction of disabilities during the training process is the degree to which cognitive and emotional behavioral disturbances are present. Depression is particularly important in limiting the commitment to use the leg or arm movement that remains. The assessment of motor system impairments differs from the assessment used for anatomic localization if one is now concerned about functional consequences. For example, the distribution of weakness within the arm or leg becomes important. One cannot use the hand if the upper arm does not provide a base for action. The use of the leg for stance depends particularly on the strength of the hip and knee extensors. Problems in trunk control and balance become important in being able to get around. The type of sensory involvement rather than merely its distribution is also important. Impairment of position sense, for example, is highly pertinent to motor control. Sensory impairment to touch or deep pain has particular relevance to the management of skin breakdown in persons with SCI. Degrees of impairment in bladder sensation and patterns of sphincter control are highly important in preventing future illness due to urinary tract infections and so forth.

Nature of the Disabilities

Disability refers to the functional (behavioral) consequences of any pathology or impairments, or both. The *ICIDH* definition of disability is "any restriction or lack (resulting from an impairment) of ability to perform an activity within the range considered normal for a human being." The newer categorizations substitute *functional limitations* for the term *disabilities*, reserving the latter for the social consequences of the impairments. Disabilities can include difficulty in getting around, communicating, dressing, and so forth. They refer to the effect(s) that the impairments have in the life of the person. They are the result of the interaction between the impairments and the person who is experiencing them. As such, they cannot be deduced merely from the neurologic examination. Input from the person or caregiver, or both, is necessary for their proper identification. The specific disabilities to be ameliorated vary with the goals and the character of the person, including his or her interpersonal interactions as well as the resources available. These include the availability of caregivers and the accessibility of the physical setting.

Normal rehabilitation practice deals with this level of analysis. The aim is to reduce the degree of disability by training the actions that are unaffected so as to compensate for those that are affected and to learn to use technical aids as necessary. Many intervening variables can affect the connection between the impairments and the disabilities. One is the ability to learn compensatory techniques dependent on cognitive and emotional issues. Cognitive issues can affect learning, but emotional issues are particularly significant in affecting the willingness or ability to commit one's energy as well as ideas to the development of compensatory methods.

Treatment of the person with the disability frequently must include the training of caregivers. Often, the ongoing availability of caregivers is crucial to living in a community setting. Problems in interpersonal interaction and the need for ongoing emotional support of caregivers become particularly important, for example, in the management of persons with tetraplegia. These issues are present in varying degrees in the management of every person with chronic illness because the effects of illness extend to the family and other systems such as the workplace. It is clear that the proper treatment of persons with chronic neurologic illness must provide not only continuity of care but also comprehensive care involving emotional as well as physical issues.

The interaction between the impairment and the subsequent functional limitation or disability is most easily illustrated by the different impact of weakness on one side of the body or the other depending on the handedness of the person. For example, the finding of weakness on the left side is important in helping to identify the site of injury to be the right side of the brain when one is operating on the level of analysis of the disease or pathology. When one operates at the level of analysis of impairment, then one becomes concerned about the degree and distribution of the weakness; whether the arm, hand, or both are affected; and to what degree. However, when one operates at the level of the functional limitation or disability, one needs to become aware as well of the personal characteristics that can help determine the effects of that weakness in this previously left-handed person.

Nature of the Handicap

Handicap is the social and societal consequence of the disease and refers specifically to the personally relevant consequences. It is the degree of handicap that, from the person's perspective, determines the real severity of any illness. The *ICIDH* definition of handicap is "a disadvantage of a given individual, resulting from an impairment or disability that limits or prevents the fulfillment of a role that is normal (depending upon age, sex, and social and cultural factors) for that individual." Areas recommended for review include "orientation, physical independence, mobility, occupation of time, social integration, and economic self-sufficiency." It is fundamentally judged in reference to the individual's own immediate social context. Examples include loss of a job or marital breakdown that arises as a result of the disabilities. An example of the relationship between disability and handicap is as follows: A handicap arises in the social context without a disability necessarily being present in a man who had a visual field defect (impairment) that did not interfere with his driving but now has a handicap when the documentation of his field defect by a physician disqualifies him from driving.[15]

The use of the WHO classification in respect to handicap becomes problematic as reflected in the example given above. Discriminating between disability and handicap merely on the basis of societal consequences is difficult. One criticism leveled at the concept of handicap is that which arises from persons with disabilities.[21] Environmental factors that are normally beyond the control of the person with disabilities, such as social expectations and prejudices, inaccessible physical settings, and the legal framework, can limit the achievement of full citizenship and participation in social roles. For example, training in the use of a wheelchair may solve the problem of mobility for a person with paraplegia but not in public places where stairs block entrances. Passage of the Americans with Disabilities Act (ADA) in the United States represents a major effort to deal with these issues, but problems remain, particularly in the areas of employment.[22]

This criticism has led to the modification of the terminology as expressed by the more recent formulation of the *ICIDH*.[16] The "level of participation" achieved is now considered to be the result not only of the person's health condition and the consequent limitations that may reside in the person but also the context in which the person lives. Derived from the principle of "equalization of opportunity" for persons with disability, a relationship should be established with the norm of expected levels of participation of persons without disabilities. Qualifiers for this aspect include contextual components, which, if present, could serve as facilitators.

The difficulties in dealing with the long-term effects of disability have led to the formulation of a concept that attempts to describe the entire spectrum of effects. Some recommend measures that include elements of physical health, reflecting the disease process and the resultant impairments; functional health, reflecting the disabilities that arise from those impairments; social health, reflecting the handicaps; and psychological health, incorporating the person's response to those other aspects.[23] *Quality of life* (*QOL*) refers to the emotional or personal response of the person to the perceived difference between his or her actual and desired activities. It reflects the sense of loss of autonomy or freedom to have choices about one's life. It is thus necessary to measure both actual performance and expected performance. Major technical problems arise when trying to assess this broad concept that is so personal and individualistic. However, it is perhaps the most useful in that it can contribute to decision making by the person with the problem. There are methods for establishing value or utility to various alternative treatments that have great promise.

Any approach to the management of persons with chronic neurologic illness that affects QOL must be responsive to the "independent living" concept as advanced by disabled persons. The issues are not the degree to which one can care for one's physical needs. One can use caregivers as necessary. The issue is the degree to which one has regained or achieved the ability to make the decisions about one's life. In a survey of persons who had stroke but who are now living in the community, their measures of QOL clustered in the following three areas: (1) opportunities in their environment, such as accessible transportation, exercise, and the ability to carry on their interests; (2) opportunities to do meaningful work, whether paid or voluntary; and (3) being treated as intelligent people, able to make their own decisions and to be allowed to think as well as do for themselves. It is clear that the process by which the management of persons with chronic neurologic illness proceeds can enable the development of such self-management skills or at least the recognition that they already exist.

The distinctions made in the *ICIDH* model between pathology or disease and their impairments and between the impairments and the consequent disabilities are useful to emphasize the full range of areas to be explored. It is important to deal with each of these aspects. Important opportunities exist to deal with treatment at the level of the disease process or pathology. The advances in the treatment of MS is one such area to be pursued. Other examples are from the area of pain and management of headache. Once the pathologic diagnosis has been reached and treatment provided, it is necessary to move to the development of a plan to deal with the results in the person. The focus changes over time from the disease and the subsequent impairments to the disabilities and then to the reduction of the handicaps or, more precisely, the reduction in the barriers to fuller participation.

The distinction made between impairments and disabilities or functional limitations is particularly useful. The impairments may remain relatively constant, but the disabilities, the functional consequences, can be improved by means of training and the use of various assistive aids. Alternative methods permit the person to continue to carry on and to accomplish goals, albeit by different means. As one moves along this continuum, the shift is from the person to the interaction between that person and the environment. The latter is subject to changes as well as the use of different technical aids, which are developed to alter the interface between the person and the environment. The focus also shifts from that which can be related to norms to that which is personal and individualistic in character. If properly done, the concomitant shift also occurs to independence in decision making and the ability to manage one's own life after injury, from professionals to the persons involved.

Meaning of Illness

The management of persons with chronic neurologic illness requires that one define each of the terms. Central to our discussion is the concept of "illness," which presupposes the experience of persons about themselves in the context of a disease. It is the subjective experience that one seeks so as to treat the impact of the disease as well as the disease itself. An important distinction should be made between "disease" and "illness." *Disease* is primarily defined in terms of the body and its systems. *Illness* is the entire complex that involves not only the sick person's body parts but also the person and the group. The obligation of the physician must be to relieve the suffering of the person who is experiencing the illness.[24]

The concept of the person has undergone changes over the years. In the Cartesian model of mind-body dichotomy, the body is assigned to medicine. The mind is not identifiable in objective terms. The only remaining site for the person lies in the mind, which remains subjective, not within medicine's domain, and is not "real." The experience of suffering being subjective is therefore not within medicine's domain. This dichotomy must be rejected. It is not possible to treat sickness as something that happens solely to the body without risking damage to the person. Because of this division, physicians may, in concentrating on curing the body, cause the patient as a person to suffer.

One must distinguish between *pain* and *suffering*. Although extreme pain can cause suffering, the two are not synonymous. One can have pain, as in childbirth, without necessarily having a sense of suffering; rather, one may find the experience uplifting. Pain is associated with suffering when it is perceived as a threat to one's continued existence, not merely to life but to one's integrity as a person. In general, suffering occurs when a person experiences a sense of impending destruction and loss of hope; it continues until either the threat of destruction has passed or the integrity of the person can be restored in some other way. One can understand the effects of a stroke or SCI as creating this sense of suffering because of its sudden onset and devastating consequences. It is one of the purposes of the rehabilitation phase to reduce the degree of disability by retraining and, in so doing, simultaneously restoring that sense of integrity and a new sense of self, thus reducing the degree of suffering that results from the injury.

Suffering can be relieved even in the presence of continued pain by making the source of pain known or by changing its meaning as well as by other techniques by which one can achieve a sense of control over the pain. One such instance was the presence of severe pain below the level of injury in the legs and groin of a man with SCI. Pain was almost constant and interfered with his ability to accomplish tasks and to get around. When asked what troubled him the most about the pain, his answer was that he was unclear as to what was causing it. Before the injury, he considered pain to be a signal that something was wrong, and that he needed to do something about the source of the pain. He really wanted to know whether this was the case with the pain he was now experiencing. Once reassured that the sensations were not the signal of something serious, he said that he felt that he could live with it. This case illustrates the importance of the person's past experience as an important component in dealing with the element of suffering.

The person brings to his or her condition character; past life experiences, particularly as related to illness and doctors; cultural norms; and social roles. One woman who "suffered" a cerebral hemorrhage when in her 30s continued to experience depression. She described her image of anyone using a cane as crippled and as being like a man she used to see who stood begging on a street corner. Those who had a stroke were to be pitied, she believed. She also felt an incongruity between what she saw in the mirror and what she felt herself to be. Everyone has a relationship to one's body. In the presence of disease, that relationship may be altered. The body is no longer considered as a friend but as a burden and even as an enemy. This is particularly true if the illness comes without warning. One cannot, then, trust one's body. The effects of the loss of bodily control may be humiliating to some. One man with injury to his spinal roots was able to walk but remained tethered to his home, unable to go out, because of his concern about loss of bowel control. He was able to leave his house when he developed an effective bowel program that led to elimination at the appointed time and place.

In an elegant and eloquent way, a person with MS wrote of her experience of "illness-as-lived"[25]:

> Illness is fundamentally experienced as a loss of wholeness. This loss is the perception of bodily impairment, not so much a simple recognition of the specific impairment but a loss of a sense of bodily integrity. . . .The body can no longer be taken for granted or ignored. It has seemingly assumed an opposing will of its own, beyond the control of the self. Rather than functioning effectively at the bidding of the self, the body-in-malfunctioning thwarts plans, impedes choices, renders actions impossible. Illness disrupts the fundamental unity between the body and self. Illness is experienced not only as a threat to the body but to the self. She is no longer a "whole person" but "less of a person." There is a loss of certainty. One must surrender the most cherished assumption, of personal indestructibility. [This is so overwhelming] . . . and leads to anxiety and fear that one is unable to communicate to others.

Nevertheless, suffering in the context of chronic illness can be ameliorated. The degree of suffering also reflects the resources of the person, the availability of others in one's life, and particularly one's resourcefulness. People are able to enlarge themselves in relation to injury and grow new ways of being. One man who became paraplegic had been a champion skier. As a result of his engineering background, he was able to design a sit-ski that allowed him to ski once again at a championship level. The body may not be able to grow another part, but the person can. One can borrow from the strengths of others who have had similar conditions and have dealt with them. Support groups are an important resource. They can provide a sense of possibility and of hope but also a sense of alternatives by which one can live one's life. They can provide ideas as well as nurture.

The focus on the nervous system as a site of disease recognizes that system as a basis of disease but also recognizes the effect of the interaction between the entire person and the environment in which that person resides. That environment includes both the physical setting, whether rural, urban, or other, and the social setting, for example, whether the person is a member of an extended or nuclear family.

Structure has been the basis for thinking about disease in the nervous system with pathologic anatomy its underpinning. Techniques have led to even more effective methods for determining structural changes. Nevertheless, illnesses exist that affect nervous system function and cause illness in persons without evidence of structural change at the level we are able to measure. The abnormality exists at a different level—that of function—and the underlying changes are those of pathophysiology. This implies that disease is a process that changes over time rather than remains static and, in the instance of chronic illness, does so over relatively long periods. These processes unfold in the context of the life of the person with "their toll being human malfunction by which individuals know themselves or are known by others to be unhealthy."[24]

The mode by which suffering can be alleviated depends at least in part on the character of the patient-physician interaction. It is necessary at the outset to consider that the two parties in the interaction have had different experiences. An inability to communicate may arise based on a fundamental disagreement about the nature of illness. In attending to the experience of illness, the physician and the patient do so within the context of different "worlds," each with its own horizon of meaning; therefore, a gap exists between the patient's experience of illness and the way the physician thinks in terms of disease. Agreement can be fostered if certain basic elements are focused on that, regardless of the specific aspects of the disease, incorporate an understanding of illness-as-lived.[25] Chapter 2 describes a process by which this can be done.

The element of chronicity also implies the need for adaptation over time so that management becomes the goal rather than cure. In doing so, the principles have changed from those of acute medicine to a model that can be derived from that of rehabilitation. That model is not limited to the usual concept of rehabilitation as relatively short-term training to restore function to the extent that the person can live outside the hospital after an acute injury such as after a stroke or SCI; rather, it is ongoing over the life of the person. Such management can be in continuity with the training period. It can, however, be ongoing without any inpatient phase, such as in the case of headache, seizures, or chronic pain. The motto is "adding life to years." The aims are to maintain the person and his or her ability to function in accordance with life goals in the presence of what may be ongoing or progressive disease and to preserve or restore optimal function with preservation or restoration of autonomy and maintenance of the person's role in the family and society at large. This requires maintenance of emotional stability and positive interpersonal relationships. The concept of "disease management" requires attention to the entire spectrum over time, including primary prevention to the extent that it is possible, reduction or limitation of damage, prevention of further damage, enhancement of the function of affected systems, enhancement of the function of unaffected systems, and development and use of compensatory strategies including the use of technology.

References

1. Prevalence of mobility and self-care disability—United States, 1990. JAMA 1993;270:1918.
2. Prevalence of work disability—United States, 1990. JAMA 1993;270:1921.
3. Schneider EL, Guralnick JM. The aging of America and impact on health care costs. JAMA 1990;263:2335.
4. Bradsher JE. Disability among Racial and Ethnic Groups. Disability Statistics Abstract No. 10. Washington, DC: NIDRR, 1996.
5. Kennedy J, LaPlante MP, Kaye S. Need for Assistance in the Activities of Daily Living. Disability Statistics Abstract No. 18. Washington, DC: NIDRR, 1997.
6. Trupin L, Rice DP. Health Status, Medical Care Use and Number of Disabling Conditions in the United States. Disability Statistics Abstract No. 9. Washington, DC: NIDRR, 1995.
7. Max W, Rice DP, Trupin L. Medical Expenditures for People with Disabilities. Disability Statistics Abstract No. 12. Washington, DC: NIDRR, 1996.
8. Hoffman C, Rice D, Sung H-Y. Persons with chronic conditions: their prevalence and costs. JAMA 1996;276: 1473.
9. LaPlante M. Health Conditions and Impairments Causing Disability. Disability Statistics Abstract No. 16. Washington, DC: NIDRR, 1996.
10. LaPlante M, Carson D. Disability in the United States: Prevalence and Causes 1992. Disability Statistics Abstract No. 7. Washington, DC: NIDRR, 1996.
11. Starfield B. Is primary care essential? Lancet 1994;344: 1129.
12. ACRM Committee. Addressing the post-rehabilitation health care needs of persons with disabilities. Arch Phys Med Rehabil 1993;74:S8.
13. Kurtzke JF, Houff SA. A primary care plan for neurology. Neurology 1995;45:1052.
14. World Health Organization. The International Classification of Impairments, Disabilities and Handicaps. Geneva: World Health Organization, 1980.
15. Wade DT. Measurement in Neurological Rehabilitation. Oxford: Oxford University Press, 1992;3–14.
16. World Health Organization. ICIDH2—International Classification of Impairments, Activities and Participation. Beta Testing 1. Geneva: World Health Organization, 1997.
17. Verbrugge LM, Jette AM. The "disablement" process. Soc Sci Med 1994;38:1.

18. Brandt EN, Pope E (eds). Institute of Medicine. Enabling America: Assessing the Role of Rehabilitation Science and Engineering. Washington, DC: National Academy Press, 1997.

19. Teel C, Dunn W, Jackson ST, et al. The role of the environment in fostering independence: methodological issues in developing an instrument. Top Stroke Rehab 1997;4:28.

20. Ozer MN. Central Nervous System. In SL Demeter, GBJ Andersson, GM Smith (eds), Disability Evaluation. St Louis: Mosby, 1996;452–463.

21. Finkelstein V. Attitudes and Disabled People: Issues for Discussion. New York: World Rehabilitation Fund, 1980.

22. LaPlante M, Kennedy J, Kaye HS, et al. Disability and Employment. Disability Statistics Abstract No. 11. Washington, DC: NIDRR, 1996.

23. deHaan R, Aaronson N, Limburg M, et al. Measuring quality of life in stroke. Stroke 1993;24:320.

24. Cassell EJ. The Nature of Suffering and the Goals of Medicine. New York: Oxford University Press, 1991; 10–15.

25. Toombs SK. The meaning of illness: a phenomenological approach to the patient-physician relationship. J Med Philos 1987;12:219.

Chapter 2
Character of the Solution

Mark N. Ozer

Goals and Objectives

In Chapter 1, the nature of the problem of managing chronic illness is explored. The incidence and prevalence of chronic neurologic illness are increasing within all age groups but have a particular effect on the elderly. A concomitant major impact on health costs has occurred. Rather than paying attention only to those costs and their reduction, the opportunity is available to redirect some of the costs so as to achieve better results. Those results must include improvement in subjective QOL as well as improvement in health. The focus must change from the disease to the persons who are experiencing illness.

Evidence of the opportunity available is the significant decrease in chronic disability rates in the elderly, documented in the years 1989–1994.[1] The reduction in numbers of disabled persons from that projected for the various age cohorts caused the disabled elderly population to grow more slowly than the total elderly population. Many causes exist for this reduction. One possible factor might be the contribution by the larger number of well-educated persons who are better equipped to participate in managing relatively complex and long-term medical treatment.

The nature of the problem faced by the health professional regardless of specialty is the problem of managing illness or, more specifically, the persons with such illness over time. Therein lies the difference between cure and care. In the absence of cure, the objective must be to maintain function and to deal with the disability experienced by the persons. This approach is an alternative to succumbing to the despair that can ensue for both the health professional and the patient when the focus has been only on affecting the disease process itself. Diagnosis and prognosis remain important but are only a means to the end of managing one's life including coping with the disease process. The health professional who is schooled to deal with curing must change focus and enable the patient to do so as well. This new paradigm includes not only an understanding of illness in terms of clinically definable disease but also an understanding in terms of the existential predicament of the patient.

Several types of medical encounters exist depending on the objectives. For the purposes of our discussion, the objective of the interaction is an overall management plan for one's life in dealing with disability. In the management of persons with chronic illness, the priority aims can vary over time. In general, they are to maintain the person in his or her ability to function in accordance with life goals in the presence of what may be ongoing or progressive disease. That goal requires a plan to preserve or restore optimal function in emotional, cognitive, and physical areas with preservation of autonomy and the person's role in the family and society at large. These efforts can be translated into a number of activities defined by the categories of the *ICIDH*, described in Chapter 1. These would include plans for the prevention of further *impairment*, the ongoing reduction of functional limitation or *disability* in the context of ongoing disease, and the maintenance of participation or *QOL* in the context of community roles. Each of these overall goals would require the development of a series of plans. The concept of disease management encompasses this ongoing activity over the life of the person with the disease to incorporate prevention and ongoing care.

The enormity of the problems requires the full use of all resources, both professional and personal. To maximize the contribution of resources by all concerned to the implementation of plans, concomitant attention must be given to the contribution by those same participants to the design and ongoing review of those plans. In chronic illness, day-to-day care responsibilities fall most heavily on patients and their families. Effective collaborative relationships with health care providers can help patients and families to handle their tasks more effectively. Collaborative management is care that strengthens and supports self-care in chronic illness while assuring that effective medical, preventive, and other interventions take place. This management includes collaborative definition of problems, targeted goal setting, support, and follow-up.[2]

In accomplishing these objectives, the method proposed is to carry out a specified planning process over time. This chapter describes the planning process, including its component parts and methods for enhancing the degree to which the patient, family, or both participate in the planning. Each of the chapters in the second section of this book illustrates modifications of this basic process in response to the characteristics of the several diseases being discussed.

The planning process is a reiterative one in which a set of questions is asked again and again. Each person brings to the planning process his or her own characteristics. It is pointed out in Chapter 1 (in the section "Meaning of Illness") that the communication between the person with disabilities and the health professional may be limited because each is coming from a different set of expectations and experiences. It is necessary to reconcile those objectives and expectations. A resource trade-off technique can illustrate the differences as well as similarities between groups made up of either professionals or persons with long-standing disabilities. A comparison has been made between the utility of the various components of the Functional Independence Measure (FIM).[3] For example, although clinicians place greater value on cognitive skills, consumers place priority on physical abilities. Both groups focused on intellectual autonomy, as well as the importance of sphincter control, as central to the control of personal destiny.

In addition to the relationship between the health professional and the persons with disabilities and their family members is the relationship between the sometimes disparate persons who make up the rehabilitation team. The person with disabilities and family members must frequently interact with a number of different persons and participate in the coordination of their efforts.

Eventually, disabled persons can develop an increased ability to manage their own life—that is, to carry out the planning process themselves. They must therefore develop the ability to plan for themselves, now interacting with the professional staff as consultants in planning. This process must have continuity over time, be comprehensive in its range, be coordinated in relation to priorities, and be collaborative or conjoint with the primary persons, the patient (now considered a client), the family, or both.

Planning Process

Figure 2-1 describes the planning process. A planning cycle contains at least one review step. The initial plan consists of a set of goals, the means by which those goals are to be accomplished, and a time for review. At the appointed time, the plans are reviewed and revised. A new cycle has begun. The degree to which the original goals were accomplished can now aid in setting new goals. The methods that may have been helpful in reaching the initial goals must also be reviewed and revised in light of experience. Not only can one define new goals at this time, but one should also revise and make more appropriate the means of achieving them. For example, a particular set of exercises may have been deemed helpful in increasing range of motion or reducing pain and so forth. One can now review and possibly change the frequency, intensity, and nature of those exercises. Similarly, one may have found a particular medication regimen helpful and may adjust that regimen at the time of review.

Figure 2-1. Planning process.

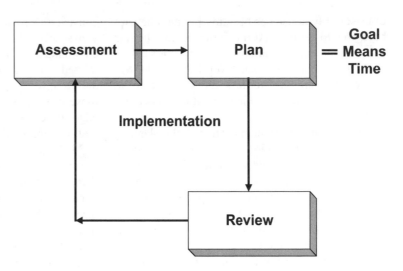

The time when reassessment takes place can also be revised in view of the rate at which one anticipates results, now also in light of experience. The frequency of evaluation can also vary with the intensity of treatment. For example, the need for monitoring progress would be greater if treatment with high intensity were given daily than if treatment were only given several times each week. This translates to team conferences on a weekly basis while the patient is in an inpatient rehabilitation program versus monthly or bimonthly review of progress while the patient is in a less intensive outpatient program.

Although the cyclical planning structure implies an explicit time interval between planning, implementation, and evaluation, it is possible to carry out the entire process in an ongoing way. At any particular time, one can choose to review the methods in use, the outcomes being achieved, and the frequency of review.

The planning process reiterates a basic set of questions. Table 2-1 describes the planning questions. Ordinarily, during the delineation of an initial plan, questions about concerns or problems and the status in relation to those problem areas precede the questions about goals. A review questions the outcomes or new status, methods, or both as appropriate some time after the initial plan is made and implemented.

One can choose to emphasize one or another question at any time. One can choose to only address the question about outcome on a daily basis and review or revise the means less fre-

quently. One can address the questions about concerns and goals more or less frequently. It is not uncommon to establish the use of certain questions before beginning to use others so that the total number of questions being addressed proceeds in stages. For example, in designing a plan for dealing with a man's chronic pain after stroke, the patient was able initially to identify the characteristics of the pain, its intensity, and its duration and then to begin to address the functional limitations that he was experiencing because of the pain. The identification of some of the functional effects provided the basis for a goal that we would evaluate on his return. The intensity of the pain limited his ability to ride in a car, along with a number of other limitations. His first goal, therefore, was "to be able to come back for the next visit."

At the time of review several weeks later, the man was able to address the question as to outcomes for the first time and the goal question once again. Because he had seen some results, however small (he had been able to return), he was now more global in stating that he wanted to be able to get out of his house and go different places. His actual statement quite graphically reflected his emotions. It was, "I want to get out

Table 2-1. Planning Questions

1. What are the concerns? What problems exist?
2. What are the goals?
3. What outcomes have been achieved?
4. What has succeeded in producing such outcomes?

of prison. My house has been my prison. I haven't been able to get out." At this initial review, he was once again able to address the question as to goals, now on a more basic level; however, he was not yet prepared to address the question as to what he had done to achieve whatever outcomes had occurred.

One measure of implementation of the planning process is a determination of which of the planning questions have been addressed and the number of times each has been addressed. One of the aims is to increase the awareness of the patient about the questions themselves. Eventually, clients can choose to ask themselves these questions independently when appropriate.

In answering any of the questions, three phases are possible. The first is *exploration*, generally asking the question three times. During this phase, it is useful to think freely without censoring one's answers. In the next phase, one can make judgments and make a *selection* as to which of the answers is highest priority or the best statement. The third phase can now include some degree of *specification*. The degree of specification sought includes defining not only the answer to "what" but also "to what degree?," "where?," or "when?" For example, in response to a question about goals, a specific answer would be, "Walk 50 ft with someone close by inside my house." Each of the questions is described in detail before the process by which they are answered is defined.

What Are the Concerns?

The initial question addressed in all medical interviews is the one dealing with problems or concerns. A working alliance must be established between the physician (or other health professional) and the client. The interview is the most powerful and sensitive instrument by which to achieve this alliance. Prerequisite to that alliance is the person feeling listened to and understood; if the patient feels understood, trust is enhanced. It is essential that the client's main concerns and fears be uncovered to the fullest extent possible rather than being terminated by pursuit of diagnostic data or by giving hasty reassurances. Reassurance should be used only after the complaint has been clarified and empathy with the concerns has been conveyed. A review of transcripts of medical interviews devoted to the specification of "empathic" communication notes that many opportunities are missed to recognize when emotions are present but are not directly expressed, to invite exploration of those unexpressed feelings, and then to acknowledge those feelings effectively so that the patient feels understood.[4]

Medical training gives priority to objective data. Physicians express their caring by conscientiously doing what they have been taught to do, that is, pursuing information related to diagnostic assessment and then treating appropriately. Patients may perceive this focus as uncaring because their need to be heard and understood is not met. Patients may feel unacknowledged; physicians may feel unappreciated. Both are hurt by a model of practice that is too narrowly focused on the biology of disease rather than on the experience of illness. As Peabody stated so long ago, "The secret of the care of the patient is in caring for the patient."[5]

In making the distinction between disease and illness, Cassell[6] notes the importance of the issue of suffering for which the person seeks relief. Expressing what one fears is often very difficult. The threat of the injury caused by a stroke may be so great that any individual can be expected to suffer; yet it is the suffering of each patient that is individual and particular. The process of defining the problem is ongoing. The answers vary with the individual's degree and type of impairment and his or her personal history and emotional state as well as the character of the environment both physical and interpersonal. The answers also vary over time as thoughts become clearer, as old problems are solved and new ones appear, and as the patient feels more trust in the person asking the questions. One can never completely know another. Ultimately, it is a question that one must recurrently ask oneself. The role of the professional can be to enable the person to answer this question as to his or her fears and concerns to the fullest extent possible.

To the extent that one enables the patient to uncover the concerns, one can begin to help the person to deal with them on several levels. The exploration of concerns can identify the specific functional consequences that the impairment has created for that person; thus, one can begin to identify the disabilities that the plan is designed to ameliorate. For example, several men with a midthoracic SCI were asked about their concerns. The question was, "In what ways has your spinal cord injury affected your life?" One young man in his late 20s was able to speak quite readily about his problems. He mentioned that getting around was not a problem for him. He said that he felt he could use his wheelchair to keep up with people. Although recently married after his injury, he denied any difficulties in his relationship with his wife. When asked again, for the third time, he prefaced his next remark by saying, "This may seem strange, but what really bothers me is that I am so short now. I used to be a tall person but when I am sitting in a wheelchair I can't reach the things I used to be able to reach." Another man in his 40s had been depressed and seemed to be unable to learn how to transfer, although he had good strength in his arms. When asked about his concerns, he was hesitant to speak. Only when offered some ideas that others had said was he able to speak of his own concerns. When told that some people expressed that "they were not the same man as they were before," he began to express his own concerns about that. "I'm not the man I was. I used to be the strongest person in my health club. When I was young, I looked weak and people would attack me. Now that I am in a wheelchair, I think that I look weak and would be attacked." Plans to deal with the problems expressed can be made much more relevant when these concerns are identified. Although the impairments remain, the possibility exists of enabling the first man to reach objects with the use of a reacher or other techniques. The second man was enrolled in a karate class that provides persons in wheelchairs with a sense of power.

By carrying out several levels of inquiry, the answers begin to reflect the person's more significant concerns. A threefold exploration is generally useful as a start. One can then establish the priority area or clearest statement of concerns within a single category. For example, the eventual answer for a woman with left-sided weakness came only after a series of questions. The first answer was general: "My left side is weak." When asked, "What problems does the weakness of your left side cause you?" she replied, "I have trouble going up and down steps." When asked again, she made her problem even more explicit. "I don't know how I'll be able to get up and down my steep front steps."

The problem had been transformed from the impairment in her left side to the functional limitation (disability), for which many options could be considered.

Asking this question in terms of the functional consequences of the impairment has significance in itself. The message being sent is that it is useful to go beyond the impairments such as the weakness on the left side to define the ways that one's life is affected. The transfer of focus to the functional consequences is frequently very difficult for the patient. The underlying wish is for a return to "wholeness," to be once again unimpaired. It is crucial to enable the patient to bridge this transition, to get on with life, without denying the underlying wish.

What Are the Goals?

Once the problem has been identified to the fullest extent possible, the next step is to explore the goals that, when accomplished, would indicate that the problem has been alleviated. It is common for patients to be asked about their problem as part of any medical encounter. It is far less usual to address the question of goals with the patient. Patient willingness to address this question requires a leap into the future. It may be quite difficult for persons to make that leap if they are accustomed to interactions with health professionals in which their active role is limited to the recital of problems. The message sent by this question is that change is possible. The patient is more likely to be willing to address this new question if the preceding exploration of concerns has been thorough enough to offer the opportunity for communication of empathy. At some point, the focus can now change to look toward the future. Once again, the ability to address this question varies. It is the role of the professional, now serving as a consultant in planning, to enable the patient to address this question with increasing facility.

Just as the concerns vary with the person's characteristics, so do the goals. Many of the measures used in assessment of disabilities assume that the appropriate goals include a reduction in the degree to which one requires assistance. The goal is defined as reducing that burden of help needed. This is true only in part. The assumption also exists that the items selected by such measures as the FIM or the Barthel Index (BI) encompass the universe of possible disabilities to be addressed. This, of course, is not so. For many, the goals are to be able to carry on one's work or other aspects of one's life and not necessarily to spend several hours each day trying to get oneself dressed or many days learning how to get dressed. The health professional needs to ensure that the patient can contribute to the definition of the goals and not assume what they are. One should collaborate with the person who identified the problem(s) in generating measure(s) that would give a sense of accomplishment.

For example, in the case of persons with chronic pain, the elements to be addressed include components within the three domains: biological, psychological, and social.[7] For the patient with severe poststroke pain who was described previously, goals became increasingly specific as well as far reaching, although they were related to his overall goal of getting back to life outside his house. At first, the goals were stated in the limited terms of "not becoming nauseated with pain." The goals then expanded to not only being able to ride in a car but to drive a car, including being able to twist the body while backing into a parking space and then, later, being able to travel several hundred miles to go to his son's wedding.

The process by which goals are generated can also change the character of the answers. For example, one concern may have been "pain in the left shoulder so bad that I can't sleep." Evidence that the problem is being solved would be a goal statement relevant to the concern. This would vary depending on the person who is experiencing the pain. For some, the goal might be to do away with the impairment, that is, the pain. A statement might therefore be "I want my shoulder pain to go away." In its further exploration, that statement might now change to dealing with the functional consequences on the level of its interference with sleep: "I want to be able to sleep my usual 8 hours each night." Still another level of exploration could address the functional consequences of the pain on an even deeper level in that sleep has its own functional consequence: "I don't want the pain to interfere with my rest so I can feel ready to start my day." One can thus transform the focus from the impairment to be addressed on the level of the disease process to the disability and even to the level

of QOL. The treatment plan could be quite different depending on the level at which the goal is established. As with the exploration step in answer to the question about concerns, asking the question three times has generally been satisfactory in working through the goals.

Another value of the process of exploration in the design of the goal statement is the concern that the initial goal may be too long range and unrealistic. If the person initially mentions a goal that would require a very long time commitment, eliciting shorter-term goals would be useful to indicate progress at the start. It is important for patients to be able to keep their vision in mind, their "impossible dream," while still defining some intermediate stages that could indicate progress. For example, it is common for persons with stroke to state their goal initially as "to be able to walk again." Depending on the actual status in terms of mobility, the initial short-term goal might be to be able to stand or sit or to be able to go from sitting to standing, and so forth. All these shorter-term goals are compatible with the longer-term goal of walking and should be related to it. There would be a greater likelihood of at least producing one goal statement to which both the professional and the patient can agree if several different goals or the different shorter-term stages in relation to any one long-range goal are explored.

Many people have difficulty distinguishing between *goals* and *means*. The goal statement relates to outcomes, the results, the ends to which any intervention is to be directed. The ends to be achieved can be addressed at different levels of complexity. Ultimately, the highest level is that of the function of the organism in one's total environment in achieving one's life goals. An example at this level is the complex set of actions encompassed within locomotion or getting food. Goals at this level can include earning or otherwise acquiring the means of getting food, shopping and making the selection, food preparation, and eating. To accomplish this complex set of actions, some activities are necessary at the level of organism. Several organ systems are coordinated such as that of locomotion and planning. Locomotion, in turn, is an organ system that includes coordinated actions of the trunk, arms, and legs. A still lower goal level would be at the organ level, such as the coordinated stepping of one of the limbs.

It is at the level of the organ or weak leg that one tends to begin to focus. If the focus remains there, then the goal can be to strengthen that leg. However, that action is merely contributory to the higher-level goals. The lower level is but a means to an end. The weak leg may have deprived the person of walking as a means of getting around. It is important to recognize that what has been lost is a means and not the ultimate goal. Mobility in the service of the organism is the aim to get to work or to shop for food, for example. Doing so by walking has obviously been important; it is the normal way. It is not, however, the only way by which one got around in the past, and its unavailability does not preclude getting around in the future; however, that fact is not easily accepted. Being clear in one's own mind of this important distinction can aid in developing a sense of alternatives in the client. One can continue to achieve one's life goals even if the means need to change.

The goal statement should therefore build on the basic identification of what is important to the person. It is important that the statement(s) eventually generated are specific enough so that their accomplishment can be measured by the person involved along with the professional. The answers to the goal question can thus serve as the basis for addressing the next question.

What Outcomes Have Been Achieved/What Is the Present Status?

Addressing this question begins the review process and the completion of a cycle. It makes the connection between the present status and the previous leap of faith into the future. It can thus confirm the validity of having addressed that previous question. Longer-term commitment depends on seeing results. At times, the previous goal statement may have been too far reaching despite the efforts to make it less so. Some would emphasize the importance of setting only easily accomplished goals at the start. However, one critical criterion has been that the goal be meaningful to the client. The process of goal setting is recurrent so that one can now begin to adjust one's sights on the basis of experience.

The threefold exploration step once again can affect the perception of those involved. The first answer to the question may be a global statement that nothing has been accomplished. It may be necessary to increase the awareness of some of the intermediate steps that have been achieved even if the entire goal was not met. One may find that many more small incremental steps need to be achieved. Alternatively, larger or unanticipated accomplishments may have occurred. It is also helpful to relate the present status in relation to the goal that had been established previously.

For example, a woman with marked flexor spasticity of the left arm after a stroke was treated with botulin toxin so that her arm would become less spastic. After treatment, when asked about the outcome, her first answer was, "I can't see any change." Her reference was that she still could not use the arm as she had before the stroke. When she was then asked whether she could now do anything more easily, her answer became more specific and more positive. "I can get my clothes on a little easier, I can use the arm to hold things down." These more functional goals may have been identified with her before the botulin toxin was given but perhaps only fleetingly. They now need to be recalled to her by the health professional. Failure to define these more limited goals before the use of a costly treatment such as botulin toxin makes everyone dissatisfied and prevents proper evaluation of effectiveness of any treatment.

It is necessary for the professional to help the client address this question several times before a sense of accomplishment and greater hope for the future can arise. Recital of at least three statements concerning accomplishments seems to be useful to establish that sense of possibility that there may be other accomplishments. One can now go on to address the future goal again. If the initial problem continues to exist, a new set of goals can be defined in relation to that problem, now in the light of experience. The time line for re-evaluation can also now be adjusted in light of experience. If the initial problem has been resolved, one can identify a new concern and set a new goal as a mark of its resolution.

The monitoring of progress is an integral part of the entire management process.[8] Follow-up is critical. To the extent practicable, the goals have been defined so that they can be measured by the client along with the professional. For example, in the implementation of plans for the management of risk factors to reduce the likelihood of recurrent stroke, the problem generally is not the identification of the risk factors or the appropriate treatments. What is problematic is the degree to which a person with hypertension, as an example, adheres to the regimens recommended. In such a long-term commitment, it is critical that the client can monitor on an ongoing basis the results that are achieved. Knowledge of one's goal in terms of blood pressure control provides the opportunity for easy measurement with an automatic monitor. The recurrent process of review that goes on in most rehabilitation settings at the team conference is another mechanism. The methods by which patient participation can be accomplished within clinical settings is discussed later in this chapter.

What Has Worked?

A plan consists of not only a set of goals and time for evaluation but also the means or treatments to be done to help achieve the goals. This question is even less commonly asked of the patient than the others, but it is potentially the most helpful. The treatment procedures, equipment, or medication regimen that have been put into place also can be reviewed at the completion of a cycle. Onc can seek the answer to this question in the context of the recital of the several accomplishments. It is the relationship between the outcomes and the means that is important. What is being sought is the efficacy of the treatments and a validation of their appropriateness. Any treatment has its costs. It takes time and effort on the part of the client and, frequently, additional professional commitment. If medication has been recommended, it frequently has additional costs in terms of possible side effects. For an activity to be considered efficacious, it must be viewed as having the power to produce a desired effect. The general efficacy of a drug, for example, may have been established as a prerequisite for its dispensation; however, its value must be confirmed in the mind of the persons involved for it to be continued. It is in the answering of this question that the treatments can not only be validated but modified so that they are tailored to the individual person.

It is particularly helpful to question what may have worked in the context of actual outcomes. In the context of having achieved some outcomes, one can consider what might have contributed to such achievements. It is sometimes necessary to evoke the actual setting in which the successful outcomes occurred ("when, where, who was there?"). In the case of the man with severe post-stroke pain, he was able to review on one occasion several instances when he was "freed from the prison" of his previous existence. These included "traveling to my son's house, taking a graduation trip," and "being able to back my car into a parking space while turning my body." It was in the context of having had several such experiences compatible with his stated goal that he was now able to consider for the first time what may have worked. By being willing to address this new question, the person with the problem has now changed his perception of the situation. He has begun to entertain the notion that actions exist that would possibly be efficacious, and he has become more aware of what some might be. Moreover, it is an awareness of actions that one has taken oneself that can help create a sense of self-efficacy. After exploring several alternatives, one can ask the client to select an action that was particularly outstanding that could then be specified in terms of where or when it occurred, and so forth.

Some of the strategies were specific, others were more generic. For example, the patient with chronic pain mentioned that while riding in the car, the pain was lessened when he would use a pillow to hold up the affected arm so that it would not be jolted. Another idea that seemed to work was to ensure that he sat supported while in a chair. Another more generic idea was that it was helpful to keep track of the times he went out or did other things that represented an accomplishment for him. The very process of keeping track was helpful in reminding him of what had happened. The question of how all the progress that had been made came about was asked of persons with stroke who were being discharged home from an inpatient facility. Many of the answers reflected the process of "knowing my goal, knowing what I am trying to do, knowing that I am reaching my goals."

Not only are specific strategies important, but the realization that a number of strategies exist is important as well. The threefold exploration step can once again be useful to establish the sense that a number of ways exist to deal with one's problem. If one way does not work, there are usually others that one could use. What that can convey is that alternatives are available. This sense of options, of alternative ways of doing things, is part of the message that needs to be conveyed to the person living with chronic illness. The old and "normal" ways of doing things may no longer be possible. It is necessary to consider that alternative ways exist and that one can use them to accomplish one's life goals. Ultimately, there must be acceptance at some level that, by being different, the alternative means that now remain available are not necessarily worse.

The focus on problem-solving strategies emphasizes the ongoing nature of the problems being faced. The problems and outcomes can vary over time, but the strategies for solving problems usually have more general application. The application of strategies in a number of different settings can aid in generalizing the strategies. The most generic application is the very process of asking the question as to what may have worked.

In describing the questions in this section, the assumption has been made that they are addressed in their entirety and in a particular set sequence. That is not necessarily true. However, it has been helpful to consider the questions as sets of pairs. For example, it is the relationship between the definition of the problem and the next step of looking to the future by setting a goal that is important. Similarly, it is the relationship between the previous goal and the question of the outcomes that is important as validating a connection between the commitment to thinking about the future and the actual accomplishments. Once again, it is the relationship between the results achieved and the actions taken and strategies used that serves to validate actions that might have required considerable effort and commitment.

The planning questions have been presented thus far as part of an ongoing relationship between the health professional as a consultant in planning and the client. The goal is for the patients to become aware of the value of asking themselves such questions. When considering how to reduce costs of management of persons with chronic illness the issue arises as to the value of an ongoing monitoring of patients in conjunction with the health care professionals. One attribute of the approach being described is that added value is created. Successive interactions can lead to an increment in the patient's self-knowledge about the ability to use the planning questions to manage his

or her own life. A method for enhancing the development of such self-knowledge is the subject of the next section.

Conjoint Planning

The planning process is based on a set of questions that are recycled again and again. In the context of this reiteration, the opportunity is available for increased awareness of the questions that one may eventually ask oneself. An ongoing process exists in which the answers to these questions can also become increasingly those of the client. An accompanying increase can therefore occur in the degree to which the answers become more salient to the person, with greater self-awareness. One can become more aware of one's problems and then the goals. One can become more aware of the present status the progress achieved and what actions were useful.

Self-awareness can increase to the degree that one hears oneself speak. The participation scale to be described reflects the level of verbal participation. As one speaks in the context of another person who gives evidence of listening, one can better hear oneself. The verbal behavior is also considered to be a basis for subsequent action. By optimizing the ownership of the replies to the questions, one is affecting the state of mind and increasing the commitment to potential action. The process therefore is to enable the person to speak for him- or herself. The role of the professional as a consultant in planning is to optimize the conditions for that to occur.

The consultant's use of questions as a means of involving the client has a definite purpose. MacKay[9] emphasizes that the grammatical form used in a discourse changes the character of the discourse. By asking a question, one signifies two things. First, the content of the question indicates what the questioner considers important. The questioner is giving information to the listener that has the potential of changing the listener's perception. For example, the question "What worked?" causes the listener to consider that some actions may have been useful. Second, the use of a question rather than a statement indicates something apart from the content; it invites the listener to contribute, to help, to participate.

MacKay goes on to state that, in a social unit established by any dialogue, "meaning" is a relative concept, different for the originator of the message and its recipient and dependent on the grammatical form used. An indicative statement attempts to affect the recipient's state of mind. For example, the indicative statement "it is raining out" has the potential to affect the recipient's state of mind, and possibly his actions, in respect to going out or using an umbrella. A question has both an interrogative and indicative function. It combines both an invitation and an indication. The question "Is it raining out?" is an invitation for the recipient of the message to affect the originator, by filling in what is missing in the mind of the originator. It is an offering by the originator to have his or her state of mind potentially modified by the recipient. Both the indicative statement and the question can modify the orientation of the participants in a dialogue. The direction of the effects is mainly on the recipient's state of mind in the case of the indicative statement and on the originator's state of mind in the case of the question.

A request or command claims control over the recipient. The originator seeks to directly control the recipient's actions, not merely his or her state of mind. "Don't go out because it is raining!" has an indicative quality as describing the goals of the originator, but its imperative nature seeks to control the actions of the recipient. Thus, the meaning of a message is governed by its grammatical form, reflecting the degree of control sought by the individual over another. Both the indicative statement and the question seek to affect the recipient's state of mind, with the question representing a lesser attempt at control by the originator. The attempt to affect the state of mind may, only by extension, affect the actions that the recipient takes. A command attempts to directly modify the recipient's actions without allowing the recipient to participate in the decision.

Because each person has different patterns of experience and different perceptions of the situation, one may perceive things that are almost beyond the grasp of the other. The originator in any dialogue has to discover and understand the state of belief of the recipient. With different sets of goal priorities, it is possible for one person to see the need for actions almost beyond the grasp of the other. The originator of any dialogue, here the professional, has to discover the order of priorities of the recipient, here the client. The use of questions provides a form of discourse in which disparate perceptions and goals can be reconciled to permit common action. With increased experience, the client can contribute to an increasing degree to the design of the ongoing treatment.

It is our premise that conscious attention by the professional to the degree to which ownership can be transferred to the client would lead to greater actual participation by the client in the planning. Greater participation in the planning signifies contribution of energy and ideas by the client, thereby enhancing the implementation of the plans so made. Nordenfelt[10] suggests that a holistic notion of health would incorporate the ability to attain the goals that are set by oneself. The value of eliciting clients' participation in the management of their health is well established in a number of settings.[11,12] It is particularly important in the management of risk factors for prevention of illness, in which situation self-monitoring of the goals originally set can aid in the maintenance of long-term plans.[13,14]

Participation Scale

A scale has been designed to measure the degree of participation in the answering of any of the planning questions. The activity is considered to be an interaction under the control of the professional. The actions of the client are therefore at least in part due to the conditions provided for participation.

Table 2-2 describes a four-point scale of participation. One may note that an additional level is outside the scale. It is placed there as a point of departure and contrast. Ordinarily, a place is not included on the scale for "compliance," which reflects a person operating under orders in which the actions are predetermined without any intermediate thought and "prescribed" as though under orders. No choice has been offered. Although widespread, the use of terms such as *compliance* and *prescription* is inappropriate in other than an acute situation or emergency.[15] The very use of these terms betrays a lack of awareness of what would be the optimal quality of the interaction in dealing with the management of chronic illness. Nevertheless, it is commonplace for the person to be told

Table 2-2. Participation Scale

	Professional	Client	Action Taken
1. Independence	—	Asks self; answers for self	—
2. Free choice	Asks open question; can agree (or disagree)	States answer for him- or herself	Accordance
3. Choice	Recommends Asks for confirmation	Agrees (or disagrees) Confirms in own words	Adherence
4. Forced choice	Recommends Does not ask	Agrees (or disagrees); nods or says yes	Adherence
No choice	Prescribes Does not ask Action predetermined	Acquiesces	Compliance

what the problem might be on the basis of assessments done by various professional staff and to have goals as well as treatments assigned without any opportunity for agreement to be sought.It is not surprising that patients follow instructions less than 50% of the time if treatment is aimed at long-term prevention. The follow-through is similar on exercise programs and in the use of prescribed equipment.[16] Such low levels of follow-through with plans seriously affect the quality and increase the costs of health care by lowering its effectiveness. Follow-through is improved when patient expectations regarding their treatment are met, which is more likely when the client and the professional have agreed as to expectations. Follow-through is also increased when the client is involved in goal setting and in monitoring progress.

Agreement

The lowest level on the scale is that of agreement. Concomitant to this level of participation would be actions by the patient at the level of "adherence" to that which has been agreed on. The professional has made a "recommendation," a single statement. The character of the interaction is quite limited in terms of options available; hence the term *forced choice* can be used to describe its quality. The client can demonstrate agreement (or disagreement) by nodding or indicating assent. The principle of this level of participation is that the actions are not predetermined; there is an opportunity to affirm the thought before the action.

This level of participation can be in answer to any one or other of the planning questions. Eliciting this as the highest level of participation is commonplace in interactions with health professionals.

Much of medical care of persons with chronic illness operates at this level, at which the client has not truly been asked but an answer is given in the form of a recommendation. This level of participation can be considered to be minimal. The aim is to move up the scale to the extent possible. During the course of the client's interaction over time, the degree of participation can be expected to rise on the basis of increased experience with one's life in dealing with the chronic illness and as a result of increased experience with the process of planning itself. A patient who has difficulty in expressing him- or herself due to language problems may be able to interact only at this level. It was found, for example, that persons with stroke could participate at this level provided that they were able to be consistent with yes or no. One man with expressive language difficulties was nevertheless able to convey his disagreement with a recommendation made by a therapist concerning his goals by shaking his head. One can meet the criterion of agreement by other nonverbal means. For example, one could check off something that is written.

Confirmed Agreement

The next level of participation is that of "confirmed agreement." The principle of this category is that the participant expresses in some way that which had been agreed on. For example, if a recommendation had been made to which the patient had agreed by nodding or saying yes, confirmation would consist of putting that which had been agreed on "into their own words." It is not intended that the ideas agreed on merely be parroted but, rather, made part of the person in some way. A major change occurs when the person must actively produce a statement rather than take the more passive role of merely nodding or assenting in some other way. The professional has invited some further participation by now asking for confirmation. It is not uncommon for the statement so generated to be somewhat different from the original yet quite appropriate. Now a change has been made by the client to which the professional can now choose to agree (or disagree).

It is important that the new wording that has been negotiated be used henceforth. This level of participation differs from the level of agreement in that the expression of offered ideas has occurred. It differs from the next level, *statement*, in that the ideas do not initially arise from the client but have been offered by the professional. The mode by which one can confirm agreement may vary. One option is to speak aloud; another is to read aloud from a previously offered list; still another is to write out from a list what was agreed on. "Putting into one's own words" can also be expressed by gesture. In all these instances, the principle has been followed of having the person organize herself enough to express the statement that has been recommended and agreed on. By saying it aloud, the most common method, the person hears it for himself and can integrate it to a greater degree than when it had merely been agreed on. The client actions taken in relation to this higher level of agreement remain at the level of adherence. The likelihood of adherence can be expected to be greater than when a person merely agrees because there has been some modification of the ideas by the patient's contributions. The client now has taken a role in making the entire effort fit him or her.

The value of this step can be illustrated in the case of an elderly man with balance problems secondary to recurrent strokes that affected the brain stem and cerebellum. He had trouble using a walker, which could help him to maintain his balance while walking. He could not seem to remember to keep his feet the proper distance apart despite having been shown and actually having his feet placed apart. The concern expressed by the therapist was that his cognitive impairments secondary to his widespread vascular disease and age would prevent him from learning what was needed. He could be described as "noncompliant." An alternative was to focus the interaction so that the

instruction would be modified to derive from him, at least in part.

The overall goal had been clearly agreed on. He understood and agreed to his need to be able to get around on his own without falling because he lived alone. He was asked, "How would you know how far apart your feet should be?" His answer was to point to the knobs on the top of the walker as helping him to estimate the proper distance. His balance then improved immediately by his using the instruction he had just modified. He had not contributed the strategy in its entirety; it had been recommended to him. However, he had made it work for him by modifying it in part, by specifying it. In so doing, it appeared to become more effective for two complementary reasons: It had become more precise, but also it had been made his and thus was more likely to be followed. By virtue of the interaction, the entire issue of the need for a wide base had been made more explicit and more likely to be followed independently. Eliciting his participation allowed the slight increment in ability to use the strategy that was apparently sufficient to make it effective.

Confirmed agreement can be the level of participation that is sought. It is, for example, an objective in some programs in the management of persons with SCI for patients to instruct their caregivers about their skin care management plan. Doing so from their written notes or printed material provided by the staff would be acceptable evidence of their having learned their set of procedures. The use of these notes would be an example of reaching the confirmed agreement level of performance. By reading aloud in interaction with another, one is better able to hear oneself.

Statement

An even higher level of participation is when one makes a statement in response to an open-ended question. The patient has been given a "free choice." The principle of this category is that the person has generated de novo the answers to any of the planning questions without any recommendations. The professional has enabled this level of participation by asking open questions to which no predetermined answers have been provided. Any actions taken would be in accordance with the freely made statements. Whereas *adherence* infers being a follower, the distinction is made that now the person is acting in accordance with his or her own ideas. The professional has merely acted as a consultant by asking the questions. The professional can now, in turn, agree (or disagree) to what has been proposed by the client. It can be expected that the client, by contributing freely to the plan, also owns that which has been produced to a greater degree, with greater likelihood of commitment to the subsequent actions.

Once the level of making statements has been reached, the professional has the option of asking the client to meet the criterion of specificity described earlier. This has been scored as "specific statement" in some scales. It would include defining not only answers to the question of what was to be the statement of the problem, the goal, or the measure of status, and so forth, but also meeting the additional criteria such as "to what degree?" and so forth. Greater specificity can contribute, for example, to clarity in evaluating the degree to which one has met the goal. Additionally, the clearer one is about what one is trying to accomplish, the more likely it is that one can keep it in mind and strive to accomplish it.

The man described previously who had major difficulty in expressive language was nevertheless able to act at the statement level of participation by gesturing to communicate the goal he wanted to meet. When the therapist made a recommendation for him to continue to proceed with a goal of dressing his upper body, he shook his head vehemently in disagreement. Rather, he pointed and grunted to his thigh, indicating his interest in doing something about his lower body. In response to his gestures, it was possible to put into words what he seemed to be saying. He nodded his agreement when he was offered the idea of dressing his lower body. He met the criterion of this category of statement by generating his own answer to the question of goal, albeit by unusual means.

The connection between the statement and the commitment to the action to be taken is illustrated in the case of a woman with long-standing weakness of the right side of the body due to a stroke. The question of what works was being addressed. Her concerns dealt with her difficulties in getting in and out of bed from her wheelchair without the aid of her husband. The goal she stated on her own was to be able to stand without her husband's aid.

In practicing with her therapist, she was able to slide forward in her chair to bring her weight more directly over her legs; however, she had difficulty in pulling herself up to a standing position because of previous surgery to her knee that prevented full range of motion. She was given the recommendation of instructing her husband to "lift!" when she was ready. He would then raise her to a standing position. She agreed to do so. When first putting the recommendation into action, she used her own word by saying "up" rather than the word *lift* that had been recommended. The important point is that she was no longer being lifted without her participation. The husband was asked to wait on her instruction and to repeat it before acting on it. The aim was for her to give herself the command along with giving it to her husband. At first, she was primarily giving the instruction to her husband. After a number of trials, she was giving the instruction to herself with commitment of the energy required to overcome the difficulty with her knee. She would say "up!" The additional increment by virtue of her contribution to phrasing the command and her commitment of force were actually bringing her to a standing position. When asked further about what had worked, she stated, "I was afraid I would fall. I could see that I could do it and it was I who was doing it." Rather than saying the command "up!" aloud, she would now say it to herself. She had internalized the instruction.

To illustrate the eventual outcome, an additional level of participation, *independence*, is displayed in Table 2-2. This is the level at which clients ask questions of themselves as well as provide the answers. This option is the eventual goal at which patients are now acting as their own planning consultant.

The specific level to be reached in relation to any of the planning questions can vary. One can focus on gain in level of participation rather than any specific criterion. For example, in one plan for persons with head injury, the objective is for the client to be able to address the question as to the status of his or her long-term goals at the time of discharge. The level was to be an increment from that of admission to the outpatient transition program. The objective of another plan is for the person with stroke to be able to address the question of goal at a statement level by the time of discharge when addressing the question of postdischarge goal. Still another plan has as its objective for

Table 2-3. Development of Independence

Stage	Professional	Patient	Goal
Acute	Asks the questions via neurologic assessment; focuses on signs	Relatively passive	To determine impairment
Rehabilitation	Asks the question via an interview	Collaborative	To determine disabilities
Continuing care		Independent; asks questions of self	To determine need for professional care

patients with SCI to address the question of outcome by being able to record their status and determine whether they had met the goal agreed to in reference to bladder function and skin integrity.

During the various phases of life after the onset of chronic illness, the role of the client vis-à-vis the professional can change. In the acute phase of any illness, the level of participation in general may be at the no choice or forced choice level, depending on the acuity of the illness. During the ongoing training or rehabilitation phase, an opportunity and a need exist for the relationship to move toward greater degrees of freedom in decision making in the context of one's life plans and their implementation. This becomes even more significant during the ongoing life of the person living in the community, where one of the objectives to be met is to address the questions on one's own and establish the criteria for when professional help is needed. Table 2-3 illustrates this development in relation to the question concerning the existence of a problem. Similar development occurs in relation to the several other questions. For example, in becoming independent, when addressing the question as to results the person with the problem has learned how to monitor him/herself as a basis for evaluating the degree to which goals have been achieved.

The aim of any healing relationship, in Pellegrino's words,[17] is to "restore wholeness, or if this is not possible, to assist in striking some new balance between what the body imposes and the self aspires to." If full restoration is not possible, amelioration, adaptation, or coping becomes the goal of the healing relationship. It is essential that the actions taken not only be technically correct but also ultimately "good" for that patient. *Good* healing actions refer to those that the individual patient perceives as worthwhile and that are personally derived from and incorporated into the patient's life. Pellegrino goes on to emphasize that the "unequivocal criterion of a good decision is one

which . . . leads to an enhancement of the patient's moral agency" even if this is contrary to the physician's opinion. This principle of the patient's empowerment underlies the whole process of conjoint management of the problems faced by persons with chronic illness. The goal is to catalyze and energize the person's capacity for life.

Coordinated Planning

The problems faced by persons with chronic illness cannot ordinarily be encompassed within a dialogue between a single professional and a single client. Several clients are generally present, including the spouse and other family members. Within the total bio-psycho-social matrix are usually several areas to be evaluated that involve several different professionals with varying focus. Comprehensive treatment generally focuses on the various dimensions of performance, such as cognitive, motor, or psychological. For example, the psychologist may intervene for the patient's feelings of hopelessness or in relation to demonstrated memory problems, or both. The speech therapist may offer training in communication issues. The nurse can offer training in areas of health promotion and sphincter control and instruction concerning medication. Various therapists may offer training in mobility and activities of daily living. The social worker may be concerned with the organization of the caregiver training and dealing with the availability of equipment. The physician may be concerned with medical issues and the overall administration of the plan.

The planning system must be adapted to a group process, at least within most inpatient programs. Just as growth must be present in the degree of conjoint planning over time, the primary participants—the client or family, or both—frequently must develop the ability to participate in the coordination of the planning team.

Any discussion about the planning team must start with the question as to its continued use within rehabilitation. What has been one of rehabilitation's most salient characteristics has been under attack in terms of its efficiency in the use of resources as well as its effectiveness in creating a focused approach to treatment and thus enhanced outcomes. Long taken for granted, it is now being analyzed as deserving of continuation in respect to its characteristics.[18]

The useful distinction has long been made between the use of staff representing the multiple disciplines appropriate for the manifold problems and the principle of the more coordinated interdisciplinary team.[19] Diller[20] has advanced the principle that "transdisciplinary" teams would, by cross training, transcend their specific professional identities to function in their roles within a work team. These distinctions reflect the efforts to deal with one of the stresses inherent in the structure of the rehabilitation team. One issue has been the basis on which the members of a team are selected. Are members chosen primarily on the basis of their personal characteristics—to contribute to the effectiveness of the team function—or are they chosen simply because they are professionals who represent a particular discipline?[21]

Rehabilitation teams attempt to strike a balance between the personal and the professional. Without the diversity of professionals, the team does not exist. It was this diversity of skills that inspired the formation of teams. This same aspect can undermine the effectiveness of the team to do its job. In most instances, the strength of the bond that holds the professionals together as team members appears to be weaker than the reference group of their professional discipline. One solution that is being advanced to deal with this issue is that the focus of the team's effort be clearly linked to patient outcomes rather than to activities alone. "Fit" between the patient and the team can be most clearly established when the patient is brought onto the team. By doing so, the patient can direct the team toward strategies that can lead to outcomes that are realistic and of greatest personal value.[22]

Another issue to be considered relates not so much to the organizational structures or role identification as to coordination in the design and implementation of the actual treatments.[23] The patient's presenting conditions provide the content of the team. Although some overlap may occur, each of the disciplines has a domain that represents its primary interest. Problems arise when coordination between disciplines dealing with similar domains is poor, or clarity, in terms of priority between domains, is lacking. For example, although it is common for nursing staff to deal with problems of incontinence, it may not be clear how that issue may interact with the therapist understanding the priority to be attached to training for toilet transfer in this particular patient. Dressing may be taught differently by nursing staff, responsible on certain days, and the therapist, working on other days. All staff have occasion to carry out transfers from bed to wheelchair yet would not necessarily take the opportunity to reinforce the techniques used by the physical therapist who is ordinarily assigned responsibility for training that activity. One option is for the patient to be the central carrier of the information concerning his or her status and the technique to be followed.

Each discipline carries out its activities without focus on common interests. Bridging the gap between disparate priorities can be aided when one involves the patient. At the level of the patient, the problem domains are not clearly delineated. They overlap and are far more fluid according to changing conditions. Each discipline is expert in general problems within its selected domain, the problems that may be common to all patients of a particular type such as a stroke that affects one or the other side of the brain. It is the particulars of the situation—of this person's stroke, in this life and in this time—that must be understood. The blending of the expertise of the professional with the specific needs and expectations of the patient can bring about the necessary focus on what may be appropriate interdisciplinary plans.

The activities of the team in planning must incorporate communication, coordination, and problem solving. The crossing of boundaries within the team and the development of shared priority goals depend on the patient being enabled to become central to the team process. Many different techniques may be useful to make this happen. In a program for persons with stroke, for example, the patient is normally present at all the team meetings, with the caregiver also present when necessary. In a program for persons with SCI, the patient is physically present in each of the team meetings after the initial one. In a program for persons with TBI, the caregiver is normally present and the patient is only occasionally there during the inpatient phase, but the patient is always present during the outpatient phase of treatment. In other settings, a person is identified as a coach and is responsible for communicating to the patient the results of the meeting. This obeys the letter of the law in that the person with disabilities is informed, but this method fails to implement the possibilities inherent in actual presence. It is important to recognize that the eventual aim is for the patient to contribute to the planning and, if possible, to develop the capability to direct it.

The mere physical presence of the patient does not necessarily constitute participation. The patient should not be spoken *about* in his or her presence but spoken *with*, and the person eventually should speak for him- or herself. This requires some preparation for the patient to be able to contribute in the assigned role of bringing focus and unity to the team planning process. How can the patient be enabled to carry out this role?

The physician can have an active role in bringing about the unity of the team, now enlarged to incorporate the patient or family members, or both. As the team leader, that person can also be assigned the role of patient advocate in ensuring the patient's opportunity to participate in the group planning. Each of the members of the team has the additional role of ensuring patient participation in the planning dealing with each of the particular domains as well as contributing his or her knowledge to the overall priorities of the team at the meeting. It is at that meeting that the team leader in the role of patient advocate can ensure that documentation occurs of the level of participation within each domain. However, the entire team, in each of its interactions, must support this effort. For example, many therapists would review informally the goals with the patients and their progress at the end of each day's session and do so consistently just before the weekly team meeting.

An example of integration of the patient into the successive team meetings has taken place in a program for persons with stroke. The nursing staff had the role of reducing risk factors for recurrent stroke such as hypertension and hyperlipemia as part of a health plan. The therapists were responsible for implementation of the plan for reducing the degree of disability as evidenced by a rehabilitation plan. The details of that program are described in Chapter 4. Common interdisciplinary interests were dealt with at the team meeting as well as review of the plans being carried out by each of the several therapists. Activities were coordinated at the weekly team meetings. Table 2-4 describes a prototype management plan that increases patient participation in planning rehabilitation as measured during the inpatient stay and subsequent follow-up sessions.

Each of the plans was put into effect after an initial assessment period. The first of the team meetings occurred within 72 hours after the completion of the assessment carried out by the therapists. At the end of each of the initial assessments, the appropriate planning questions were to have been addressed with the patient by the various team members. The initial team meeting was concerned with the coordination of the various plans and the formation of any interdisciplinary plans that required more than one staff member for their implementation. The team meeting was also the opportunity for documentation of the degree to which the patient had been involved thus far. In the context of the recurrent team meetings, the patient had the opportunity, being present, to become more aware of the questions addressed in the planning process as well as becoming more aware of the answers by virtue of contributing to them.

Evaluation of Implementation

The process of individual planning requires ongoing review and revision. The implementation of an overall program-wide plan dealing with groups of patients similarly requires ongoing review and revision. The effective implementation of any plan with an individual patient requires that attention be paid to the level of participation elicited. Similarly, attention needs to be paid to achieving commitment by the staff to such an effort. Participation is encouraged in modifying the methods used as well as setting goals for successive programmatic level changes. For example, the implementation within a stroke unit can require agreement for a coordinated approach by several physicians and their teams, made up of a number of different therapists. It has

Table 2-4. Stroke Recovery Program

	Days 1–3 Assessment	Day 4 Initial I/P Team Meeting	Day 11 Interim Team Meeting	Day 18 Discharge Team Meeting	(Varies) Initial Ambulatory Team Meeting	(Varies) Interim Ambulatory Team Meeting(s)	(Varies) Discharge Team Meeting
Activities	Rehabilitation plan designed	I/P interdisciplinary plan completed	I/P rehabilitation plan implemented, reviewed, revised	I/P rehabilitation plan reviewed, revised. Ambulatory rehabilitation plan designed	Ambulatory rehabilitation plan completed	Ambulatory rehabilitation plan implemented, reviewed, revised	Ambulatory rehabilitation plan implemented, reviewed, revised
Objectives	1. Rehabilitation problems identified 2. Goals established	1. Status reviewed 2. Priority goals established	1. Status established 2. New goals established	1. New status established 2. What worked established 3. New goals established	1. New status established 2. What worked established 3. New goals established	1. New status established 2. What worked established 3. New goals established	1. New status established 2. What worked established 3. New goals established

I/P = in-patient.

been particularly helpful in eliciting increasing commitment to do so via a low-cost method for data collection and consistent feedback of data reflecting degree of implementation. The principle has been to make data collection intrinsic to the clinical efforts.

The goals set for any programmatic level plan such as on a stroke unit can specify two aspects. One is the questions to be addressed; the other is the degree to which the patient, a family member, or both are enabled to answer those questions. The degree to which the total set of planning questions is being implemented in concert with the patients can be established for the entire program. One or another of the questions might be addressed. One can recall that the wording of the questions can send a message. Overall, by considering any of the questions, patients have opportunities to change their perspective. For example, the use of the question of concerns is designed to move toward an awareness of functional limitations rather than impairments and so forth. The culture of a program begins to change as one begins to consider goals

and outcomes and "what works" throughout the staff. The more often the question is addressed, the greater the likelihood that the question and the message it can convey arise in the patients' minds as a useful issue to be considered.

Figure 2-2 describes the format used for team meetings. Data to be used for evaluation were thus documented within the context of providing patient care. The larger box contains the answers to the planning questions addressed during the team meeting. One may note that categories are identified that reflect the areas that are ordinarily reviewed for persons with stroke in an inpatient program. The categories vary depending on the content of the program. For those with SCI, for example, the areas could focus on other issues. A notation in these boxes signifies that the question was addressed and could be used for documentation for that purpose. A notation in the smaller box indicates that the question was addressed with the patient. Thus, the use of the question is documented with the patient. Secondarily, the specific notation (derived from the participation scale) signifies the

	Status/Progress	Goals	What Works/Cues
Mobility	□	□	□
Self-care	□	□	□
Health	□	□	□
Communication	□	□	□

Figure 2-2. Form for team conference.

level of participation by the patient in answering that question. Notation in both boxes thus documents the implementation of planning with the patient. The specifics of the notation in the smaller box document the actual participation level reached. An "A" reflects agreement; "C," confirmed agreement; "S," statement; and "SS," specific statement. Figure 2-3 illustrates the actual data that might become available at an initial team meeting. At that time, the first opportunity would be available to review the progress in plans dealing with both incontinence and intelligibility of speech that were established on the first day of the patient's stay.

The objectives can vary. A target level of participation can be established in relation to any of the questions at any of the opportunities offered. For example, one objective can be for the goal question to be answered at a statement level by the time of the discharge conference and the status question to be answered at the level of at least confirmed agreement. One can monitor and document various degrees of implementation. The principle is that measurement would be conducted during the team conferences, and scoring would be carried out by team members themselves as a way of raising the awareness of all team members of the level of participation achieved. The team leader or other team member would be initially trained to score the level of participation. Interrater reliability is achieved by having the team members score their own individual interaction with the patient during the team meeting along with the team leader scoring that same interaction.

Phase One

Several phases were involved in the implementation of this approach in a pilot clinical program. The first phase was limited to seeking patient participation in rehabilitation planning only. Participation in planning for health needs would await further training of nursing staff. Limitations existed in the questions to be posed to the patient by the rehabilitation team. The question concerning goal identification has been well established in the lexicon of the therapist and patients in this program. Therapists were accustomed to setting rather specific goals using the FIM as a model. The first phase of implementation was thus to share goal setting with the patient at the initial team meeting. It was also consistent with the therapist's previous experience to address the question as to status in relation to the previous goals at the time of the interim and discharge team meetings. The staff agreed to elicit patient participation in both the status and goal questions at those times. The staff was not prepared to elicit patient participation in respect to addressing the "what worked" question during this first phase.

Figure 2-3. Data that might become available at an initial team meeting. A = agreement; C = confirmed agreement.

	Status/Progress	Goals	What Works/Cues
Mobility	Transfer with moderate (50%) assistance [A]	Transfer with minimal to moderate (35%) assistance [A]	
Self-care	Dressing upper body with moderate (50%) assistance [A]	Dressing upper body with minimal (25%) assistance [A]	
Health	Continent of urine during day [A]	Continent of urine (100%) [C]	Use of every 2-hr toileting schedule [A]
Communication	Intelligibility (60%) [A]	Intelligibility (85%) [A]	Take a deep breath [C]

Table 2-5 describes the limited objectives during this first phase of implementation. The level of implementation reflects the number of times a question was to be addressed. At the time of the initial team meeting, only the goal question was to be addressed in three possible problem areas by the appropriate team members. These were ordinarily mobility; self-care; and communication, swallowing, or both. At the interim and discharge meetings, each of the appropriate staff would address the question of status and new short-term goal. At the discharge meeting, the team leader would incorporate the "what works" question but only in relation to the overall progress that had occurred. Thus, during a typical inpatient stay, a total of nine opportuni-

ties would ordinarily occur for addressing the goal, six opportunities for addressing status, and one opportunity for addressing "what works," and that in relation to general issues. All three planning questions were to be addressed at the initial ambulatory visit in review of the plans made at the time of discharge from inpatient services.

The level of participation sought was even more limited. The objective was for the patient to verbalize the goals (either confirmed agreement or statement) at the time of the discharge meeting. This objective was based on the principle that the discharge conference would be a useful opportunity or the patient to participate indefining appropriate goals to work on at home given the

Table 2-5. Stroke Program: Patient Self-Management Objectives, Phase One*

	Initial Team	Interim Team	Discharge	Initial Ambulatory
Status	—	×3	×3	×3 Confirmed agreement
What worked	—	—	×1	×3 Confirmed agreement
Goals	×3	×3	×3 Confirmed agreement	×3 Confirmed agreement

*Figures indicate the number of times a question was addressed.

Table 2-6. Phase One Evaluation

Level of Implementation		
Questions Addressed	**First Quarter***	**Second Quarter***
Goal	188/360 (52%)	202/288 (70%)
Status	135/240 (56%)	230/288 (80%)
What worked	2/40 (5%)	10/32 (30%)
Level of Participation		
Questions Answered at Confirmed Agreement or Better at Discharge	**First Quarter**	**Second Quarter**
Goal	30%	27%
Status	—	25%
What Worked	—	—

*Numerators indicate the opportunities used by staff for patients to address the planning questions. Denominators indicate the number of opportunities possible.

idiosyncratic quality of each person's environment. One could now begin to call on the patient to be a more active participant given that opportunities have been available throughout the inpatient stay to become aware of the process of planning—the questions and possible answers. At the time of the first postdischarge visit, the objective was to aim for a level of at least some verbalization such as confirmed agreement in answer to the other planning questions including status and any new goal.

Phase one also provided an opportunity to determine the feasibility of the entire effort. It would be necessary to incorporate the patient at the team meeting while maintaining the existing time constraints and to establish a baseline as to the level of participation that could be achieved. Once the feasibility could be established of having the patient present and able to address these questions, one could begin to increase the degree to which the entire approach could be implemented.

Feedback to the staff during this first phase is illustrated in Table 2-6. The level of implementation reflects the degree to which the questions were addressed with the patient. The numerator indicates the opportunities actually used by staff for patients to address the planning questions. The denominator indicates the number of opportunities possible. This figure reflects the number of patients multiplied by the number of possible planning sessions. Data are included from the several planning teams to reflect the activities carried out under the auspices of the several medical team leaders.

The overall objective for implementation of the planning questions during this first phase for the entire stroke program encompassing the three physician-led teams was 75% implementation of the goal and status questions. The data indicate that the degree to which these questions were actually implemented improved during the two quarters, eventually achieving the program objectives. No initial objective was set for the "what works" question during this first phase. Although the number of times that question was addressed increased, the level of implementation was still quite low. A baseline had been established; however, analysis of the several physician-led teams indicated uneven implementation within the total stroke program staff and use primarily on only one of the three teams.

Table 2-6 also describes the level of participation achieved. The objective was to attain some degree of verbalization in respect to the goal statement. During the second quarter, feedback was given about the degree to which verbalization was achieved with respect to the other questions. Some participation, albeit limited, was achieved at the discharge conference that could serve as a baseline for further improvement.

The actual responses elicited in respect to the "what works" question at the discharge meeting are listed in Table 2-7. All statements were recorded and collated. The answers are generic because they were elicited in elation to the overall progress rather than to any specific area. The majority of statements reflected patient commitment. Other

Table 2-7. Responses to "What Worked?"

Awareness of progress (15%)
   Positive attitude/seeing progress/having hope
Awareness of goals (25%)
   Knowing what my goals were/had a goal
What works (5%)
   Using adapted clothes/medication/diet
Commitment (50%)
   Push myself/determination/desire to get better

responses included some of the very activities being carried out during the process of patient participation such as goal setting and monitoring progress.

Phase Two

The objectives of the second phase of implementation are described in Table 2-8. This table describes both the level of implementation to be achieved (i.e., questions addressed) and the level of participation on the part of the patient (i.e., answers). The nursing staff began to initiate a health plan immediately on the patient's admission, with the first review at the time of the initial interdisciplinary team meeting at 72 hours. A minimum of four plans were now made with the patient. These changes increased the number of times the planning questions were addressed but also marked the extension to the entire professional team.

The number of times that the various questions were to be addressed also increased. The status question was now to be dealt with at the initial team meeting by the rehabilitation staff along with the goal question as before. A major new commitment was made to addressing the "what works" question by the rehabilitation staff. It was to be addressed in each of their three areas starting with the interim conference. By incorporating a health plan, an opportunity was present at the initial team meeting to address with the patient the status of that plan's goals and what might have worked. Thus, the patient had many more possible opportunities to address the entire range of planning questions.

The level of participation to be achieved was also increased. For example, answers to the goal question were to be verbalized at the interim meeting and at a free statement level by the time of discharge. Similarly, for the first time, the objective was for some degree of verbalization exemplified by confirmed agreement at the time of discharge for the other planning questions.

Table 2-9 reflects the evaluation of phase two. The level of implementation previously reached in terms of the status and goal questions was maintained. The number of opportunities for addressing the "what works" question increased but did not reach the level of implementation of the other two questions. There had been, as expected, a marked change in the quality of the statements generated with patients in response to the "what works" question. These statements had become far more specific and could be translated into potential instructions that the patient could give him- or herself. Examples for self-care included instructions such as "put the affected arm in first while dressing." Examples relat-

Table 2-8. Stroke Program: Patient Self-Management Objectives, Phase Two

	Day 1	Initial Team	Interim Team	Discharge	Initial Ambulatory
Status		Agreement: Health plans Rehabilitation plans	Agreement: Health plans Rehabilitation plans	Confirmed agreement: Health plans Rehabilitation plans	Statement level: Health plans Rehabilitation plans
What worked		Agreement: Health plan	Agreement: Health plans Rehabilitation plans	Confirmed agreement: Health plans Rehabilitation plans	Statement level: Health plans Rehabilitation plans
Goals	Agreement: Health plan	Agreement: Health plans Rehabilitation plans	Confirmed agreement: Health plans Rehabilitation plans	Statement level: Health plans Rehabilitation plans	Specific statement: Health plans Rehabilitation plans

Table 2-9. Phase Two Evaluation

Level of Implementation

Questions Addressed	Percent
Goal	75
Status	75
What worked	28

Level of Participation

Questions Addressed at Confirmed Agreement or Better at Discharge	Percent
Goal	41
Status	40
What worked	18

ing to mobility included such instructions for transfer from bed to wheelchair as "leaning forward" or "bringing myself to the edge of the bed." In relation to issues such as slurred speech, the instructions discussed included "slowing down" and "taking a deep breath before speaking."

Concomitant with the expansion of the repertoire of the questions asked, additional criteria were established for the degree of verbal participation to be sought. Table 2-9 also describes the level of participation achieved. During the first phase, the objective had been to achieve a level above agreement only at the time of discharge with respect to the goal. The objective during this second phase was to establish the highest level possible with each of the questions. Improvement was seen in the level of verbal participation, with particular need for further attention to the level of participation in relation to "what worked."

There was agreement by the staff to maintain the objectives. Ideas were offered by various staff members as to modifications of the procedures to make the objectives more likely.

It appears that additional inservice training of staff would need to be devoted to continued implementation of the entire range of planning questions. Considerable change, however, had occurred in the behavior of nurses and therapists in relation to their patients in the team meeting. The focus had clearly shifted toward enabling the patient to understand and participate in his or her own planning. Changes in less formal interactions not as easily subject to documentation had begun to occur during the therapy sessions.

During the course of implementation of this patient self-management plan over several months and many patients, with feedback to the staff of the results achieved, it was possible for the staff to agree to seek to achieve an even higher degree of participation with respect to any one or other of the questions. Staff also began to contribute ideas to making the effort more effective while maintaining cost constraints. Once the patient self-management program (PSM) has been implemented to this degree, aided by the documentation and feedback, the opportunity is present for measuring the impact of such levels of implementation on the outcomes achieved. Chapter 3 deals with the methodologic issues inherent in such clinical efforts, reflecting even higher levels of implementation and patient participation.

References

1. Manton KG, Corder L, Stallard E. Chronic disability trends in elderly United States populations: 1982–1994. Proc Natl Acad Sci U S A 1997;94:2593.
2. Von Korff M, Gruman J, Schaefer J, et al. Collaborative management of chronic illness. Ann Intern Med 1997;15:1097.
3. Stineman MO, Maislin O, Nosek M, et al. Comparing consumer and clinician values for alternative functional states: application of a new feature trade-off consensus building tool. Arch Phys Med Rehabil 1998;79:1522.
4. Suchman Al, Markakis K, Beckman HB, et al. A model of empathic communication in the medical interview. JAMA 1997;277:678.
5. Bellet PS, Mahoney MJ. The importance of empathy as an interviewing skill in medicine. JAMA 1991;266:1831.
6. Cassell E. The Nature of Suffering and the Goals of Medicine. New York: Oxford University Press, 1987.
7. Talo S, Rytokoski V, Hamalainen A, et al. The biopsychosocial disease consequence model in rehabilitation: model development in a Finnish "work hardening" programme for chronic pain. Int J Rehabil Res 1996;19:93.
8. Wagner EH, Austin BT, Von Korff M. Organizing care for patients with chronic illness. Milbank Q 1996;74:511.
9. MacKay DM. The Informational Analysis of Questions and Commands. Information, Mechanism and Meaning. Cambridge, MA: Massachusetts Institute of Technology Press, 1969.
10. Nordenfelt L. On the Nature of Health: An Action Theoretic Approach. Boston: D. Reidel, 1987;65.
11. Ozer MN. Management of Persons with Spinal Cord Injury. New York: Demos, 1988;107–109.
12. Ozer MN. The Character of the Solution. In MN Ozer, RS Materson, LR Caplan (eds), Management of Persons with Stroke. St. Louis: Mosby–Year Book, 1994;18–26.
13. Mullen PD, Simons-Morton DC, Ramirez G, et al. A meta-analysis of trials evaluating patient education and

counselling for three groups of preventive mental health measures. Patient Educ Couns 1997;32:157.

14. Leaf A. Preventive medicine for our ailing health care system. JAMA 1993;269:616.

15. Haynes RB, Taylor DW, Sackeff DL (eds). Compliance in Health Care. Baltimore: The Johns Hopkins University Press, 1979.

16. DiMatteo MR, DiNicola DD. Achieving Patient Compliance. New York: Pergamon, 1982

17. Pellegrino ED. The Healing Relationship: the Architonics of Clinical Medicine. In EA Sheps (ed), The Clinical Fabric of the Physician-Patient Relationship. Boston: D. Reidel, 1983.

18. Strasser DC, Falconer JA. Linking treatment to outcomes through teams: building a conceptual model of rehabilitation effectiveness. Top Stroke Rehabil 1997;4:34.

19. Melvin J. Interdisciplinary and multidisciplinary activities and the ACRM. Arch Phys Med Rehabil 1980; 62:51.

20. Diller L. Fostering the interdisciplinary team, fostering research in a society in transition. Arch Phys Med Rehabil 1990;71:275.

21. Strasser DC, Falconer JA. Rehabilitation team process. Top Stroke Rehabil 1997;4:34.

22. Stineman MG, Strasser DC. Team process and effectiveness: patients, families and staff characteristics. Top Stroke Rehabil 1997;4:21.

23. Falconer JA. Team process and outcome: components of treatment. Top Stroke Rehabil 1997;4:12.

Chapter 3

Measurement of Effectiveness

Kenneth J. Ottenbacher

Nature of the Problem

This book deals with the need to respond to problems faced by persons living with the effects of neurologic disease. The ongoing nature of disruption in their lives requires changes in the character of the relationship between the professionals acting within the health care system and their clients. Among these changes, as outlined in Chapters 1 and 2, is the need to include the patient or the family, or both, as integral members of the planning/treatment team. One of the principles of the participatory planning process is to consider how to improve the effectiveness of services. Viewing the provision of services as an ongoing planning process enables the review or evaluation step to be intrinsic to the clinical setting. This chapter describes how the evaluation of effectiveness can occur in the context of the requisite changes in responsiveness to individual differences.

Emphasis must be devoted to integrating and assimilating research into clinical practice with the direct goal of improving the services provided to patients and consumers. A secondary goal is to involve the patient, family, and other caregivers in this process. It may not be realistic to expect clinicians to complete complex and time-consuming research and evaluation studies based on traditional experimental procedures. Clinicians do, however, have the opportunity and obligation to assess client performance, document change, and report the results to consumers and colleagues.

Increasingly, this obligation includes providing an opportunity for the patient and family to have a role in the assessment, intervention, and evaluation process.

The ability to plan, implement, and report the results of clinical investigations is essential to keep pace with the rapidly changing health care environment and the current demands for evidence-based practice.[1] An indication of the importance of evidenced-based assessment is reflected in publications by the Joint Commission on Accreditation of Health Care Organizations (JCAHO).[2,3] In 1993, the JCAHO published *The Measurement Mandate: On the Road to Performance Improvement in Health Care*. This book begins by stating, "One of the greatest challenges confronting health care organizations in the 1990s is learning to apply the concepts and methods of performance measurement."[2] In 1994, the JCAHO published a related text entitled *A Guide to Establishing Programs for Assessing Outcomes in Clinical Settings*.[3]

In discussing the importance of assessment in health care, the authors present the following consensus statement: "Among the most important reasons for establishing an outcome assessment initiative in a health care setting are to describe, in quantitative terms, the impact of routinely delivered care on patients' lives, to establish a more accurate and reliable basis for clinical decision making by clinicians and patients, and to evaluate the effectiveness of care and identify opportunities for improvement."[3]

Character of the Population

The complexity of defining and assessing rehabilitation outcomes is frequently identified as one of the reasons for the slow progress in establishing evidence-based practice in medical rehabilitation. The difficulty, in part, is directly related to the unit of analysis in rehabilitation research investigations[4]: the individual and the individual's relationship with his or her environment. In contrast, the unit of analysis in many medical specialties is an organ, a body system, or a pathology. In fact, DeJong[4] has argued that traditional medical research and practice arc organized around these pathologies and organ systems, for example, cardiology and orthopedics. One consequence of this organizational structure is a system of assessment that emphasizes the absence of pathology in, or the performance of, a specific organ system, for instance, the use of an electrocardiogram to evaluate the function of the heart. In contrast to these organ-based medical specialties, the goal of rehabilitation is to improve an individual's ability to function as independently as possible in his or her natural environment. To achieve this goal requires broad-based measurement instruments and flexible research designs that examine individual performance in thc home, vocational, or leisure environment.

This same issue arises in the context of dealing with some of the other disease entities described in this book. The management of persons with chronic neurologic illness, like that of rehabilitation, focuses on the person with the disease rather than the disease alone. Although there is concern for minimization of the degree of neurologic impairment as a result of the disease process, the ultimate measures of effectiveness deal with "adding years to life." The goal is to enable the person to minimize the extent to which the ongoing impairments affect the function of the individual, that is, to reduce the disabilities and enhance the quality of life. When dealing with the person rather than the nervous system as the affected organ, the variety of settings as well as the variety of individual characteristics can be considered.

Traditional research designs in which a group receiving treatment is statistically compared with a similar group not receiving treatment may have limited feasibility in many clinical settings or natural environments. Such investigations, typically referred to as *experimental designs* or *randomized*

clinical trials (RCTs), are powerful methods of demonstrating relationships between variables under controlled conditions. Group-based experimental methods, however, represent only one approach to collecting and analyzing data.

Efficacy and Effectiveness

The Agency for Health Care Policy and Research (AHCPR) makes a useful distinction between efficacy and effectiveness that is relevant to the types of designs used in clinical research.[5] *Efficacy of treatment* is defined as the ability to clearly demonstrate relationships between treatment and outcomes under controlled or "ideal" conditions. Efficacy studies are characterized by attempts to use the most powerful and sophisticated research designs. RCTs are associated with efficacy research. In a randomized clinical trial, the investigator attempts to identify homogeneous groups of patients (subjects) with similar disorders, similar levels of severity, and similar demographic characteristics. The patients are assigned at random to treatment or control groups. The treatment is generally provided using a very specific protocol, and every attempt is made to keep the level and type of intervention constant across the patients receiving it. The outcome measures are determined in advance, and it is important that all patients (subjects), both those receiving the treatment and those not receiving the treatment, be measured in the same manner using the same tests or instruments. The investigator is interested in making controlled comparisons between persons in the treatment group receiving the intervention and individuals in the control group not receiving the treatment. The comparison is made using statistical tests that allow the investigator to determine the probability that persons in the treatment group perform differently than persons in the control group on an outcome measure of interest. In an efficacy investigation, the researcher attempts to control extraneous variables that might influence the performance on the outcome measure. This control is ensured by using random assignment to groups and by maintaining a high level of consistency and standardization in the administration of the treatment and the assessment of the outcome.[6] A schematic of a typical randomized clinical trial design used in an efficacy study is presented in Figure 3-1.

Establishing treatment efficacy is important as a first step in the process of integrating research into clinical practice. The second step is to demonstrate treatment effectiveness. *Effectiveness*, as defined by the AHCPR, is the ability to show that an intervention produces changes in a typical clinical or natural setting.[5] In discussing this issue in rehabilitation research, Johnston and Granger[7] make the following distinction between effectiveness research and efficacy investigations: "Randomized clinical trials (RCTs) . . . are frequently limited in their generalizability. RCTs are typically efficacy studies involving distinctly selected patient subgroups at university medical facilities. In contrast, outcomes research examines effectiveness in facilities with a staff of average competency, practical levels of funding, and the normal range of variation in patients served."[7]

RCTs used in efficacy investigations are often difficult or impossible to implement in a natural clinical setting. The practical limitations of RCTS have been discussed by Kramer and Shapiro, who note that "despite the obvious advantages and impressive track record of RCTs, clinical investigators have become increasingly aware of certain difficulties in their interpretation, feasibility, and ethics."[8] These difficulties include obtaining an appropriate sample size, random assignment of participants to groups, and the ability to provide the same type, level, or intensity of intervention to all persons in the treatment groups. Other concerns with RCTs in effectiveness investigations include the use of the same standardized measure for assessing outcome in all subjects; the feasibility of blinding the treatment measures, outcome measures, or both (i.e., the persons receiving the treatment or collecting the outcome data are unaware of whether the subject is in the treatment or control group), and ethical objections associated with denying treatment to participants who are in control or placebo conditions. The difficulty of meeting the requirements of RCTs in clinical settings has forced investigators to use modified versions of classic experimental procedures or to develop new approaches to conduct effectiveness investigations.

Patient-Centered Evaluation

For any intervention to be successful, it is essential that the clinical problem be identified and that

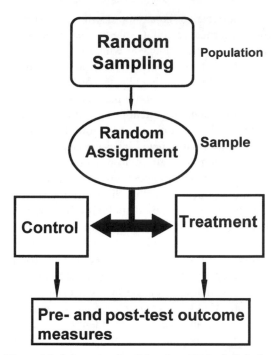

Figure 3-1. Schematic of traditional randomized clinical trial showing that sample is randomly selected from target population. Subjects from sample are randomly assigned to treatment and control groups.

behaviors associated with the problem be clearly stated. Traditionally, standardized norm-referenced tests have been used to help identify problem areas and measure outcomes. These assessments, however, may be of limited value in identifying the individual and qualitative aspects of function associated with a disability or societal limitation. Too often, standardized approaches to assessment and intervention do not adequately involve client input. Trombly[9] has described the traditional method as the "bottom-up" approach to patient assessment and treatment planning. The primary target of assessment in this approach is the level of discrete component abilities that the clinician anticipates may be affected by the patient's identified condition.[9] The potential functional impact of these component deficits may be inferred but is often not assessed by direct measurement or patient feedback. As a consequence, the link between deficits in basic abilities and the functional problems the patient experiences in daily life may never become clear to him or her. This, in turn, may raise doubts about the meaningfulness of the intervention.

An alternative is a "top-down" approach in which information about what the person needs or wants to do, the context in which he or she typically engages in these activities, and the current level of performance is collected by the treatment team. Brown et al.[10] have pioneered the use of strategies designed to identify the skills needed by persons with a disability to function maximally in their natural environments. These strategies involve the construction of an environmental or ecological inventory that includes all of the settings in which the individual with a disability interacts on a regular basis. A detailed analysis of the environment is conducted to determine the specific skills needed to maintain the highest possible functional level within each setting. The ecological inventory strategy is designed to develop, organize, and refine information that can be used to determine the exact problems encountered in the person's environment and then clearly identify the corresponding skills that are required to ameliorate functional deficits.

The top-down approach to information gathering should result in improved communication and compliance with rehabilitation treatment objectives.[11] The ability to implement a top-down approach depends on the availability of assessment instruments that are congruent with a patient-centered treatment approach, consider the person in the context of his or her natural environment, and are psychometrically sound.

Character of the Solution

This chapter focuses on alternatives to RCTs in research dealing with individual characteristics. They must meet the need for patient-centered clinically relevant (effectiveness rather than efficacy) measurement. These particularly include single-subject designs and goal attainment scaling (GAS).[12] Both of these approaches are practice based and practitioner oriented. They allow for individualized evaluation and can be used to achieve the following objectives: (1) assess a wide variety of individualized outcome measures, including physical, social, economic, and psychological function; (2) involve patients and caregivers as collaborators in the evaluation process; and (3) be adapted for use in clinical, home, or community settings.

Canadian Occupational Performance Measure

One attempt to develop a top-down, patient-centered assessment approach is the Canadian Occupational Performance Measure (COPM),[13] a criterion-based assessment developed in consultation with the Department of National Health and Welfare and the Canadian Association of Occupational Therapy.[13,14] The COPM reflects a client-centered practice philosophy of measurement and incorporates roles and role expectations within the client's own environment. *Client-centered* means that the assessment incorporates roles and role expectations from within the client's living environment using a semistructured interview approach.

The COPM encompasses the areas of self-care, productivity, and leisure as the primary outcomes being measured but can also include an assessment of performance components to gain an understanding of why the client may be having difficulty in a particular functional area. The COPM was designed to help therapists establish functional goals based on client perceptions of need and to measure change objectively in defined problem areas.[15] The COPM measures the client's identified problem areas in daily functioning. In those instances in which a client is unable to identify problem areas (e.g., a young child or an individual with dementia), a caregiver can respond to the measure. The COPM considers the importance of the performance areas to the person as well as the client's satisfaction with present performance. The instrument takes into account client roles and role expectations and, in focusing on the client's own environments and priorities, ensures the relevance of identified areas in the assessment process.

The COPM is generic (not diagnosis specific) and can be used across different age groups. The instrument is administered in a five-step process using a semistructured interview conducted by the rehabilitation professional together with the client, caregiver, or both. The five steps in the process include problem identification/definition, initial assessment, intervention, reassessment, and calculation of change scores.

First, problems are defined jointly with the client and appropriate caregivers. Once the problem areas are defined, the client is asked to rate the importance of each activity on a scale of 1 to 10. The client (or caregiver) is also required to rate his or her ability to perform the specified activities and his or her satisfaction with performance on the same 1 to 10 scale. These scores are then compared across time. The scale has two scores: one for performance and one for satisfaction. Administration time takes approximately 30–40 minutes on average.

The authors of the COPM report findings on an extensive pilot study that involved administration of the instrument to 256 clients in many facilities across Canada and in other countries, including New Zealand, Greece, and Great Britain.[13] Data gathered during this multiphase study included feedback from therapists and clients about the clinical utility of the COPM, data on the sensitivity of the instrument to change, and descriptive statistics on identified problems and client scores. Comments by therapists involved in the pilot studies were generally favorable regarding the clinical utility of the measure. Because the assessment involves an interview with clients, who are often unaccustomed to participating in the identification of their own problems, some awkwardness with administration has been reported by therapists during their initial attempts at administration. Also, because of its reliance on client participation in the assessment process, it is viewed as being of limited use in clients who have significant cognitive impairment. The perceived clinical utility of the COPM is related to its flexibility, the use of client-centered approaches in practice, and support by administrators who value the philosophy that underlies the instrument.

Research continues on the COPM, with particular attention to its validity as a bona fide measure of real changes in functional performance. Although it is a new instrument, the COPM has the potential to provide useful and important information regarding functional skills. Unique features of the COPM include the quantitative emphasis on client satisfaction and the focus on active patient participation in the goal-setting process.

Participatory Planning System

Ozer et al.[11] have also outlined a comprehensive, patient-centered approach to top-down treatment planning. The planning approach includes two essential elements that build on and contribute to the identification and definition of the problem. First is the emphasis on input and feedback from the patient and patient's family in the determination of both interventions and outcomes. Second is the reliance on information from all members of the rehabilitation team in the planning process. The general model of treatment planning proposed by Ozer et al. is presented in Figure 2-1 and described in detail in other chapters in this text. This approach to treatment planning is easily operationalized in single-subject designs and GAS, as described below.

The model developed by Ozer et al.[11] and the COPM use a patient-centered approach to assessment but do not directly address how to implement or assess intervention. Single-subject designs and GAS represent methods of outcome evaluation that allow for individualized goal setting and also provide the opportunity to incorporate patients in the process of goal setting, assessment, intervention, and reassessment.

Goal Attainment Scaling

GAS was first presented by Kiresuk and Sherman[16] in a study of mental health practitioners. The procedure they described included two basic steps. The first was to construct a plan for each client based on the desired or expected level of performance. This was called a *goal attainment guide*. The second step was to use this guide to rate the client's performance at a predetermined time after intervention. Kiresuk and Sherman[16] developed a goal attainment guide, illustrated its use in a clinical setting, and presented a formula for computing a goal attainment score.

Since the original description, the method has been successfully used in psychotherapy and mental health,[17–19] education,[20] mental retardation,[21] and general rehabilitation.[22,23] The method, however, is not widely known or used by rehabilitation professionals. The purpose of this section is to describe and illustrate the use of GAS as a method of clinical effectiveness research with relevance to medical rehabilitation. For additional information, the reader should refer to *Goal Attainment Scaling: Applications, Theory and Measurement*, by Kiresuk et al.[12]

Goals

The basic idea of GAS is not a new one. The practice of setting measurable goals for intervention is well established. Rehabilitation goals are often vague or global without defined time frames, making evaluation and measurement of success difficult. As a result, goals may end up being irrelevant, immeasurable, or unattainable. Goals are also frequently determined unilaterally by one professional with little input from the client, family, or other team members. This raises the issue of whose goal is being pursued. Goals should have social and functional validity. That is, they should be established in relation to the client's home, work, and community environments.

GAS provides the framework for developing program goals that are measurable and attainable, and are socially, functionally, and contextually relevant. In addition, GAS produces a quantitative index of client progress that can be used to compare performance of one individual over time or to compare performance across clients in the same program.

A major component of GAS is establishing the desired or expected level of client performance. The desired or expected level of performance is used to construct a goal attainment guide or plan. Information related to the expected level of client performance is best collected from multiple sources. The accuracy of this information, and, hence, the accuracy of the GAS score, is enhanced when data are collected from the client, family members, and other service providers.

The first criterion for a goal is that it must consist of observable and recordable behavior. In addition, goals should be time limited. The goal should provide the clinician, client, and family with an identified time line for expected performance. At the termination of the specified time, the scale is scored and the goals can be changed to meet a new set of expectations or a new (revised) intervention program.

Establishing Goals

The process of establishing goals can be accomplished in eight interrelated steps. To illustrate these steps, a GAS is developed for a hypothetical client with acquired brain injury who is enrolled in a program designed to teach skills necessary for community living and competitive employment.

Step 1. The first step is to identify an overall (general) objective. In the present example, the rehabilitation professionals, the family, and the client all agree that community integration with part-time employment in a competitive (nonsheltered workshop) environment is the overall program goal.

Step 2. The second step is to identify specific problem areas that should be addressed. This involves prioritizing areas and then reducing them to observable, reportable components. For example, improving social interactions and reducing weight are possible areas for change. The important component in this step is to identify problem areas in which a measurable indication of performance can be obtained.

Step 3. Step 3 is to identify what behaviors or events indicate improvement in each of the areas selected in step 2. The purpose of this is to provide the operational detail required to make the scale a useful instrument to evaluate performance. For example, if social relations have been identified as a problem area (see Step 2) then the number of appropriate verbal contacts between the client and other participants in the training classes might be selected as one (measurable) indicator of improvement.

Step 4. After the operationalization of the goals in step 3, the clinician must determine the methodology to be used to collect the desired information. In this step, a plan is developed to determine how the information is to be collected, who is to collect it, and in what setting the evaluation data are to be gathered.

Step 5. Step 5 involves selecting the expected level of performance. This step relies on professional judgment and realistic appraisal of the client, which is simultaneously one of the strengths and liabilities of the evaluation method. If the expected levels are at variance with actual performance, this inaccuracy is reflected in the GAS score. This step is based on the assumption that experienced clinical practitioners are able to "predict" treatment outcome with input from the client, family members, and other health care providers.

Table 3-1. Goal Attainment Scale Including Levels of Predicted Attainment and Operation Criteria for Two Goals

	Goals	
Predicted Attainment	**Social Relations**	**Weight Loss**
Most unfavorable outcome (−2)	Speaks to no one except therapist during 3-hr session	Gains 5 lbs over 1-mo period
Less than expected (−1)	Says "hello" or other greeting to fellow workers during 3-hr training session	Maintains current weight over period of 1 mo
Expected level of outcome (0)	Holds sustained, interactive conversation of 200 words (or 10 mins) with one other worker during 3-hr session	Loses 5 lbs over 1-mo period
Greater than expected outcome (+1)	Holds interactive conversation of more than 200 words (10 mins) with two or more workers (independent or simultaneous) during 3-hr session	Loses 10 lbs over 1-mo period
Most favorable outcome likely (+2)	Holds interactive conversation of 500 words (or 20 mins) with three or more workers during 3-hr session	Loses 15 lbs over 1-mo period

For example, if the clinician and others judge that it is realistic that the client lose 5 lbs in a month, then this is a satisfactory operational criterion for the goal of weight reduction. This operational criterion relies heavily on the therapist's (and others') knowledge of the client, the weight loss program, and the environment.

Step 6. Step 6 involves identifying the most favorable outcome, the least favorable outcome, and intermediate levels of client performance. Kiresuk et al.[12] suggest that the evaluator develop five levels of performance, ranging from the most favorable to the least favorable outcome. Activities identified at the five levels represent a continuum of behaviors (or events) with no gaps or obvious overlaps in behavior. The five levels of performance are used in the scoring of the GAS. The focus is on realistic outcomes. The most favorable outcome, for example, should reflect what the client could accomplish if everything in the program goes smoothly. In the weight loss example, the operational criterion of this goal may indicate that if all goes smoothly the client could lose 5 lbs in 1 month. On the other hand, the least desirable outcome would be that the client gains 5 lbs during 1 month of intervention.

Table 3-1 lists the behaviors and levels for the two problem areas identified in step 1, social relations and weight loss. Each of the five levels is operationally defined and assigned a numeric value, with 0 indicating the expected level of performance and −2 and +2 indicating the least and most favorable outcomes, respectively.

Step 7. Once the goal attainment guide has been completed, it should be checked for overlapping levels, gaps between levels, or more than one indicator in a problem area. The scale should also be checked to make sure that the definitions of behaviors are clear and that instructions on how to collect data are not ambiguous.

Step 8. The final step in establishing the goals for the GAS is to ascertain the current status of the individual and determine when the client can be evaluated again to document whether she or he has progressed. The selection of the time period between evaluations is related to several factors, including the type of intervention provided, the expected level of performance, and external criteria imposed by third party payers, accrediting agencies, and others. In the example, the client might be weighed before program implementation and the weight recorded. The clinician and others would then determine when the client would be weighed again.

Scoring the Goal Attainment Scale

Several options are available to score the GAS. It is important that the option selected is used consistently across all protocols so that comparisons can be made across individuals. The most commonly used system of scoring, proposed by Kiresuk et al.,[12] relies on a five-point scale of performance (see Step 6), with scores ranging from –2 to +2 for each scale. In this scheme, a rating of –2 is associated with the least favorable outcome; –1, less than expected outcome; 0, expected level of performance; +1, greater than expected outcome; and, +2, most favorable outcome. These ratings are used for each of the levels across all goals (see Table 3-1).

In scoring the GAS, relative weights are assigned to each of the goals identified for the client. No standard procedure exists for determining how each goal is weighted. The weighting is (ideally) achieved by consensus among the patient, clinician, family members, and other persons concerned with the patient's performance. Generally, the weighting simply reflects a prioritizing or ranking of the goals. If four primary goals are prioritized, for example, then the most important goal is given a ranking (weight) of +4 and the least important goal a weight of +1. For example, a goal of reducing self-abusive behaviors may be identified as very important and given a ranking of +3. The goal of social relations might be identified as important and given a ranking of +2, whereas weight loss is least important and is ranked +1. The weights (rankings) must be determined in the goal-planning stage and not in the evaluation phase. If goals are weighted during the evaluation, the weights might reflect the priorities of the patients or clinicians as they look back on the outcome of the program and its strengths and weaknesses. This would introduce the possibility of systematic error or bias into the evaluation process.

After the intervention has been administered, the weights for the goals and the rating of each level of performance are used to compute a GAS score. This score represents a numeric index of the client's improvement (or lack of improvement).

The following formula is used to compute the GAS:

$$T = 50 + \frac{(10\Sigma W_i X_i)}{(1 - r)\Sigma W_i^2 + r(\Sigma W_i)^2}$$

where X_i represents the outcome score for each behavior (a value from –2 to +2) and W_i represents the weighting for a particular goal. The r value in the formula reflects the estimated average intercorrelation between outcome scores. Kiresuk et al.[12] argue that an r value of .30 can safely be assumed

and used as a constant in the formula. Finally, the T value is a standardized score with a mean of 50 and a standard deviation of 10.

The formula can be demonstrated through an example. Table 3-2 presents information for a participant with developmental disability enrolled in the program described in Step 1. Four goals were identified and weighted from 1 to 4 as depicted in Table 3-2. The table also includes the outcome score for each of the goals obtained at the final evaluation along with other information needed to generate the T score from the formula presented above.

When the information from the table is included in the formula, the following results are obtained:

$$T = 50 + (10 \times 7)/(.70 \times 30) + (.30 \times 100)$$
$$T = 50 + 70/51$$
$$T = 50 + 1.37$$
$$T = 51.37$$

A T score of 50 corresponds to the 0 point on the original profile, that is, the expected level of performance ranging from –2 to +2. A T of greater than 50 represents performance above the expected level, and a T of less than 50 reflects performance below the expected level. In the example, the score of 51.37 indicates that the client has had slightly "above average" overall performance after involvement in the program.

The T score is a better reflection of client performance than the simple raw score because it combines the outcome scores for all the goals to provide an overall measure of client improvement (or lack of improvement).[24] Another advantage of the T score is that it allows the weighting given to the individual goals to be incorporated into the final outcome.

GAS is a flexible set of procedures for evaluating individual (or group) performance in a variety of areas. An advantage of the system is that it is not bound to any theoretical orientation or particular type of treatment or outcome measure. Another strength is that goals can be individualized and are specifically designed to represent realistic expectations concerning client performance. Along this line, the GAS strategy actively encourages cooperative goal setting. Input from clients, family members, and other health service providers is important in establishing and prioritizing (weighting) the goals and in determining realistic levels of expected performance.[25]

Table 3-2. Data for Four Goals Including Weight and Score for Expected Level of Performance

Goal*	Weight (W_i)	Outcome (X_i)	W_iX_i	W_i^2
1	4	0	0	16
2	3	+2	+6	9
3	2	+1	+2	4
4	1	−1	−1	1

*Possible goals: (1) percent productivity, (2) self-abusive behaviors, (3) social relations, (4) weight loss.

The major advantages of the GAS method are its flexibility and the fact that goals can be individualized. GAS can be used with selected individual clients or with groups. It can be used in a relatively informal evaluation context or in the context of effectiveness research in which clients are assigned to groups and intervention is carefully manipulated.[12,26]

It is important to emphasize that GAS is not a research methodology. It represents a set of procedures designed to assist professionals in assessing client change. As Smith[25] accurately notes, "Goal attainment scaling can, quite properly, be viewed as an accountability system." The procedures associated with GAS can, however, be incorporated into many standard research designs. If GAS is used in a research context, then attention must be devoted to ensuring the internal validity of the investigation by appropriately assigning clients to groups, blindly recording the outcome measure, and establishing the reliability of the dependent measures. Lewis et al.[26] provide valuable suggestions and guidelines to clinicians interested in using GAS in a research context.

In evaluating the advantages and limitations of the GAS methodology, it is important to recognize that GAS is not a measurement instrument designed to determine the status of clients relative to a particular trait of interest such as gross motor performance or ADL. Rather, it is a methodology designed to measure change. The focus of GAS is on process (measuring change), not product (determining status).

From the perspective of standardized normative assessments, the construction of identical goals across raters is an important psychometric requirement. From the GAS perspective, however, the construction of similar goals and weights across raters is not of primary importance or concern. In fact, insistence on identical goal construction

would eliminate the ability of GAS to provide individualized assessment.

The issue of reliability is an important one in relation to the actual measurement of the client's performance and the GAS score. Estimates of the inter-rater reliability should routinely be computed and reported. Because the goals are individualized, the inter-rater reliability of assessing client performance must be established for each distinct goal. The process of establishing inter-rater reliability for the outcome measures used in GAS is similar to that required by other idiographic procedures such as single-subject designs (see the following section).

Another important component in using the GAS is how the data are going to be collected. To reduce bias and help ensure the integrity of the GAS score, it is ideal that the measurement of the goals be done blindly; that is, the person collecting the final outcome information should not be aware of the client's initial status or of the group to which a client was assigned (if groups are used in the study).

Despite the limitations already described, GAS represents an improvement over the subjective and anecdotal evaluations that often typify clinical assessments. It is a flexible evaluation methodology that can address the documentation and accountability concerns facing health care providers. GAS is a method that is practice oriented, practitioner based, and patient centered. Single-subject designs also include these characteristics and provide another method of individualized patient evaluation.

Single-Subject Designs

Bloom et al.[27] argue that single-system designs, also referred to as *single-subject, small-N, single-*

case experimental, or *N of 1* clinical trials, represent the preferred method of evaluating clinical change in many human service environments. The methods provide continuous assessment and outcome information that can be used by the clinician to monitor patient progress and even adjust the intervention, as indicated based on data interpretation. The flexibility of single-system evaluation methods allows the clinician to modify the treatment, depending on the individual needs of the patient or situation. This is generally not possible with more traditional group comparison designs in which the treatment remains the same throughout the investigation. The single-system methodology permits the clinician to achieve two major goals: (1) monitor patient progress and (2) determine individual intervention effectiveness. The basic components of and steps followed in using single-system designs to achieve these goals are outlined in the remainder of this chapter.

Specifying the Problem and Developing an Intervention Plan

It is important that the clinical problem be clearly stated and that the behaviors associated with the problem that can be observed and measured are able to be identified. Traditionally, standardized norm-referenced tests have been used to help measure research outcomes. Standardized norm-referenced assessments, however, may be of limited value in identifying the individual and qualitative aspects of function associated with a disability. Brown et al.[10] pioneered the use of strategies designed to identify the skills needed by persons with a disability to function maximally in their natural environments. These strategies involve the construction of an environmental or ecological inventory that includes all of the settings in which the individual with a disability interacts on a regular basis. A detailed analysis of the environment is conducted, including input from the client and family, to determine the specific skills needed to maintain the highest possible functional level within each setting. The ecological inventory strategy is designed to develop, organize, and refine information that can be used to determine the exact problems encountered in the person's environment and then clearly identify the corresponding skills that are required to ameliorate functional deficits.

Selecting an Evaluation Design

The interpretive logic of single-system designs rests on a comparison between phases when the intervention is and is not present or when two or more treatments are compared.[27] This comparison is generally made over time within one subject (or a small group of subjects). The sophistication of single-system designs has increased dramatically over the past decade. The discussion of various designs presented here is meant to be illustrative rather than exhaustive. Clinicians who wish to employ single-system designs as a method of evaluation research should consult one of the excellent resources now available for more detailed information.[28–31]

AB Designs. The AB design is the most basic form of single-system design. *A* represents the baseline or nontreatment condition (phase A). Subsequent interventions are indicated by different letters of the alphabet. If an intervention baseline is repeated, then the same letter is used to represent the repeated phase. For example, Figure 3-2 displays the effect of an exercise intervention program on the weight gain of a cardiac patient. Phase A represents the baseline period in which the patient's weight was recorded on a weekly basis. A program of graded exercise was initiated at the end of the ninth week of baseline and represents phase B. The vertical axis of the graph indicates the patient's weight in pounds.

The AB design illustrated in Figure 3-2 is the simplest single-system design. Other design variations are easily developed from this basic design pattern. Bloom et al.[27] advocate the AB design as the cornerstone for conducting single-system evaluation research. These researchers contend that the fundamental step in becoming an accountable professional is to start counting with the AB design.

Variations of the AB Design. An extension of the AB design, in which the treatment is withdrawn in the third phase, is the ABA design. The withdrawal of the intervention provides greater confidence in determining the effect of the treatment based on what Barlow and Hersen[29] label "the principle of unlikely successive coincidences." In other words, it is possible that a data pattern could change as a result of something other than the treatment that is

Figure 3-2. Example of single-subject AB design, where A is the baseline and B is the intervention period.

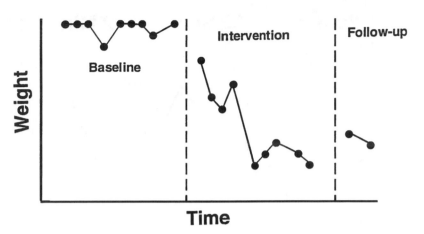

coincidentally affecting the problem at the same point at which the treatment is introduced. However, with each successive pattern change corresponding to the introduction or withdrawal of the treatment, it becomes increasingly unlikely that the change can be attributed to such a coincidence. One disadvantage of the ABA design is that the patient is left in an undesirable state, that is, the absence of intervention. Therefore, another treatment phase (phase B) can be added to reintroduce the intervention effects, resulting in an ABAB design.

Another alternative is to begin with the treatment phase, withdraw it, and then reintroduce it so that the design becomes a BAB pattern. This design may be particularly useful when it is not possible to collect baseline data initially. However, after the treatment has been introduced, a baseline phase (without treatment) may be justified to see if the intervention effects can be maintained.

More complex variations of the AB design are possible. One common example is the changing criterion design, which allows the patient to demonstrate sequentially higher performance. During the initial intervention, a criterion of successful performance is established. After successful achievement of this performance level across several trials or after achieving a stable criterion level, the criterion increases. In the next phase, a new and more difficult criterion level is established while the intervention is continued. When behavior reaches this new criterion level and is maintained across trials, the next phase, with a more difficult criterion, is introduced. Figure 3-3 demonstrates a patient's progress in developing independent standing ability. In phase A, the criterion was 20

seconds of independent standing. In phase B, the criterion was raised to 60 seconds, and in phase C, the criterion was 120 seconds. The changing criterion design is useful in monitoring patient change but is limited in determining why the change occurred.

Multiple-Baseline Designs. In some cases in which the treatment or intervention cannot be withdrawn or when withdrawing the treatment would not result in a return to preintervention performance levels, a multiple-baseline design may be appropriate. In this type of design, baseline and intervention data are collected on several individuals for a similar behavior or setting. The most common version of this design is the multiple baseline across subjects in which data are collected across several different individuals.[27] In a multiple-baseline design, the intervention phase is generally introduced in a staggered manner across individuals, behaviors, or settings. For example, Figure 3-4 illustrates a multiple baseline across subjects (individuals). The intervention is introduced to each subject in a sequential staggered manner, and the outcome measure is recorded. The consistently increasing performance of each individual as the intervention is introduced indicates the effectiveness of the procedure across the three patients. The multiple-baseline design across subjects is a particularly useful single-system design because it does not require the withdrawal of treatment and has the additional benefit of including replication of the finding across at least three subjects.

As noted previously, the design examples presented in this chapter are meant to be illustrative.

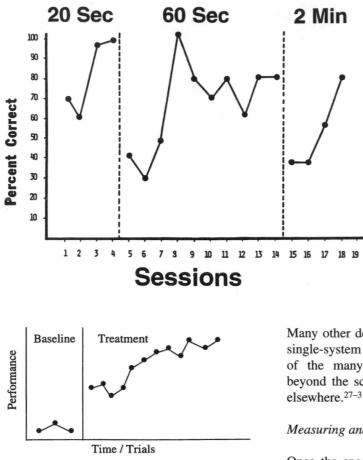

Figure 3-3. Example of changing criterion design in which level or criterion of performance is raised at each phase.

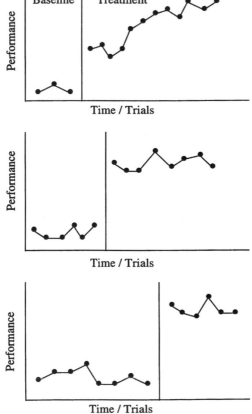

Figure 3-4. Example of multiple-baseline design across subjects. This design shows three subjects with staggered introduction of the intervention in each B phase.

Many other design variations are possible using a single-system framework. A detailed examination of the many possible design modifications is beyond the scope of this chapter but is available elsewhere.[27–31]

Measuring and Recording Behavior

Once the specific patient skills or outcome measures have been identified, these skills must be broken down into units of behavior that can be observed, counted, or measured in some way. The ability to measure the patient's repeated behavior or performance is essential to implementing the single-system approach. Each behavior unit can be defined in terms of how often it occurs (frequency), how long it occurs (duration), and also in terms of qualitatively desirable components.[18]

Two other issues closely related to recording patient performance are the training and reliability of the rater. It makes little sense to develop a sophisticated system of recording performance if the person doing the recording is poorly trained or unreliable in his or her recording. The behavior to be recorded must be clearly defined, as noted previously, and the rater must be familiar with how, when, where, and how long the behavior should be observed and recorded. Various procedures have been developed to train raters and observers to determine the consistency and accuracy of their recording efforts.[29–32]

Analyzing Data Collected

Graphic analysis and visual inspection are the traditional analytic tools used to present and interpret the results of single-system evaluation research.[27,30,31] Kazdin[31] has observed, however, that, as single-subject designs have become more popular in the applied research areas, the emphasis on the need for statistical analysis of the collected data has increased. The use of various statistical procedures with single-system designs is a controversial topic.[27] Several authorities believe that it is inappropriate to use statistical techniques with single-system designs and argue that the application of such procedures confuses the issue of clinical and statistical significance.[31] Barlow and Hersen[29] present an excellent overview of the arguments surrounding the issue of clinical significance and statistical significance as they relate to single-system designs.

Data collected in single-system designs are generally of a repeated nature; that is, measurements on a variable are taken repeatedly based on the performance of an individual or small group over time. The fact that repeated measurements are gathered from a patient means that a degree of serial dependency or autocorrelation may exist within the data collected. *Serial dependency* refers to the fact that sequential responses emitted by the same individual will be correlated. The result of this serial dependency is to reduce the variability in the observed responses and thereby bias the estimates of behavioral score properties such as stabilities, variabilities, or averages.[27,30]

The presence of serial dependency within data adds to the interpretive difficulties based solely on visual analysis. We agree with the position of Elashoff and Thoresen,[33] who argue that statistical and visual methods should be partners in the analytic endeavor. These researchers contend that statistical and visual analyses should be used jointly to provide a clearer interpretation of single-system evaluation research.

References

1. Rosenberg W, Donald A. Evidenced based medicine: an approach to clinical problem solving. BMJ 1995;310:1122–1126.
2. Joint Commission on Accreditation of Healthcare Organizations. The Measurement Mandate: On the Road to Performance Improvement in Health Care. Oakbrook Terrace, IL: JCAHO, 1993.
3. Joint Commission on Accreditation of Healthcare Organizations. A Guide to Establishing Programs for Assessing Outcomes in Clinical Settings. Oakbrook Terrace, IL: JCAHO, 1994.
4. DeJong G. Medical Rehabilitation Outcome Measurement in a Changing Health Care Market. In MJ Furher (ed), Rehabilitation Outcomes: Analysis and Measurement. Baltimore: Paul H. Brookes, 1987;261–272.
5. Hibbard H, Nutting PA, Grady ML. AHCPR conference proceedings. Primary Care Research Theory and Methods. Washington, DC: Agency for Health Care Policy Research (AHCPR), U.S. Department Health and Human Services Publication No. 91-0011, 1991.
6. Keppel G. Design and Analysis: A Researcher's Handbook (2nd ed). Englewood Cliffs, NJ: Prentice-Hall, 1986.
7. Johnston MV, Granger CV. Outcome research in medical rehabilitation: a primer and introduction to a series. Am J Phys Med Rehabil 1994;73:296–303.
8. Kramer MS, Shapiro SH. Scientific challenges in the application of randomized clinical trials. JAMA 1984;252:2739–2745.
9. Trombly C. The issue is—anticipating the future: assessment of occupational function. Am J Occup Ther 1993;47:203–209.
10. Brown L, Nietupski J, Hamer-Nietupski S. Criterion of Ultimate Functioning. In MA Thomas (ed), Hey Don't Forget about Me. Reston, VA: Council for Exceptional Children, 1976.
11. Ozer MN, Materson RS, Caplan LR. Management of Persons with Stroke. St. Louis: Mosby–Year Book, 1994.
12. Kiresuk TJ, Smith A, Cardillo JE. Goal Attainment Scaling: Applications, Theory and Measurement. Hillsdale, NJ: Lawrence Erlbaum, 1994.
13. Law M, Baptiste S, McColl MA, et al. The Canadian Occupational Performance Measure: an outcome measure for occupational therapy. Can J Occup Ther 1994;57:82–87.
14. Law M, Polotajko H, Pollock N, et al. Pilot testing of the Canadian Occupational Performance Measure: clinical and measurement issues. Can J Occup Ther 1994;61:191–197.
15. Law M. Evaluating activities of daily living: directions for the future. Am J Occup Ther 1993;47:233–237.
16. Kiresuk T, Sherman R. Goal attainment scaling: a general method of evaluating comprehensive mental health programs. Community Ment Health J 1968;4:443–453.
17. Greenspan SI, Sharfstein SS. Efficacy of psychotherapy: asking the right questions. Arch Gen Psych 1981;38:1211–1219.
18. Grey ME, Moore LS. The goal attainment scale for psychiatric in-patients. Q Rev Bull 1982;8:19–23.
19. Lewis AB, Spencer JH, Haas GL, DiVittis A. Goal attainment scaling: relevance and replicability in follow-up of inpatients. J Nerv Ment Dis 1987;75:408–417.
20. Garwick G. Recent findings on the use of goal-setting in human service agencies: the implementation flexibility and validity of goal attainment scaling. Goal Attain Rev 1974;1:1–4.

21. Bailey DB, Simeonsson RJ. Investigation of use of goal attainment scaling to evaluate individual progress of clients with severe and profound mental retardation. Ment Retard 1988;26:289–295.

22. Clark MS, Caudrey DJ. Evaluation of rehabilitation services: the use of goal attainment scaling. Int Rehabil Med 1983;5:41–45.

23. Goodyear DL, Bitter JA. Goal attainment scaling as a program evaluation measure in rehabilitation. J Appl Rehab Counsel 1974;5:19–26.

24. Clark MS, Caudrey DJ. Evaluation of rehabilitation services: the use of goal attainment scaling. Inter Rehab Med 1986;5:41–45.

25. Smith A. Goal Attainment Scaling: A Method for Evaluating the Outcome of Mental Health Treatment. In P McReynolds (ed), Advances in Psychological Assessment. San Francisco: Jossey-Bass 1981;5:424–459.

26. Lewis AB, Spencer JH, Haas GL, DiVittis A. Goal attainment scaling: relevance and replicability in follow-up of inpatients. J Nerv Ment Dis 1987;175:408–417.

27. Bloom M, Fisher J, Orme JG. Evaluating Practice: Guidelines for the Accountable Professional (2nd ed). Boston: Allyn and Bacon, 1995.

28. Barlow DH, Hayes SC, Nelson RO. The Scientist Practitioner: Research and Accountability in Clinical and Educational Settings. New York: Pergamon, 1984.

29. Barlow DH, Hersen M. Single-Case Experimental Designs: Strategies for Studying Behavior Change (2nd ed). New York: Pergamon, 1984.

30. Ottenbacher KJ. Evaluating Clinical Change: Strategies for Occupational and Physical Therapists. Baltimore: Williams & Wilkins, 1986.

31. Kazdin AE. Single-Case Research Design: Methods for Clinical and Applied Settings. New York: Oxford University Press, 1982.

32. Johnston JM, Pennypacker HS. Strategies and Tactics of Behavioral Research (2nd ed). Hillsdale, NJ: Lawrence Erlbaum, 1993.

33. Elashoff JD, Thoresen CE. Choosing a Statistical Method for Analysis of an Intensive Experiment. In TR Kratochwill (ed), Single-Subject Research Strategies for Evaluating Change. New York: Academic Press, 1978.

Part II
Applications

Chapter 4

Management of Persons with Vascular Disease

Mark N. Ozer

Nature of the Problem

Extent of the Problem

Incidence

Cerebrovascular disease leading to stroke is a principal cause of morbidity and mortality in the United States and in other developed countries.[1] Estimates of the incidence in the United States vary depending on the population sampled, but the most general estimate is 550,000 Americans hospitalized each year; of those, 150,000 die.[2] Samples drawn from a biracial population suggest that the overall incidence is substantially higher, with approximately 730,000 hospitalized.[3] This is attributed, at least in part, to the substantially higher (two times higher) incidence for blacks, both male and female, as compared with their white counterparts.[4]

Although the incidence of stroke has been decreasing for many years, it has not continued to do so as of 1995.[5] Stroke still represents the third leading cause of death after heart disease and cancer. Incidence of initial stroke is related to age. Data collected in 1975–1976 show a doubling in each decade between 45 and 85 years of age.[6] Other data continue to show the median incidence of stroke (excluding subarachnoid hemorrhage) in the decade of 60–70 years.[7] For thrombotic stroke, somewhat greater than two-thirds of patients are in the age group of 61 years or older. Despite this

relationship to age, stroke in persons younger than 65 years has substantial impact. One measure used to calculate the effects of such loss is the years of potential life lost before 65 years of age. The loss is in the range of 250,000 years for cerebrovascular disease.[8] Here again, the disparity between blacks and whites is particularly great for black men (four times) in the working age cohort (45–59 years).[4]

The case fatality rate during the first 30 days after a vascular event varies with the type of stroke.[9] As expected, it is considerably higher for stroke associated with hemorrhage. It is 67% for intracranial bleeding. The overall rate for cerebral embolism and brain infarction is approximately 15%. Age-adjusted mortality in 1995 was 1.2 times higher for men than women. It was 1.8 times higher for blacks than whites. For black men in particular, mortality is approximately twice that of white men.[5] This variation was confirmed with persistent high mortality in the southeastern portion of the United States (so-called Stroke Belt) for both blacks and whites, men and women.[10] The management of persons with stroke must be responsive to such statistics.

Prevalence

Prevalence can also serve as a measure of severity. The number of stroke survivors exceeds 2 million.[11] Its prevalence in the population appears to be increasing, due at least in part to increased survival after stroke. Such survivors have a high likelihood of recurrent stroke with consequent increased impairment as well as death. Data as to the incidence of recurrence derive from the National Survey of Stroke carried out in the mid-1970s, when 400,000 persons were discharged from acute care general hospitals with one-fourth treated for recurrent stroke.[6] In the 45–64 age group, the attack rate for initial stroke was 180 per 100,000, with an average rate of recurrence 15 times that. For persons older than 65 years, the initial rate of 1,000 per 100,000 had a recurrence rate seven times that. A community-wide study in Britain established a recurrence rate over 5 years of 30%, approximately nine times the risk of stroke in the general population. The risk was highest (15 times the general population) in the first year, with an average annual risk of 4% after that.[12]

The Framingham Heart Disease Study offers a more specific prospective sample of the age-adjusted incidence of stroke and its recurrence.[13] "Strokes" include both transient ischemic attacks (TIA) and completed strokes. The latter included atherothrombotic infarction (ABI), cerebral embolism, and intracerebral hemorrhage (ICH). Long-term survival was reported only for the ABI group. After early survival, those with ABI who were free of hypertension and cardiac comorbidity had 5-year survival equivalent to their age group. For men with both these risk factors, the cumulative survival rate was reduced from 85% to 35%. Hypertension alone reduced the survival rate to approximately 50%; cardiac comorbidity alone reduced the survival even more to approximately 40%. For women, the effect was somewhat less; however, in the presence of both factors, reduction from 70% to 55% was seen in 5-year survival.

Stroke recurrence after ABI was also affected by these risk factors. Men experienced a 42% 5-year recurrence rate, which was reduced to 28% by excluding those with both risk factors at the time of the initial vascular episode. A similar exclusion in women had considerably less effect, reducing the incidence from 24% to 19%.

Thus, among long-term survivors, cardiovascular disease is a leading contributor to death. Cardiovascular disease and hypertension are also important factors leading to recurrent stroke, at least in men. The extent to which treatment of risk factors can contribute to reduction in stroke mortality has been calculated particularly for hypertension.[8] Based on data from 1986, it is estimated that almost one-third of the 150,000 deaths from stroke might be eliminated by maintaining systolic blood pressure below 140 mm Hg. Deaths caused by coronary heart disease would be substantially reduced by lowering cholesterol levels, another potentially treatable risk factor; the reduction is projected to be approximately 40%. The management of persons with stroke must be responsive to opportunities for reducing the rate of progression of vascular disease with treatment of risk factors such as hypertension, hyperlipidemia, and cardiac arrhythmias. Although criteria for treatment and the appropriate treatment are well known,[14] management remains problematic because of a lack of adherence to recommended regimens.[15]

Data as to mortality and incidence of stroke reflect only the broadest outlines of the problem. The associated morbidity is more difficult to delineate, particularly with respect to the resultant functional disabilities. The degree of disability and the care required to carry on one's life vary with the severity of the injury and the specific impairments that have occurred. The burden of care also varies with the availability of family and community resources that can help supplant or at least mitigate the need for institutional care.

Burden

The economic burden of stroke is measured in terms of both the direct medical costs and the indirect costs associated with lost productivity and earnings. Some prevalence-based studies in the United States are derived from 1991 Medicare records (thus reflecting persons older than 65 years who were hospitalized with stroke). A large-scale sample of persons with ischemic stroke showed an average cost of $15,000 during the first 90 days. The total figure was $6 billion. This 90-day period incorporates the stay in rehabilitation hospital programs in most instances because more than one-half of those discharged from acute hospitals were treated somewhere other than their home. It is unclear whether such data derived from Medicare also capture other costs for home-based services and outpatient care.[16] The estimate for total direct costs was $17 billion; additional indirect costs of $13 billion led to a total of $30 billion for stroke in the year 1993.

An alternative method for determining economic burden is based on incidence and resultant lifetime costs.[2] This method is helpful in reflecting the effects of prevention methods and other interventions on the course of the disease. Data are drawn from first strokes that occurred in 1990 with projected costs based on both survival and recurrence rates. Direct costs include the full range of treatments; indirect costs reflect loss of productivity. Such costs vary with the type of stroke. For hemorrhagic stroke (excluding subarachnoid hemorrhage), the average lifetime direct costs are $124,000, with $91,000 for ischemic stroke. The aggregate projected cost associated with these 400,000 first strokes is $41 billion, with $30 billion attributed to ischemic stroke. One may note that these disparate studies merely reflect the magnitude of the problem and are not strictly comparable.

Costs include not only financial expenditures but also the price paid in human terms. For those who require institutionalization, a loss of independence occurs; for society and family, the burden of providing care must be met. Both emotional and physical distress are common among caregivers.[17] For many, the prospect of being severely impaired and unable to live independently is so devastating that they would prefer not to live at all. Many families make major sacrifices to maintain their loved one at home, as in the following case.

A not uncommon story is that of a 78-year-old woman who had a brain stem stroke that affected her swallowing and speech as well as motor control. She had previously lived on her own and had been active in community life. After her stroke, she was initially transferred to a nursing home for low-intensity rehabilitation after her stay in an acute care hospital. She had been discharged from rehabilitation services and now lived in a nursing home, assigned to what appeared to be maintenance care only. Both her son and daughter, particularly the latter, were dissatisfied with relegating their mother to what they called a "dust bin." Brought to her daughter's house, the patient required two persons to help transfer her from the bed to the wheelchair or toilet. She was fed entirely via a gastrostomy tube. Her speech was unintelligible, although she could indicate yes or no. A hired caregiver was available throughout the day and the daughter was present during both day and night. The daughter soon developed back problems, and

the mother was returned to another nursing home. Her condition further deteriorated, and her family decided once again to bring her home. Over the next year, she improved considerably. She can now be transferred by the one full-time hired caregiver. She maintains her caloric requirements via oral feedings and uses the gastrostomy tube for fluids only. She is able to communicate her needs with gestures as well as respond to questions. Her daughter, after several attempts, has found a nursing home with which she is satisfied to use for respite care several months each year.

The severity of the problem of stroke is likely to increase because the incidence of initial stroke is related to age, and the age distribution of the population shows a steadily increasing elderly fraction. The present and projected growth of the oldest age groups are illustrated in Figure 4-1.[18] The projected population of persons older than 65 years (using the Census Bureau middle mortality series) will rise to 52 million by 2020, 57 million with lower mortality. Projected increase in the group older than 85 years is even more impressive: The middle mortality projection forecasts 6.7 million by the year 2020. The dramatic impact of these figures becomes clear when one considers the likelihood of the increase in disability and concomitant institutionalization. The burden of care resulting from disability in 1985 is based on data concerning those who need nursing home care and those who need help from another person although they live at home. Figure 4-2[18] describes this. For those older than 85 years, a majority of women (62%) and a substantial proportion of men (46%) either reside in nursing homes or require assistance to live at home. The specific contribution of stroke to this pattern of disability is undoubtedly large. The incidence of morbidity and the burden of care will certainly increase, and at least some of those effects will be due to stroke. The prevention of stroke, the reduction of the burden of care, and, most particularly, a reduction in number of those who require institutionalization must be seen as a major concern. The goal must be to postpone disability until later in life, if at all, and to minimize the degree of such disability, particularly loss of independence. The identification, training, and ongoing support of caregivers, both family members and others, must be an integral part of treatment of persons with stroke to maintain community living.

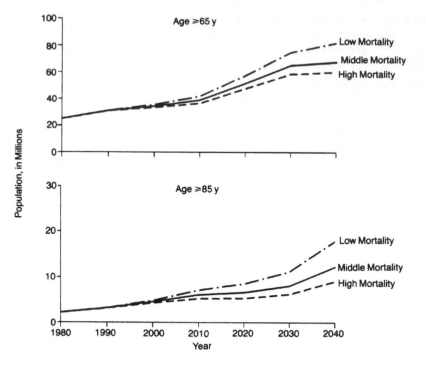

Figure 4-1. Projected growth of population aged 65 years and older and 85 years and older. Projections are based on low (series 9), middle (series 14), and high (series 19) mortality assumptions from the U.S. Bureau of the Census. (Reprinted with permission from EL Schneider, JM Guralnik. Aging of America. JAMA 1990;263:2335.)

Nature of the Disease

Thus far, we have addressed the overall problem of stroke with recognition of some of the differential effects of hemorrhage versus infarction. Stroke is not a unitary disease, and its manifestations are not the same regardless of age, sex, or race-ethnicity. It can be helpful to recognize that one can define the problem on several levels. The first is that of the cerebrovascular disease process. The occurrence of a stroke is the relatively sudden expression of an underlying disease process that involves, in the case of infarction, the distribution of nutrients to the brain via the vascular system. In the case of hemorrhage, the effect is of destruction or interference with function by the blood. The suddenness of the onset can obscure what has been a long-standing development over the lifetime of the person of effects due to hypertension or atherosclerosis, or both. The disturbance in blood supply to the brain is also a specific manifestation in the cerebral circulation of more diffuse vascular disease, frequently affecting the coronary arteries as well as those elsewhere. Even when one considers the cerebral circulation itself, the disease process is not limited to any one vessel.

Cerebrovascular Insufficiency

Vascular insufficiency can appear in the anterior (carotid) or posterior (vertebral-basilar) circulation and in any one of the arteries in either of those systems. Blockage of vascular supply to any one portion of the vascular tree is but one factor that affects the distribution and extent of injury to the brain. Vascular insufficiency in any portion of the vascular tree reflects not merely the vessel that has presumably been affected. The effects also result from the degree to which the vascular system can respond by continuing to provide nutrients to the brain via alternative collateral routes. Herein lies the relative frequency with which brain injury occurs by occlusion of the small end arteries feeding the basal ganglia. The diffuse nature of atherosclerotic disease in the elderly also affects the ability of the hardened vessel walls to respond to obstruction in any one component of the vascular tree. The rate at which obstruction occurs can further modify the degree to which collateral circulation can respond—hence the major effects of even quite small emboli from the heart or elsewhere. A slower onset of obstruction can mitigate the degree of insufficiency through the development of collateral circulation.

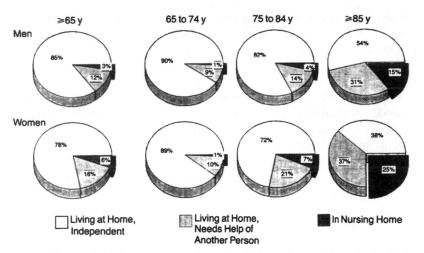

Figure 4-2. Percentage of the population by age group and sex who (1) live at home independently, (2) live at home but require the help of another person, or (3) reside in a nursing home. The percentages of older persons in nursing homes by age group are from the 1985 National Nursing Home Survey. The percentages of persons living at home and needing assistance are from analyses of data from the Supplement on Aging to the 1984 National Health Interview Survey, applied to the total population. Assistance is defined as needing help with one or more of the following activities: eating, dressing, bathing, transferring from bed to chair, using the toilet, walking, cooking, shopping, managing money, using the telephone, and performing light housekeeping. (Reprinted with permission from EL Schneider, JM Guralnik. Aging of America. JAMA 1990;263:2335.)

Brain Injury

The next stage in the evolution of a stroke is for the vascular insufficiency to proceed to actual injury because of infarction or destruction of brain tissue caused by extravasation of blood. Thrombolytic treatment soon after onset of occlusion attempts to lessen the degree to which vascular insufficiency leads to actual infarction or death of tissue. A number of other treatments are under intensive study for use to mitigate the extent of injury at this early stage of treatment. The degree to which infarction occurs with subsequent impairment in neurologic function reflects a sequence of metabolic events after the loss of nutrients that are normally provided. Modifying in some way these metabolic derangements, minimizing the amount of edema due to death of tissue, and lessening the degree of lactic acid formation are all efforts to maintain the viability of brain tissue that has not yet been completely destroyed.[19] The management of persons with stroke requires that knowledge of early signs of stroke be widespread and that early treatment be readily available.

Another opportunity to affect the degree of eventual functional impairment lies early in the course of recovery. The mechanism for this early recovery of neurologic function is not entirely clear. Disruptions in function may reflect a physiologic change without permanent destruction of tissue. *Diaschisis* is the term given to these relatively temporary distant effects.[20] Activation of the healthy hemisphere after a focal injury can contribute to early recovery as measured by Doppler ultrasonography.[21] The time since the onset of stroke is an important variable in that "spontaneous" recovery occurs. Such functional recovery may also be enhanced by the avoidance of drugs that have an influence on the brain, such as benzodiazepines, anticonvulsants, and other drugs that affect central mechanisms.[22] Alternatively, drugs such as dextroamphetamine that enhance the activity of the norepinephrine system reduce impairment when accompanied by retraining.[23]

Whether the anterior or posterior circulation is affected, the extent to which the disease process is intracranial or extracranial, and whether the disease implicates the heart as well as the rest of the vascular system are all important variables. Some of the opportunities for management of persons with stroke relate to treatment of the heart to lessen the likelihood of arrhythmia and to prevent the formation of blood clots as a source of emboli. Surgery is available to diminish obstruction if present within the extracranial carotid arteries. The neurologic model emphasizes the importance of determining a specific diagnosis and the prognosis in terms of its natural history. The rate of recovery varies, and thus the timing of intervention is important.[24] Also relevant are the extent and distribution of the brain injury, whether diffuse, multifocal, or focal.

Determining the stroke mechanism[19] initially requires differentiation between the two major subtypes: hemorrhagic or infarction (ischemic). The former includes ICH or subarachnoid hemorrhage (SAH). The nonhemorrhagic stroke category includes both thrombosis that affects the larger arteries (ABI) or small penetrating arteries (lacunes) and cerebral embolism either from the heart or other arteries. To establish the mechanism for any particular person, it is helpful to consider not only the mode of presentation but the person in whom the stroke has occurred in terms of the risk factors present. Age is one factor. For example, cerebral infarction in young adults (ages 15–44 years)[24] has a somewhat different distribution of risk factors. Those for whom probable cause was found had a higher incidence of hematologic disease and a lower incidence of small vessel disease. Illicit drug use was determined in approximately 10%.

Still another factor is race-ethnicity in establishing the pathophysiology of the stroke. For example, using overall mortality figures, Hispanics in the United States have a higher percentage of deaths from hemorrhage than do non-Hispanic whites.[25] The percentage of patients with stroke due to ICH who were admitted to the hospital in northern Manhattan was also higher in Hispanics as well as blacks when compared with non-Hispanic whites.[26] In this same geographic area, in cases of cerebral infarction, a greater proportion of intracranial atherosclerotic disease and lacunes was found in both Hispanics and non-Hispanic blacks than in whites.[27] A preponderance of intracranial occlusive disease in Chinese persons as opposed to whites in an area in Boston drawing from both populations has also been documented.[28] Compared with extracranial stenoses, intracranial stenoses do not

correlate as well in this Chinese population with the typical atherosclerotic risk factors of peripheral and coronary arterial disease such as male gender and hypercholesterolemia. One can postulate that the disease process loosely called *atherosclerosis* differs in those with intracranial large vessel occlusion from those who are found to have extracranial carotid involvement.

Nature of the Impairment

In these several ways, the character of the cerebrovascular disease process delineates different patterns of prognosis and early treatment as well as methods for prevention of recurrent stroke. The next or second level of analysis of a person with stroke relates to the actual impairments in neurologic function that now exist as a result of the brain injury. The patterns of impairment reflect the extent and site of the brain injury.[19] Neurologic deficits in the brain influence all aspects of a person's life, including sitting, standing, walking, turning, speaking, seeing, and thinking. Deficits associated with motor and sensory systems are most obvious and are easily used for localization purposes, but cognitive and behavioral changes may also be present[29] and can have significant impact on the person's ability to learn how to use those functions that remain, and thus on eventual outcome.

Anatomic Localization

Significant differences exist between lesions, reflecting involvement of the posterior circulation (vertebral-basilar) as opposed to involvement of the anterior circulation (carotids). In the former, effects are evident in the posterior fossa including the brain stem and cerebellum as well as the visual system. Vascular disease generally causes intramedullary lesions within the tissue of the brain stem as a result of infarction or hemorrhage. The classic pattern of involvement represents ipsilateral cranial nerve involvement and contralateral sensory or motor involvement, or both, on the body (crossed syndrome). The specific cranial nerve nuclei affected can help determine the level at which the brain stem is involved with cranial nerve III (oculomotor) and IV (trochlear) in the midbrain; V (trigeminal), VI (abducens), VII (facial), and VIII (vestibular) in the pons; and IX (glossopharyngeal), X (vagus), and XII (hypoglossal) in the medulla. Lesions that affect the lateral portion of the brain stem are more likely to cause difficulty in the sensory tracts; more medial lesions can cause problems in motor action on the opposite side of the body. Although the posterior cerebral artery arises from the posterior circulation, it provides nutrients to the occipital lobe and can be considered in relation to the cerebral hemispheres. Resultant impairments can affect the person's ability to eat and swallow, to speak clearly and loudly, to coordinate eye movements to prevent double vision, to maintain balance, and so forth.

Impairments in cerebral function secondary to involvement of the large arteries of the carotid system differ depending on which hemisphere is affected, whether the impairments are in the distribution of the anterior or middle cerebral artery, and whether they are focal or diffuse. A 1998 study once again explored the effect of the side of the injury on eventual outcome.[30] Functional outcomes in ischemic stroke were found to be better in left- than right-sided lesions regardless of site within the hemisphere. Others have found no difference in outcome related to hemisphere.[31] Similarly, the outcomes achieved in terms of ambulation and self-care vary in hemispheric lesions depending on the extent of impairment in the presence of motor deficit alone, motor plus sensory, and motor plus sensory and homonymous visual deficits.[32]

In addition to injury affecting the cortical areas, the other major area is injury in the basal ganglia, which is generally attributed to small vessel disease leading to occlusion or hemorrhage. Persons with stroke can present with varying degrees and various combinations of impairment. For example, in a report from the Northern Manhattan study,[33] lacunar syndromes (generally approximately 20–30% of ischemic strokes, twice as common in blacks and Hispanics as in whites) included pure motor hemiparesis, pure sensory syndrome, mixed sensorimotor syndrome, and ataxia-hemiparesis. Prognosis as to outcome varies with these various syndromes, with pure motor hemiparesis having the best result. The classic presentation of focal involvement of motor, sensory, and visual systems opposite to the side of injury can come about as a result of cortical, basal ganglia, and internal cap-

sule (BG) or combined cortical, internal capsule, and basal ganglia (COM) involvement.[34] The outcomes for these several groups of patients with comparable impairments varied, depending apparently on the site of injury. Persons with only cortical lesions had the least damage demonstrated on imaging studies and also did best. However, the COM group did better than those with BG lesions alone. This was despite the greater size of the lesions in the combined group. Detailed study of the BG group demonstrated persistent impaired balance and persistent hypotonia. It is these specific findings that, if present, may perhaps account for the differential functional outcomes.

Specific Impairments

As with subgrouping based on the disease process, subgroups based on anatomic localization provide only partial explanation for the eventual outcome. The clinical neurologic examination assesses motor actions and sensory inputs primarily to determine the site of the brain injury. This determination has considerable value for establishing in a rather global fashion the pattern of impairment. For example, the effects of injury to the left side of the brain in a right-handed person versus effects of injury on the right side of the brain might have significant implications. Although originally designed to measure strength in reference to lower motor neuron injury, the Medical Research Council (MRC) Scale provides the basis for quantifying a selection of specific motor actions to provide a motoricity index.[35] Even more significant can be the degree to which a combination of impairments (impairment load) determines the degree to which those impairments affect the person's ability to carry on his or her life.[36]

Modifications in the clinical neurologic examination have been necessary to meet the need for reliability for the purpose of prognosis and measurement of treatment effects. Measures of degree of impairment of greater precision such as the National Instititutes of Health Stroke Scale (NIHSS) have evolved for evaluating the effects of treatment during the early poststroke stage.[37] This measure of severity of impairment has also been useful through the next stage of medical rehabilitation.[38] The NIHSS is discussed in greater detail in the last section of this chapter.

Global measures of neurologic impairment have only partial prognostic value. One must assess the impairments in the individual case to develop a treatment plan for enabling the person to once again establish a sense of control over his or her body and life. Moreover, impairments can vary over the life of the person who has experienced a stroke. Impairments commonly affect the motor and sensory systems but also affect cognition and affective states. Depression can be an early problem and remains so. Control of sphincters can also be an early problem. Pain may become a major problem after stroke.

The needs of the professional concerned with early diagnosis and management of the person with stroke differ from those of the professional who deals with the patient during the rehabilitation and continuing care phases. In the latter phases, the need for precise anatomic localization for determining the plans to be made is less. The assessment process must reflect this new focus. To begin with, in an elderly person, previous impairments may have affected performance. The person may have needed to use a cane for ambulation as the result of a previous stroke or musculoskeletal problem or a wrist splint for an old carpal tunnel syndrome. Overall, how the person is able to move and what his or her insight and goals might be are crucial findings. Particular attention must be paid to the affective and cognitive state. A process of adaptation to the impairments that exist would be necessary. Learning of new skills must go on to enhance the function of the unaffected systems and the development of compensatory strategies to deal with those aspects that remain impaired. Memory, especially immediate and delayed recall, is important because there may be a lot to learn. With impairments in memory, the patient may be able only to reacquire some already learned premorbid skills.

Recovery is strongly affected by family, particularly spousal presence and support. Their assurance of an eventual return home provides emotional strength and confidence. It is rare that a person with a projected discharge to a nursing home demonstrates a will to improve. The relationship between the patient and spouse as caregiver frequently reflects a reversal of roles, leading to stresses in the marriage. The formerly dominant spouse is now dependent. Many did not expect to have to work as hard as they are now in a rehabilitation program, where they are involved in learning "new tricks." These new efforts may need to be ongoing. The management of persons with stroke must reflect the need to re-establish and maintain a sense of hope that one can regain control over one's body and life. Necessary also but difficult to accept is a sense that alternatives exist by which one can function.

A sense of loss leading to depressed mood or even major depression is common.[39] This aspect can be missed if a communication problem exists as well. The sense of loss is compounded in elderly persons, who may feel that they have finished many of their life tasks and are looking forward to relaxing and enjoying the fruits of their labors. Their dreams have been shattered.

A case illustrating the devastating nature of the impairments is that of a man who had anticipated retirement from dental practice. One of his preparatory activities had been collecting notes for a book dealing with his professional experiences. While undergoing surgery for treatment of a cervical syrinx, he became quadriplegic as the result of a brain stem infarct. Instead of happily leaving his work and continuing his friendly rivalry with his Dallas Cowboy–loving brother, he is now totally dependent on his family, hired assistants, and a power-driven wheelchair. He requires help for all his daily activities, including personal ones, such as controlling his saliva. A major part of any rehabilitation program must be aiding him to cope with the vast differences between what he had been expecting for himself at this time of life and his current status. Being an invalid is contrary to his entire previous lifestyle.

Insight may be impaired, making any new learning unlikely. Persons who have had a stroke may not agree with the younger professional that their balance and left leg strength are not good enough for them to safely transfer out of bed and walk to the toilet. Safety awareness and judgment are necessary if one is to be able to leave the patient without the need for constant supervision. The goal is to prevent falls while still enabling the person to try to recover the ability to get in and out of bed when needed. In assessment of visual-spatial skills, signs of "neglect" would include better attention and following of directions when approached from the unaffected side or food spilled or undiscovered on the affected side. Neglect can contribute to the problem of poor insight.

In assessment of the cranial nerves, the presence of a field defect and the degree of inattention in the affected field can have impact on reading as well as driving a car or propelling a wheelchair. Problems in extraocular movement can be associated with diplopia and difficulty in reading. Weakness of the facial musculature can have importance for pocketing or dribbling of food. A weak voluntary cough, coughing within 1 minute after swallowing water, and vocal quality changes after swallowing liquid are suggestive of possible aspiration. The ability of the tongue to carry out rapid alternating movements can be associated with the degree of slurring of speech. Voice quality and degree of slurring are assessed as relevant to the ability to communicate by speaking.

Motor impairments are usually but not necessarily unilateral and are generally more severe at the periphery involving the ankle and the hand. Proximal-gross motor control is more likely to return than is more distal-fine motor control. Muscles and functions that have strong bilateral upper motor neuron innervation, such as swallowing, bladder control, and trunk control, are likewise more likely to return. Most people who have experienced a stroke place a very high value on being able to walk. This fact, coupled with the high level of automaticity in the ambulation motor program, enables a high frequency of eventual success.

Muscle weakness can be assessed by the MRC Scale, but problems extend beyond weakness to issues of motor control in the presence of the upper motor neuron site of injury. It is appropriate to assess the strength of major joint movements on a scale of less than or more than action against gravity. Particular attention would be paid to the ability to carry out hip extension and knee extension as helpful for achieving stance. Hip flexion and ankle dorsiflexion are relevant to ambulation along with some measure of balance that can be assessed by attempts at tandem gait. Distribution of weakness in the upper extremity is of interest. Is the prerequisite support of the hand present by adequate strength of the proximal upper limb? The pattern of preserved limb movement is generally but not necessarily one of enhanced flexor synergy in the upper extremity and extensor synergy in the lower extremity. The extent of such synergy can

be assessed as a measure of the motor control problem. For example, the ability to extend the index finger while maintaining a flexed elbow has functional consequences that reflect discrete motor action outside the upper extremity flexor synergy pattern.

In a stroke that affects cerebellar action, strength may be preserved, but the patient has difficulty in controlling movement in open kinetic chains. Providing resistance may compensate for the problem by closing the kinetic chain. Ataxia during spontaneous movements of the limbs indicates how this problem can affect the patient in carrying out natural movements. The finger-nose test adds information but is an artificial movement. When transferring from a supine position to a seated position, one can observe balance by how widely the person places the feet apart on the ground. Difficulty of this kind suggests a higher level of impairment of balance and the necessity for support if any attempt is made to carry out movement from sitting to standing.

The most important sensory modality for the stroke survivor is proprioception. Preserved position sense can enable the person to use the limb without visual input. The absence of position sense disables the person from carrying out actions such as dressing that require bilateral movements. The presence or absence of response to pinprick has implication for the development of central poststroke pain. Light touch and temperature are also important for protecting the limb against traumatic injury in the presence of neglect or in the use of an orthosis.

The musculoskeletal system is an important factor affecting the use of the motor system. Contracture can be acutely acquired during the early recovery phase due to improper positioning and inadequate use of passive range of motion or be chronic due to pre-existing arthritis or injury. Resistance to passive range of motion or increase in tone may occur after initial flaccidity and is considered to be part of the process of reorganization that occurs after upper motor neuron injury. It becomes important to preserve the range of motion of the various affected joints while the tone is increased so that contractures and later pain do not develop. It is vital to maintain at least 90 degrees of shoulder abduction and of external and internal rotation to be able to groom one's hair and don a pullover shirt.

The typical flexor posturing of the hemiplegic arm held tightly against the trunk, the elbow flexed, and the hand fisted causes foreshortening of the muscles and tendons, which is necessary to carry out activities. The chronically fisted hand becomes difficult to clean, and the contractures become fixed. It becomes difficult to thread an arm into the sleeve of a shirt under these conditions.

In the lower extremities, recovery of an efficient and normal-appearing gait pattern is compromised if the hip external rotators are allowed to develop permanent contracture in the externally rotated toes-out position in which a hemiplegic leg tends to rest. Full internal rotation of the hip during the swing phase of walking is critical to proper placement of the foot during heel strike.

Selective measures of impairment have been found to be helpful in prediction of functional outcomes. Examples such as upper limb motor function, proprioception, and postural function have been found to be useful in predicting the ability to go home after stroke in those patients selected for treatment in a stroke unit.[40] Motor impairment defined by an MRC rating of 4 or below and limb placement as a measure of hemihypesthesia predicted outcome as to functional ambulation in a group of patients with subcortical lesions.[41] Admission motor score on the Fugl-Meyer Assessment (FMA), a measure of impairment, was a predictor of discharge functional status in terms of mobility and self-care in a group of patients admitted to a stroke rehabilitation facility (RF).[42] Even more specific findings that support the ability to become community ambulators include proprioception but also the ability to maintain knee extension.[43]

Although stroke-related impairments and their functional consequences (disabilities) are significantly correlated with each other, reduced impairment level alone does not fully explain the reduced degree of disability that occurs in the context of rehabilitation.[44] Therein lies the opportunity offered by rehabilitation in which, even in the presence of continued impairment, training in the use of the unaffected portion and the learning of compensatory strategies including the use of assistive devices can lead to satisfactory outcomes in re-establishing community living.

Different degrees of impairment do not translate to equivalent degrees of disability. Each person has his or her own emotional and cognitive reactions and coping skills for the motor problems, sensory disturbances, swallowing, and communication problems that the stroke has induced. The anatomy of the neurologic injury and the resultant impairments do not inevitably cause the same degree of disability. Anatomy does not equal destiny.

Nature of the Disability

Although measures of impairment have some overall predictive value, a third level of analysis is necessary. One must determine the disabilities, the functional consequences of the impairments. It is not surprising that the levels of function at admission to stroke treatment programs are in most instances the best predictors of those same functional measures at discharge. Functional status measures (FSMs) assess the functional consequences of the impairments and are the outcomes that have greater applicability to issues of rehabilitation focused on discharge home.

Particularly relevant is the issue of mobility. Can the patient get out of bed, then get to a toilet, then move about the house, and then get out of the house? The clinical assessment of function is an analysis of whether the person can move with or without assistance and also the quality of those movements. In rising from supine to sitting, how well is the affected arm or leg included? Once sitting, can it be done unsupported or must one prop oneself up? Can one maintain sitting balance while using the unaffected limb for some action? Next, in moving to standing, how much assistance is needed? The range of assistance can vary; generally, the patient must contribute approximately 75% of the effort or require only "contact guard" to be managed at home with a caregiver. Is assistance required for impaired balance, for impulsiveness, or for weakness of the leg or trunk, or both? Once standing is achieved, is support required to maintain stance? If toileting is to be possible, it is necessary for the person to maintain stance without the support of another person for a short period. Crucial to the achievement of mobility is being able to rise from sitting to standing and to pivot or otherwise move to a toilet or wheelchair. Later, gait should be assessed.

Functional Status Measures

A number of FSMs have been developed that can lead to a score. The FIM incorporates a basic set of measures that then represent an outcome at discharge correlated with functional status necessary for community life.[45] Each item is scored on a seven-point scale on the basis of degree of support needed by the person to carry out activities such as dressing, feeding, walking, or communicating. Key aspects of the continuum reflecting burden of care are a score of 5, indicating the need for supervision, versus a score below that, signifying the need for varying degrees of physical assistance. The total score has been used to quantify a global level of function, severity of disability, or burden of care.

The quality of the disability reflects the exact type of functional status deficits. The more specific the profile, the more related to the actual result. The motor subscale contains 13 items and excludes the 5 items that measure communication and social cognition. It has been particularly predictive to the assessment of performance directly relevant to the ability to function at home as measured by LOS in RFs.[46] The person's motor FIM score on admission was the single strongest predictor of discharge motor FIM. In a similar way, a subset of six items has been useful for determining status at the time of discharge from an acute care hospital. These items include bathing, bowel control, toileting, social interaction, dressing the lower body, and eating.[47]

Alexander[48] attempted to stratify appropriate selection of patients into acute inpatient rehabilitation settings as a reflection of the interaction of functional level and age. This retrospective study measured admission FIM (A-FIM) and FIM gain as well as age and eventual placement. Although highly predictive, the relationship is a complex one. Younger persons (younger than 55 years) and those with high A-FIM (older than 80 years) regardless of age almost invariably went home and might therefore have been appropriate for discharge directly to outpatient settings. Even those with a low A-FIM (less than 40) in the 55- to 64-year-old group had a high likelihood of discharge home. It is not surprising that the degree of improvement during the rehabilitation stay contributed to the eventual outcome in this group as well as in the age group of 65–74 years. Persons older than 75 years, however, were less likely to return home even if A-FIM scores were somewhat higher (40–60) and substantial functional improvement occurred. It is suggested that such persons go directly to less intensive (and less costly) rehabilitation settings.

Age herein reflects a number of variables, including endurance and medical comorbidity, but even more importantly can also serve as a marker of the availability of caregivers and their health. Measures of functional level have enhanced predictability of community living outcome when coupled with social factors such as the availability of caregivers. It is clear that the identification of caregivers and their training and support must be an integral part of any program to manage the effects of stroke. The case described earlier illustrates how the availability of necessary resources and the commitment of the daughter to her mother's care enabled community living despite severe impairment.

Groupings (functional related groups, or FRGs) derived from the FIM (FIM-FRGs), reflecting both the motor and cognitive subscales, have been stratified into three bands with implications both for eventual disposition and LOS.[49] This effort at more precise analysis of FIM scores can serve to select patients for more efficient use of resources as well as provide benchmarks for outcome based on severity of disability. The lower band with the most severe motor or cognitive disabilities, or both, had the longest LOS and the least but still considerable likelihood of community discharge (approximately 50%). Concomitantly, the median performance was at the level of requiring supervision in relation to what might be considered to be relatively basic functions, such as eating, grooming, and sphincter control. Age 75 years or older was an additional variable that contributed to membership in this band. The middle band consisted of persons with either moderately severe or milder physical disabilities coupled with more severe cognitive problems. At discharge, they required no help in the basic functions but low levels of assistance in transfers and dressing compatible in general with a high likelihood of community discharge. The upper band had the least severe physical disabilities and high function in the cognitive area with problems limited to mobility. By almost universal discharge home, this group required only some consideration as to safety but were generally independent in walking and tub transfers.

Although more highly predictive, these measures of functional status have only actuarial (group) significance and weakly predictive power for individuals. For example, the FIM-FRGs explain 54% of the variance in discharge motor FIM scores, which in turn only partially explain the variance in eventual discharge home. Moreover, it is less clear how to use these facts to construct programs for individual patients or for groups at any given level of severity. The determination of the disabilities that require remediation is only partially encompassed with the items within the FIM. Although compatible with items that have significance for community living, they do not contain the range of items that may be necessary. For example, the ability to deal with a telephone or transportation may be highly important. It is necessary to go beyond outcome measurement at the time of discharge home from an inpatient facility to measure outcome that extends into community life. Continuity of measurement into outpatient or home treatment is thus necessary for adequate management of the person with stroke.

Specific Disabilities

More fundamentally, the determination of the effects of any impairment on the life of the person depends not only on its severity and scope but also on its significance to that person. An impairment such as weakness of the left hand varies in its importance depending on whether the person is right or left handed. A problem such as a hemianopsia has far different consequences for a 53-year-old man whose entire work history has been as a truck driver than for an older retiree. The consequences of that same impairment vary for the older retiree who has access to a substitute driver or for whom public transportation is readily available as an alternative to driving a car. The disabilities—the functional limitations that result from the impairments—vary with the person's perceptions, goals, and the idiosyncratic environment in which that person needs to operate. The development of a rehabilitation plan appropriate to the person requires the definition of that person's priorities. Those priorities reflect not only the impairments but the person and his or her environment.

Data must be generated as to the physical characteristics of the patient's home. Does it have stairs or an elevator? Where are the bedrooms and toilets? How wide are the doorways if one needs to use a wheelchair? What kind of rugs are on the floors? What kind of bath or shower is in the home? Who is available as a caregiver and to what extent? Is someone available only to drop in and do the shopping? Does the caregiver work and on what shifts? Are services such as Meals on Wheels available in the community? Does the person qualify, amid the tangle of regulations, for outside services and to what extent, for how long, and so forth? Does the patient have other resources?

The identification of the problem is the first step in the development of a series of plans for life after stroke. Such information cannot be assumed a priori. Input is required from the person with stroke or family members, or both. A collaborative approach that enables those persons to contribute to the definition of the problem and to do so increasingly must be part of a truly effective set of plans.

In designing plan(s) for rehabilitation and continuing care phases, the factor of changes over time must be recognized. Impairments may worsen or improve; moreover, priorities may change. Particularly important is the possibility of changes in the environment in which the person with impairments needs to operate. The availability and nature of caregivers can change, and the physical setting can vary in its accessibility, and so forth.

In summary, the problems presented by cerebrovascular disease are extensive and likely to increase due to an enlarged aging population. The nature of the disease varies but is generally progressive with exacerbations. The progressive nature can be modified by reduction of risk factors specific to the person and his or her racial-ethnic group. Methods for prevention are well known but not applied universally. Some segments of the population remain particularly at risk. Methods for increasing commitment to ongoing stroke prevention regimens remain problematic. The degree of brain injury varies as do the resultant impairments in function because of the sites and extent of injury. The site of injury and the ultimate outcome of return to community life are not directly correlated. Rather, that outcome is more highly correlated with the actual functional effects of the impairments. Those functional consequences (disabilities) in turn only partially explain the outcome of community living. The physical setting and the availability of caregivers are significant factors. In addition, the character of the services provided to aid in the management of the person or caregiver, or both, can enhance the likelihood of a good outcome. The next section of this chapter deals with ways in which the organization of services can lead to the optimization of results in recognition of these multiple factors.

Character of the Solution

Overall Plan

The management of the person with stroke is an example of the management of a person with a chronic neurologic illness. Care of the person with chronic illness is considered to be an ongoing planning process. Problems are identified, goals set, activities designed, and time established for review and revision of the initial plan. At the time of review, the progress is identified and the process by which those results have come about is discussed before a new plan is made once again. The structure of this cyclical planning process is exemplified by the recurrent team conference, which serves as a planning conference. This reiterative process is described in detail in Chapter 2.

Continuity of Care

The stroke survivor is in recovery for the rest of his or her life. One component is therefore to provide continuity of care over time. The life of the person after stroke is divided into three phases of unequal duration wherein the frequency and intensity of the planning process vary along with the implementation of the plans made. The initial acute care phase lasts for hours to days. A team or planning conference may occur once or twice during the course of the stay. Initiated by the relatively sudden appearance of the impairments, the goal is to limit the degree of impairment and to establish medical and neurologic stability. An initial plan is made for the next phase of retraining or rehabilitation.

The next or rehabilitation phase lasts for weeks to months with the goal of re-establishment of community life by reducing the degree of disability and establishing a support structure to the extent necessary. A planning conference may occur weekly or biweekly, becoming monthly as intensity diminishes. For example, services may be provided within inpatient settings of varying intensity and then subsequently in outpatient day programs. Recovery from impairments may become maximal after several months, but recovery from the disabilities can vary considerably. Improvement can continue dependent on the emotional and cognitive resources, with a much diminished role of the professional staff. A plan is made for the next phase after discharge from rehabilitation services. The continuing care phase lasts for months to years with planning conferences occurring intermittently but perhaps yearly. This is the point for which the patient must be amply prepared to prevent regression into a lower level of functional independence. It may be necessary to enable the patient to carry on his or her own self-rehabilitation program with only distant supervision from a therapist or rehabilitation physicians. The overall goal is to maintain the person with stroke in the least restrictive environment for the longest possible time by reducing the likelihood of further impairment from recurrent stroke and by maintaining the support structure for community living. Problems and goals can change and new opportunities can arise.

The case that follows has "value added" in ongoing management that addresses medical and prevention issues in the context of dealing with reduction of disabilities. The caregiver was able to serve as the patient's coach, after training sessions with the physical therapist. A subsequent short series of sessions with a physical therapist took place only after many months of independent work by the patient and her caregiver.

An example is the case of a 68-year-old overweight woman with long-standing type II diabetes and hypertension who had experienced a stroke that affected her left side. Before her stroke, she had injured her left knee in a fall, and she was fearful of having another one. She lived with her retired husband, who was in good health, in a one-story house. Although her speech was somewhat slurred, this presented no difficulty to her. Her major concern was her continued problem with mobility, particularly her transfer from bed to toilet or wheelchair. She had received a series of physical therapy sessions without improvement in her functional problem. This remained bothersome because her husband needed to get up to help her the several times each night that she needed toileting. Her difficulties in straightening her leg to bear weight were a result of her old injury but were compounded by her excessive weight. An early goal, therefore, was to concentrate on that which she could do something about—that is, her weight. She stated that her goal was to reduce her weight to 160 lbs so as to increase her mobility. She was successful in losing a substantial amount of weight over the next few months. She reported that she was particularly pleased because she now no longer required insulin for control of her diabetes. Her blood pressure also came under better control, requiring a lower dose of medication. She could now address the goal of independent transfer. Her husband was trained to be her coach in using the strategies she already knew but had not been able to put into effect. She was indeed now able to transfer without need for physical assistance. The next set of plans dealt with her getting around the house, walking to the toilet with her husband merely observing. She needed now to be fitted with a new orthosis, for which she received several sessions with a physical therapist to aid in meeting her new goals.

A further value of ongoing management is the more consistent use and generalization of what had already been found to work. An example is a 55-year-old right-handed man who had experienced a stroke several years before that affected the right side of his body and his ability to express himself. He was soon able to get around with the use of a cane. His language difficulties continued to be disabling, particularly when he attempted to communicate with strangers. While working with a speech therapist, he found several strategies that were helpful when he had difficulty in finding the words he needed. One that was particularly useful was to write out the word he wanted. Once he had done so, he was able to read it, and in reading it aloud, he could then say it at other times. Although he was aware of the strategy, he found it cumbersome to carry around a small notebook and did not choose to use this method on his own. He preferred to try to communicate with gesture or some of his other less effective strategies that were based mainly on oral language. He was no longer eligible for intensive speech therapy. The issues were now to enable him to generalize the use of the strategies he already knew. The overall goal was to build his vocabulary and fluency. He agreed to write each day in his notebook at least one word that was problematic for him. He found that he was able to order a taxi on the telephone when he wrote out beforehand what he wanted to say. He also found that he did better when he felt less rushed. He agreed to tell his sometimes impatient brother or others, "I have a problem with language. Please give me more time." He also agreed to make what he needed to say as short as possible by thinking it out beforehand. After he returned to the speech therapist several months later, he estimated that his fluency had improved approximately 50%. He could now begin to consider some volunteer work that he had not been willing to try before.

Comprehensive Care

The professional components of the planning team vary depending on the phase and, therefore, the range and severity of the problems. Coordination of a comprehensive range of interdisciplinary services is generally required, at least at the start. The entire biological-social-psychological matrix in which the person must act needs to be considered. Three major efforts are described. First, health promotion is an integral part of any program for stroke survivors, with particular attention to the management of risk factors so as to reduce the likelihood of recurrent stroke. Another major effort is training the survivor to reduce the degree of functional disability in a functional treatment plan. This effort must frequently be coupled with the training and ongoing maintenance of caregivers.

In the case of stroke, one must deal with the medical and health issues throughout the several phases, with the greatest intensity during the acute phase. During rehabilitation, professionals on the planning-treatment team in addition to a physician and nurse ordinarily include therapists who deal with mobility, ADL, and speech and language. The interdisciplinary planning team has been a major component of the rehabilitation process. Its continuation remains desirable. Methods for enhancing its performance are discussed in Chapter 2. These other rehabilitation professionals may participate only rarely or intermittently during the continuing care phase. Psychological services are frequently necessary during the rehabilitation phase in conjunction with cognitive and adjustment problems.

Ongoing need may exist during continuing care, particularly as related to the maintenance of the caregiver relationship. Social worker services are necessary to support plans for community living starting in the acute phase and with greater intensity during the rehabilitation phase, with subsequent ongoing intermittent need.

The person with stroke and any family caregiver are part of the planning team from the start. A major component in the management of persons with chronic illness is the training that goes on in the context of ongoing planning to enable these primary participants to eventually become better able to manage for themselves. In the case of stroke, participation leading to self-management must occur in both the health promotion and functional rehabilitation areas. Continuity can be provided by a physician or nurse, who must act with recognition of the broad context of health care. The role of the primary or principal physician can be supplemented by specialty physicians, depending on the constellation of problems.

Cost-Effective Care

The intensity and duration of overall services and, thus, costs also vary with the phase and the LOS within each. Coupled with concern about costs should be concomitant measurement of outcomes to optimize cost-effectiveness. The treatment of persons with stroke has been in the forefront of efforts using evidence-based models of care.[50] The AHCPR developed guidelines for the appropriate selection of levels of rehabilitation services. Alternatives include ambulatory rehabilitation services in a clinic or at home or inpatient care within an acute care facility or a less intensive subacute care facility. The latter is likely to be provided within a nursing home rather than a hospital-based facility. Selection for the higher-cost acute model would normally be based on the greater need for medical supervision and the ability to maintain a relatively intensive schedule of 3 hours or more of interdisciplinary treatment. Another factor that supports this additional effort is the likelihood of a caregiver being available.

Stroke is one of the areas that has been most affected by the emergence of managed care.[51] Patients who are "managed" are more likely than those under fee-for-service plans to receive their rehabilitation care in nursing homes, where the intensity and comprehensiveness of care are likely to be less than the other alternatives. The criteria established by ACHPR still remain in effect when one distinguishes between those who should receive their rehabilitation within inpatient versus outpatient sites. What has happened is that the character of treatment in those sites has changed. Those who receive care within the community are more likely to receive treatment outside rather than in the home. Transportation is thus an added cost, mainly borne by family members. Those who receive inpatient care are more likely to be treated in less intensive subacute settings. Although reduced costs may have been paid by the insurers, it is less clear that overall costs have been reduced when one considers overall effects on the families as well as the patients. Crucial to any analysis are the choice of outcome measures and the duration of follow-up.

Kane et al.[52] compared differences in outcomes of Medicare patients with strokes discharged to RFs with those of individuals discharged either to rehabilitation nursing facilities or nursing homes. The two nursing home levels of care were differentiated on the basis of staffing patterns. This was a prospective study carried out during 1988–1990 in Minneapolis–St. Paul, Houston, and Pittsburgh. Data collection went on at the time of discharge from the acute care hospital and at 6 weeks, 6 months, and 1 year. A complex ADL scale was used to measure outcome. Those who went to RFs did significantly better than those discharged to the other facilities, with no significant differences between the two others. The ADL score served to stratify those who were "healthier" and "sicker." Both strata sent to RFs did better, with the healthier doing particularly well, showing substantial improvement maintained throughout the year. The sicker sent to RF had improvement, although deterioration occurred during the course of the subsequent year. In contrast, those who were healthier and sent to the other facilities showed little change in functional level, and the sicker not only had little improvement initially but showed increased disability on follow-up.

These findings were in general confirmed in a larger-scale study carried out in 17 states during 1991–1994.[53] Once again, rehabilitation services of varying levels of intensity were identified.

Medicare costs, intensity of therapy, and physician visits were available. Outcome measures included community residence and ADL score mainly derived from the BI. A 6-month follow-up was carried out. Those who went to the more costly RFs were more likely to have caregivers and to be at a somewhat higher functional level. They were also more likely to return to the community and to have improvements in ADL score. The relationship of the increased costs to the results cannot be easily calculated because these were measures of effectiveness and were not measured in dollars.

Costs will undoubtedly come under ever-increasing scrutiny, and LOS, already reduced, will become even shorter with care further rationalized. Outcome measures will continue to be based on minimization of degree of disability manifested by community living with the lowest possible burden of care. Improvements in the cost-effectiveness ratios can still occur. One opportunity is to focus efforts on health promotion with the outcome measures to include freedom from illness and satisfactory QOL. Another opportunity already discussed is to support maintenance within a community setting by support for caregivers. The third major opportunity now to be discussed is a change in the mode of interaction between the professional and the primary participants. The opportunity lies in changing the quality as well as the quantity of the interaction.

Collaborative Care

Underlying the overall management plan is the development of the capability for self-management by the primary participants. The planning process must be a collaborative one, leading to conjoint contribution of both energy and ideas. Although the management of stroke is similar to that of other chronic illness, some attributes are specific to the disease process. The event that one calls a *stroke* appears to be sudden and of unknown source. The impact of this mode of onset extends beyond the sometimes quite devastating functional impairments that affect basic functions, such as mobility, self-care, and communication. The person can have a fundamental impairment in the sense of self, in self-confidence, and a sense of self-efficacy. This is the impact of what has been the almost instantaneous nature of the transformation from an independent, free-thinking individual to someone who is unable to perform such functions as moving out of bed, controlling one's bladder, and so forth. Passivity must eventually be counteracted. The re-establishment of a sense of control over one's body and life must be integral to the process of management.

Participation in the planning process can aid in this process of reintegration. The details of this process are described in Chapter 2. Under the auspices of the rehabilitation team, participation is maximized for contributing to the identification of the disabilities and goals. Hope is engendered to the extent that the person becomes aware by participation in the review process, addressing the question as to progress made in relation to his or her goals. Self-efficacy is enhanced by awareness both of the accomplishments and the relationship between the results and the actions of the person. It is the ability to begin to address the question as to the actions taken ("what works") that is crucial.

When the person with stroke is able to live in the community, he or she enters the phase of "independent living," a principle that must be clarified. It is not defined by the degree to which a person with stroke is independent of the need for extrinsic support; rather it is the degree to which the person with stroke is able to manage his or her life, including caregivers. In the rehabilitation phase, disabilities are alleviated by the learning of compensatory strategies and the design of modifications in the environment. Assistive devices must frequently be selected or designed; these ideas are usually provided by professional staff. The re-entry into community living is a first step on the road to independent living. Thereafter, the primary participants must deal with an environment that is both more variegated and changing over time. They must learn a broader range of strategies as well as responses to unforeseen circumstances. The goal is to have a sense that alternative strategies exist; if the usual way no longer works, another is generally available. The relatively predictable environment of the rehabilitation setting is replaced by a setting in which caregivers are not always available, inaccessibility is present, and public benefits are not readily put into place. Therefore, one must be able to generalize compensatory strategies learned during the rehabilitation phase to new and varied settings. Not only must existing strategies be implemented, but new strategies must be found as new problems surface. For example, major issues about family life may surface that were less evident earlier. One must also contribute not only the answers to the planning questions but also be able to ask oneself the questions, for example, whether a problem exists, so as to determine when to seek professional consultation.

In summary, the characteristics of the management plan for persons with stroke must include continuity over time and the coordination of sometimes very comprehensive interdisciplinary services that are subject to ongoing evaluation as to both costs and outcomes. The ultimate product can be to learn how to manage one's own health and life after stroke in concert with the professional staff. The next portion of this section illustrates the application of these principles at a programmatic level and in the case of individual patients.

Health Promotion Plan

Nature of the Problem

Stroke is ideally suited for prevention. Risk factors have been identified, and criteria have now been established for treatment. These include the ongoing use of medication as well as changes in lifestyle, such as diet, exercise, and cessation of smoking.[14] Particularly disturbing is the incidence of recurrent stroke leading to further impairment in persons who may have recovered sufficiently to lead independent lives. Long-term survival and recurrence rate can be significantly affected by treatment of risk factors. Yet fewer than one-half the patients who had experienced a TIA or stroke were apparently made aware of the risk of recurrent stroke and the value of managing risk factors.[54] Major problems remain in the degree to which regimens established to treat risk factors are actually carried out.[15]

The medical rehabilitation setting immediately after stroke is ideally suited for training in stroke prevention, particularly if relatively difficult changes in lifestyle are to be recommended. The opportunity arises during what is usually a several-week period to establish new behaviors when a greater likelihood of concern also exists both on the part of the survivor and the family members. The problem is the degree to which one can establish adherence to

any regimen toward changes in managing one's health. Innovative approaches are needed that go beyond traditional methods of patient education. The training process must lead to both the ability to carry out a regimen and the commitment to independent implementation after discharge. Studies of the conditions for maintenance of regimens for the management of chronic illness emphasize the importance of patients' participation in the design of their program plan, the ability to monitor results, and the value of ongoing follow-up.[55]

Goals

A health promotion plan should be integrated within the rehabilitation of persons with stroke. A plan should be developed, implemented, and evaluated with maximal patient participation as a means of increasing the likelihood of ongoing adherence to the regimen.

Methods

The health promotion plan, if integral to the entire rehabilitation process, supports that process. It provides an area for the person to re-establish a sense of control over his or her body in a relatively clear fashion because the goals are specific and can be measured regularly. Table 4-1 describes such a plan for implementation during the course of a several-week stay on a rehabilitation unit. Comparable plans can be generated for varying LOS and in outpatient settings. Possible problem areas are identified on admission in terms of blood sugar, hypertension, and hyperlipidemia, as well as the use of anticoagulants (INR). Priorities are established, and at least one specific subplan is generated for implementation during the first few days and is reported on at the initial team conference. Review and revision of the health component goes on in relation to the weekly interval team conference, which provides the basic structure of the reiterative planning cycle.

Each plan includes a goal and means by which the goal is to be met along with a frequency of review. Hypertension is an example. Elevated blood pressure is identified as a risk factor that contributes to the likelihood of recurrent stroke; the value of control is in reducing this likelihood. The problem has thus been identified by the health

Table 4-1. Health Promotion Plan

	Day 1	Day 2	Day 3 Initial Team	Day 8 Interim Team	Day 15 Discharge Team	Day 30 Postdischarge
Objectives	1. Establish IP HP plan	1. Implement HP plan	1. Establish interdisciplinary HP plan	1. Review and revise HP plan 2. Implement CT plan	1. Review IP-HP plan 2. Establish postdischarge HP plan as appropriate	1. Review implementation HP plan
Activities	1. Identify HP problems/priorities (BS, BP, INR, LDL) 2. Identify goals 3. Provide educational material 4. Identify equipment needs (BP, BS) 5. Schedule training groups 6. Establish CT plan	1. Evaluate outcome 2. Evaluate what works	1. Evaluate outcome 2. Evaluate what works 3. Identify goals 4. Evaluate patient participation	1. Evaluate outcome 2. Evaluate what works 3. Identify goals 4. Evaluate patient participation 5. Initiate CT as needed for implementation of HP plan	1. Evaluate outcome 2. Evaluate what works 3. Identify goals 4. Evaluate patient participation 5. Evaluate caregiver component	1. Evaluate outcomes 2. Evaluate patient participation
Evaluation	1. Physician's HP 2. Physician's orders 3. Nursing assessment 4. Nursing care plan	1. Progress notes, physician/nurse	1. Team conference report	1. Team conference report	1. Team conference report 2. Patient planning form	1. In-out visit session report

IP = inpatient; HP = health promotion; CT = caregiver training; BS = blood sugar; BP = hypertension; INR = anticoagulants; LDL = hyperlipidemia.

professional. Agreement from the patient is sought on the existence of a problem and the willingness to pursue a plan for management. This agreement extends to knowing the goal, monitoring that goal along with the health professional, and then using a blood pressure monitor on one's own and keeping a log. In addition to monitoring the degree to which the goal is being met, agreement is sought to address the question as to the means or methods that are working to maintain control. This might include a list of medications, their names, dosage and frequency, and so forth. The methods might also include the diet and exercise program that was being used.

The blood pressure goal may vary from 140/85 to some other figure compatible with the patient's age and previous level of blood pressure. The monitoring process can be reinforced at least twice a day when blood pressure is normally measured. Educational material is provided along with at least one group meeting. In accordance with the overall planning structure, a report on this health plan is made by the patient along with the staff at the team conference concerning the level of goal accomplishment and the methods in use. Any changes in the plan are addressed. At the successive team conferences before discharge, the reports can be of the initial area such as hypertension or of any new health plan. For example, blood sugar or use of INRs also can be monitored by the patient.

Measurement is of the degree that the goals such as blood pressure are being met and also the degree to which the patient is describing his or her own status and what is working. By discharge, the intent is for the patient or caregiver, or both, to be able to describe the answers to the questions being addressed, namely, goal, status, and methods. This is preparatory to the ability to carry out this process more independently at home. In the model shown, the follow-up of primary health surveillance is normally the province of the primary physician. Therefore, only one follow-up visit is available to the rehabilitation staff. It is at that time, generally within the first month after discharge, that one can evaluate the adherence to the plan. This is determined by the existence of a log that is brought in, the ability to use the blood pressure device correctly, and the ability to answer the question as to what is working. These answers can include the list of medications, any changes in the diet, and so forth.

This same procedure can be followed with plans dealing with blood sugar, in which instance the concept of frequent monitoring with the use of a glucometer is well established. It is frequently possible to initiate a process of weight loss and commitment to a weight reduction diet. This can enable many individuals to bring their blood sugar under adequate control without the need for insulin or with less hypoglycemic medication.

The importance of self-management in the use of anticoagulant medication along with awareness of the vitamin K content of foods is illustrated when recurrent stroke occurs with either too low or too high an INR.[56] The primary physician and the patient are encouraged to work together in a similar format. They can now agree on a new goal and establish the criteria for review and revision of the plan. The frequency of follow-up can vary. The patient or caregiver, or both, now have the ability to monitor their own status along with the professional.

Evaluation

Documentation goes on during the team planning conference. The health promotion plan is reviewed along with the other reports being made. Questions that are addressed include the goal and the status of meeting that goal as well as what may be contributing to the accomplishment of the goal. One is also measuring the degree to which it is the patient speaking by use of the scale described in Chapter 2. A log sheet is kept at the bedside comparable to one that patients will keep on their own at home.

The overall program is evaluated in accordance with the format described in Chapter 2. For example, the degree of implementation is measured by documentation on the team conference report (see Figure 2-2). A second level of evaluation, once again as documented in the small box on the team conference report (see Figure 2-3), is the actual degree of patient participation achieved at the various team conferences, at the time of discharge; and at the time of follow-up visit. A third level of evaluation is the long-term incidence of actual implementation and its effect on stroke recurrence.

Functional Treatment Plan

Nature of the Problem

The process of recovery of function after stroke is concerned with both the prevention of further impairment and reduction of the functional consequences of the impairments that remain. Although one can have spontaneous improvement in the degree of impairment, that is not a specific goal of retraining, and recovery to the level before the stroke is not often ever complete. Yet it is that aspect that is most prominent in the thinking of most people. It is illustrated in the often expressed goal to walk again, to be like one was before this sudden event happened without warning. It is at the level of impairment that most focus. It is necessary to go beyond the impairments to the level of their functional consequences. Much can be done to reduce disabilities even if impairments remain. It is necessary to address those functional consequences and clarify, for example, the distinction between the goals of "getting around" and the means by which one could do so.

The means might need to be different from those used previously. For example, walking may no longer be possible as a means of getting around one's house. Transfer out of bed to a wheelchair may be necessary at least initially. Using methods that are alternatives to what one has done throughout one's life is difficult, particularly for the elderly. A willingness to do so can be based on an ability to consider moving the focus from the impairments to their functional consequences.

In addition to being willing to consider alternative ways of doing things that are by their nature

Table 4-2. Functional Rehabilitation Plan

	Preadmission	Day 1	Day 2–3 Initial Team Meeting	Day 8 Interim Team Meeting	Day 15 Discharge Team Meeting	Time Varies Outpatient Team Meeting(s)
Objectives	1. Identify level of care needed	1. Initiate RP	1. Establish inpatient IDP	1. Review and revise IDP	1. Review IDP 2. Establish PDP	1. Review and revise PDP
Activities	—	1. Identify rehabilitation problems 2. Identify rehabilitation team	1. Identify priorities 2. Identify status, goal in priority areas 3. Schedule treatment	1. Evaluate status 2. Evaluate what works 3. Establish new goals	1. Evaluate status 2. Evaluate what works 3. Establish new goals 4. Schedule treatment	1. Evaluate status 2. Evaluate what works 3. Establish new goals 4. Schedule treatment
Evaluation	1. Preadmission report	1. Physician's orders	1. Team conference report 2. Physician's orders	1. Team conference report 2. Physician's orders	1. Team conference report 2. Physician's orders	1. Outpatient team conference report 2. Physician's orders

RP = rehabilitation plan; IDP = interdisciplinary plan; PDP = postdischarge plan.

abnormal is the problem of the additional effort that is required. Not only is it necessary to learn new ways of doing things that require an additional investment, but the methods that one learns themselves may necessitate more effort. A higher degree of organization is usually required. That which came naturally no longer does, and the alternatives frequently require more effort. More energy is needed and over long periods. One must be able to both sustain a commitment of energy and to consider alternative ways of thinking.

Emphasis on cost-effectiveness has led to reduction in the intensity, complexity, and duration of professional services available to the retraining of persons with stroke. It becomes ever more necessary to enlist all possible resources. The resources of the patient both in terms of energy and problem-solving ideas are to be enlisted along with the professional staff. Shortened inpatient LOS requires coordination of staff focused on interdisciplinary activities based on priorities defined collaboratively with the patient or family, or both.

Goals

The goals are to reduce the degree of disability (burden of care) by retraining, including the use of assistive devices. Overall, one aims to restore the person's sense of self, the ability to regain control over one's body and life, by maximizing patient participation in the planning-treatment process.

Methods

The process of training is considered to be an ongoing planning process that focuses on the maintenance of hope and a sense of inquiry into alternative ways of doing things. The patient is to be enabled to become an active member of the planning team. Ozer[57] describes in detail the implementation of such a program. Table 4-2 describes the overall process. An initial assessment by each of the appropriate staff leads to identification of problems and goals, with patient agreement sought to the answers to these questions. The initial team meeting leads to a coordinated interdisciplinary team plan based on the identification of priorities that affect discharge from inpatient services. One can also project planned discharge date as well as assistive devices that will be necessary. Caregiver training can generally be scheduled to take place at the time of the next team meeting. Short-term goals can be established and level of staff commitment in terms of individual and group treatments prescribed. The patient is present at each of the successive team planning sessions. At the minimum, agreement is sought in reference to the short-term goals. This commitment then provides the basis for participation at the subsequent team meeting in assessing the degree to which the goals are being met. At that time the opportunity is also available to address the question as to what actions may have contributed to the results achieved, and new goals are set for the next interval before discharge. Once again, at the discharge conference, status is reviewed as well as what worked before the development of the ambulatory care plan. These same questions are addressed during the successive planning sessions at the ambulatory care phase, leading eventually to discharge from rehabilitation services to the continuing care phase.

Evaluation

Evaluation is performed on several levels. The first level is the degree of implementation of the participatory rehabilitation process. This is provided by documentation on the team conference report (see Figure 2-3) of the questions being addressed in reference to the several areas listed, such as ADL, mobility, and communication. A second level is the degree to which patient participation is sought. This is documented by the existence of a score in the small box, which reflects such participation. A third level of evaluation is the actual score achieved in terms of patient participation as documented in the small box. Table 2-9 illustrates a report generated during the implementation of a sample program plan. Once an acceptable level of implementation has been achieved, still another level of evaluation is the measurement outcome achieved via the use of FIM, and so forth.

Caregiver Training Plan

Nature of the Problem

The ability of the person with stroke to live at home once again and be maintained there depends not only on the degree of disability but also on the availability of caregivers, particularly spouses, to help compensate for the disabilities. In addition to the possibility of discharge home, the availability of social supports leads to improvement in the degree of progress during rehabilitation per se and

ongoing improvement.[58] Indeed, those who perceived a high degree of support appeared to overcome the effects of more severe stroke. Conversely, social isolation can be seen as a risk factor for poor outcome. Those with the least amount of social support did not maintain improvement and appeared to decline in functional status over time.

If a caregiver is needed, the maintenance of the relationship becomes important. The concept of *burden* can be defined in two ways. Distinction is made between objective burden (amount of time spent in caregiving, financial problems) and subjective or perceived burden, with the latter having a major impact on the willingness to continue care. For caregivers of long duration, the actual objective burden of care measured by the degree of disability could explain only to a minor degree the perceived burden of care. The latter was more affected by the caregiver's feelings of unmet needs for psychosocial support.[59]

Social support is an important risk factor in prognosis and clinical management, and efforts must be made to identify and potentiate the effectiveness of caregivers as an integral part of management of persons after stroke. Caregiver training has focused primarily on knowledge about stroke and specific skills that relate to management at home. Although education of that sort has been helpful, additional counseling focused on problem solving has led to even more improved patient adjustment maintained over a year after discharge.[60] The training of caregivers must incorporate not only specific skills and information but optimally must contain a process of ongoing support. The basis for that must be established early in the course of treatment after stroke, with training in the ability to identify problems and solutions on an ongoing basis as essential for the caregiver as for the patient. The pair, both the patient and caregiver, should be considered the client.

Goals

The goals are to provide *information* concerning stroke: the impairments, prognosis for recovery, and need for stroke prevention; *skill training* in enabling the person with stroke to be cared for safely; and *problem-solving* capability, leading to self-confidence and independent initiative to access resources as needed.

Table 4-3. Caregiver Training Plan

	Preadmission	Day 1	Day 2–3 Initial Team	Day 8 Interim Team No. 1	Day 14 Caregiver Practice Day	Day 15 Discharge Team	Day 30
Objectives	1. Orientation	1. CT plan designed/ initiated	1. Interdisciplinary CT plan established	1. CT plan implemented	1. CT plan reviewed and revised	1. CT plan reviewed	1. Postdischarge review
Activities	1. Identification of caregiver 2. Establish commitment 3. Ensure presence at admission	1. Identification of problems, priorities 2. Identification confirmed of caregiver to be trained 3. PFC scheduled 4. Information provided as to acute retraining phase	1. Identification of problems, priorities, and objectives with team 2. CT schedule confirmed 3. PFC schedule confirmed	1. PFC takes place 2. Training implemented 3. Caregiver practice day scheduled 4. Information provided on community life phase	1. Caregiver practice takes place 2. Problems and priorities revised as needed	1. Review of caregiver practice and entire CT	1. Phone call 2. Review identification of problems in community life for development of new plan as needed
Evaluation	1. Social worker report	1. Presence of family member on day 1	1. Team conference report	1. Caregiver available for PF conference 2. Caregiver available for training 3. Caregiver identifies concerns and questions in respect to acute retraining phase			

CT = caregiver training; PFC = patient-family conference.

Methods

The development and implementation of the caregiver component are integral to the entire process. Table 4-3 describes a model that starts with the identification of the availability of caregivers before admission to a rehabilitation setting. This is one of the criteria used along with the degree of functional disability to determine the appropriate level of care.

At admission, the identified caregiver is familiarized with the plan including the scheduled training times and is provided information concerning stroke, particularly as it relates to the acute and rehabilitation phases. The schedule is keyed to the team conferences. At the initial team conference, the need for assistive devices determines some of the training that is to occur. For example, a blood pressure device, a wheelchair, or an orthosis may be needed. In many instances, the caregiver spouse is available throughout the patient's stay. However, when the identified caregiver is one of the patient's children, work schedules may require that a specific time be established when training is to take place. This is coordinated on a training day approximately halfway through the patient's stay at the time of the interim team planning conference to which the caregiver is invited. A patient-family conference occurs during which the physician and caseworker meet with the parties. One can then deal with the overall discharge plan, answer questions particularly regarding health issues, and make arrangements for assistive devices as needed. The information provided on admission regarding stroke is reviewed, with additional material provided concerning community life. The skills training component takes place on that day with additional time booked as needed by each of the professional team. The weekend after this training day provides an opportunity for the caregivers to practice what they had been taught earlier that week under the supervision of the professional staff. This can include safe transfers to and from bed, monitoring blood pressure with the use of a device, or carrying out a toileting schedule to prevent incontinence.

The caseworker in other contacts encourages the caregiver to identify concerns or questions and to take initiative in access to community resources. Arrangements are made concerning discharge, with follow-up visits booked for outpatient or home-based treatment and follow-up visit(s) with the physician along with transfer to the primary physician for medical care. The case manager follows up with at least one phone call concerning the implementation of scheduled treatments and so forth. A subsequent opportunity is available to continue the participation of the patient and caregiver in the ongoing review and revision of the rehabilitation plan as well as one visit for review of the health promotion plan. Counseling takes place during the ongoing team conferences as long as the person with stroke remains in the ambulatory rehabilitation phase. During this period, caregivers may convene to form a group that focuses on sharing problem-solving strategies.

Evaluation

Evaluation takes place at several levels in this particular format for implementation of the caregiver plan. The first is the degree of implementation as measured by identification of the primary caregiver and the presence of such caregivers at the time of admission and then at subsequent checkpoints, including participation in the patient-family conference and in the scheduled training. The next level of evaluation deals with the outcomes of the training per se. This is assessed at the time of the practice day and at the time of the first follow-up visit. Still another level of evaluation is available at the time of 6-month follow-up.

Measuring Effectiveness

Measurement of outcomes must be integral to the management of persons with stroke. Each of the programmatic plans described in the previous section had specific objectives. Data were generated within the clinical activity to the extent possible. Data collection and analysis were carried out on a regular basis and feedback provided as a means for staff commitment and problem solving for improvement. Such program evaluation is an example of how one can monitor the degree to which program initiatives are being implemented and make ongoing improvements.[61] This section describes the instruments available to measure outcomes given the degree to which implementation has been achieved. At least four possible levels of evaluation can be made in persons with stroke. The first is that of the disease process itself. This can include the patency of the carotid arteries, status of the vascular system, and so forth, as well as the findings on magnetic resonance imaging (MRI) and head computed tomography (CT) or positron emission tomography (PET) scans documenting the brain injury. These aspects are beyond the scope of this chapter. The major focus is on the management of persons after stroke. In accordance with the various phases of the life of the person poststroke, the effects of treatment are measured in respect to the degree of impairment, the degree of disability, and the degree of handicap. This section is designed to familiarize professionals with a sample of the major assessment tools specific to, or widely used, in persons with stroke.

Measurement of Impairments

It has been noted that the degree of impairment contributes to a major degree but only partially explains the ultimate outcome in terms of either the burden of disability or actual entry into community living. The effects of training during the rehabilitation phase contribute to the reduction of disability even as impairments may remain. The ability to live in community settings also depends on the availability of caregivers and an accessible environment. Nevertheless, interest has been renewed in the assessment of impairment using standardized neurologic testing with the advent of methods for treatment to reduce the degree of impairment in hyperacute stroke.[62]

National Institutes of Health Stroke Scale

The NIHSS has been used in clinical trials of treatment of acute ischemic stroke.[37] It is a 42-point scale that quantifies neurologic deficit in 11 categories. In addition to motor and sensory testing, level of consciousness, gaze and visual fields, facial weakness, language and dysarthria, and general attention are measured. The higher the score, the greater the deficit.[37] For example, limb strength is scored from 0 to 4, with 0 indicating no drift of the outstretched limb, 1 indicating drift, 2 indicating some effort against gravity but not full range, 3 indicating no effort against gravity, and 4 indicating no movement. The sensory domain is scored from 0 to 2, with 0 being normal, 1 indicating diminution of pinprick but touch intact, and 2 indicating that the individual is not aware of touch. Inter-rater and test-retest reliability have been acceptable.

Although the NIHSS is widely used, its organization and format lead to several concerns.[63] It was designed around the traditional neurologic examination and is effectively confined to use by medical staff. It is not an ordinal scale overall because non-assessable items are scored as 0; therefore, a ceiling exists that can be far below the theoretical. This is particularly true when aphasia or disturbance in level of consciousness is present. The NIHSS has been validated in relation to CT infarct volume and to functional outcomes at 3 months. Assessment of limb strength constitutes a relatively small portion of the total score. Because it incorporates a number of domains beyond that of motor impairment, it appears to reflect an overall degree of neurologic deficit. It has thus been found to predict 3-month outcomes in a fashion superior to that of other impairment scales when measured against broadly stated outcomes such as "alive at home," "alive in care," and "dead at 3 months."[64] A score of 13 or below identifies patients who are likely to be independent in the context of this study carried out in Glasgow, Scotland.

Attempts have been made to collapse the results of this impairment scale into an overall stroke outcome classification[65] (Table 4-4). Six domains are to be assessed, including motor, sensory, vision, language, cognition, and affect. The score reflects the total number of domains affected as well as their extent. When more than one domain is affected, the overall severity score is defined by the domain most impaired. If one were to use the NIHSS as one of the sources of data for scoring, the score would need to be collapsed as follows: If the motor domain contains a score of 4, then the impairment rating of that domain would be C, severe; if the score is 1–3, then the score is B, moderate; a score of 0 would lead to a severity score of A. Similarly, when assessing the sensory domain, one could use the NIHSS in which a score of 2 reflects a severity score of C, 1 translates to a B, and 0 leads to an A. It is recommended that other standardized assessment scales be used for cognition (Mini-Mental State Examination) and for a language assessment as well as a depression scale. The total number of domains affected and the domain with the greatest severity determine the score for impairment.

This scheme has certain benefits in that it is semiquantitative, giving a relatively global measure of the overall burden of impairment. This is further coupled with a score based on the degree of functional disability, discussed later in this section.

Fugl-Meyer Assessment

The FMA[66] has long been the most widely accepted assessment tool for evaluation of impairment, particularly in research studies. It is based on a theory of motor recovery derived from the work of Twitchell[67] and thus assesses the degree of impairment in a fashion keyed to possible stages in treatment. The scale ranges from flaccidity along with the absence of movement through the development of synergistic patterns of movements en bloc with associated increase in spasticity to the point at which selective voluntary actions are present with normal muscle reflexes. When a lack of selectivity in motor actions occurs, the effects of posture become evident. FMA incorporates this aspect with a score based on posture. For example, when upper limb function is assessed, the patient must be in a seated position. In assessing lower limb actions, the patient is examined when assuming successively the supine, seated, and standing positions depending on the stage of return of motor activity. It is a very extensive examination that requires considerable training with very explicit instructions for positioning.

The FMA samples three major categories: motor abilities and balance, sensation, and passive joint motion and pain. The sequence of motor items follows the theory of return as described above. Each item is scored from 0 to 2, with 0 representing "cannot be performed" and 2 representing "can be fully performed." Within the broad category of motor function, the upper extremity, wrist, hand, upper extremity coordination, and speed are measured and then lower extremity action, coordination, and speed. Explicit instructions are given in relation to each of the actions to be sampled. For example, in assessing the upper extremity, assessment is performed at five levels: I is eliciting reflexes at the biceps, triceps, and finger flexors; II deals with volitional movement performed within the dynamic flexor or extensor synergies, or both; III deals with volitional movement performed mixing the dynamic flexor and extensor synergies; IV deals with volitional movements performed with little or no synergy dependence; and V concerns normal reflex activity. Within each of these levels, three areas are sampled. For example, within level III for the upper extremity, the actions include (1) the affected hand actively positioned on the lumbar spine, (2) the shoulder flexed to 90 degrees in a pure flexion motion, and (3) pronation-supination of the forearm with the elbow joint actively flexed to approximately 90 degrees.

Within the broad category of balance, three actions are sampled while the patient is sitting and four if he or she is standing. For sitting, these include "sit without support," with a score of 0 indicating that the individual cannot maintain sitting without massive support, 1 indicates that the individual can sit for only a short time on a stool or bed with the legs hanging, and 3 indicates that the individual can sit for at least 5 minutes without any support. The category of sensation includes mea-

Table 4-4. Stroke Outcome Classification

AHA.SOC score = Number of domains × severity × function

Number of neurologic domains (motor, sensory, vision, affect, cognition, language) impaired

Score

0   0 domains impaired

1   1 domain impaired

2   2 domains impaired

3   >2 domains impaired

Severity of impairment

Level

A   No, or minimal, neurologic deficit due to stroke in any domain

B   Mild to moderate deficit due to stroke in ≥1 domain

C   Severe deficit due to stroke in ≥1 domain

Function

Level

I   *Independent* in BADL and IADL activities and tasks required of the roles that the patient had before the stroke. Patient is able to live alone, maintain a household, and access the community for leisure or productive activities, or both, such as shopping, employment, or volunteer work.

II   *Independent* in BADL but partially dependent in routine IADL. Patient is able to live alone but requires assistance or supervision to access the community for shopping and leisure activities. Patient may require occasional assistance with meal preparation, household tasks, and taking medications.

III   *Partially dependent* in BADL (<3 areas) and IADL. Patient is able to live alone with substantial daily help from family or community resources for more difficult BADL tasks, such as dressing lower extremities, bathing, or climbing stairs. Patient requires assistance with such IADL tasks as meal preparation, home maintenance, community access, shopping, handling finances, and/or taking medications.

IV   *Partially dependent* in BADL (≥3 areas). Patient is unable to live alone safely and requires assistance with IADL except for simple tasks such as answering the telephone.

V   *Completely dependent* in BADL (≥5 areas) and IADL. Patient is unable to live alone safely and requires full-time care.

AHA.SOC = American Heart Association Stroke Outcome Classification; BADL = basic activities of daily living: feeding and swallowing, grooming, dressing, bathing, continence, toileting, and mobility; IADL = instrumental activities of daily living: using the telephone, handling money, shopping, using transportation, maintaining a household, working, participating in leisure activities, etc.

Source: Reprinted with permission from American Heart Association. Stroke Outcome Classification. Stroke 1998;29:1275.

Table 4-5. Motricity Scale Weights

Stage (MRC Scale)	All Movements	Prehension
0	0	0
1	28	33
2	42	56
3	56	65
4	74	77
5	100	100

MRC = Medical Research Council.
Source: Reprinted with permission from G Demeurisse, O Demol, E Robaye. Motor evaluation in vascular hemiplegia. Eur Neurol 1980;19:382.

surement of light touch and position sense. The latter is sampled at the interphalangeal joint of the thumb, wrist, elbow, and glenohumeral joint and in the lower extremity at the great toe, ankle, knee, and hip. Joint motion and pain are assessed for most joints of the affected limb; joint pain is assessed at those same joints with 0 indicating pronounced pain during the entire movement or severe pain at the end of movement, 1 indicating some pain, and 2 indicating no pain.

Motricity Index

The motricity index is a short, simple measure of motor loss.[68] The patient should be sitting in a chair or on the edge of the bed but can be tested while lying down if necessary. The grading is derived from that of the MRC, from 0 to 5. Weighted scores are used based on the relative difficulty found by the author in a sample of 100 patients followed for 2 months after stroke in going from one stage to another on the MRC Scale. Weights are similar for all actions other than the prehension scale. The weights are described in Table 4-5. Six limb movements are tested that have been selected both on the basis of ease and as representative of the entire set of possible actions. For example, in the upper limb, these are shoulder abduction, elbow flexion, and pinch grip. In the lower limb, they are ankle dorsiflexion, knee extension, and hip flexion. A motricity score is calculated by multiplying the MRC score by the weight. This weighted score, when divided by the three items in each limb, provides the motricity index. This serves to reflect the changes in degree of

motor impairment on successive evaluations. Its validity and reliability are proven.[69]

Measurement of Disabilities

It has been noted that the degree of functional disability only partially explains entry into community living. The ability to live in community settings depends also on the availability of caregivers and an accessible environment. In addition, disability is not a unitary global concept but ultimately is reflective of the specific priorities and resources of the person with disabilities. These resources include the ability and the willingness to continue to seek and maintain compensatory strategies.

The scales are used to monitor progress during rehabilitation and to measure overall dependence in relation to criteria for admission to or discharge from a rehabilitation setting. All these measures are of performance, not what the patient "could do." The scores all reflect the issue of *burden of care*, defined as substituted time and energy that must be brought to serve the dependent needs of a disabled individual so that a certain QOL can be achieved.

Motor Assessment Scale

The Motor Assessment Scale is an example of a scale designed to serve as a basis for planning appropriate physical therapy.[70] It is more related to training for everyday functional tasks than for the patterns of movement assessed in the FMA. It has a further advantage in ease of administration and scoring. Areas sampled include the ability to move from supine to side lying, supine to sitting, sitting balance, sitting to standing, and walking. For upper limb function, the range sampled includes upper arm function, hand movements, and advanced hand activities. Scoring criteria range from 0 to 6, with the higher scores demonstrating more independent and better performance. As an example, the scoring criteria for sitting balance, the most reliable item, range from 1, indicating that the individual sits only with support, through 3, which indicates that the person sits unsupported with weight well forward and evenly distributed, to 5, indicating that the person sits unsupported, reaches forward to touch the floor, and returns to starting position. This assessment illustrates the transition between descriptions of motor action and functional activities. It is described as having good validity and reliability and as being useful for research activities.

Barthel Index

The BI has been the most widely accepted measure of function in relation to ADL. Most studies have been based on a possible score of 100, with a score of 60 validated as consistent with community life. The BI is considered to be reliable in test-retest and between observers. Like any measure of basic daily activities, a ceiling effect exists in that it does not measure more advanced activities that may have relevance for the ability to function in community settings.

In a modified version of the scale,[71] 20 possible points are derived from 10 items. The items include bowel and bladder control as well as grooming, feeding, toileting, dressing, and bathing. Items of mobility include transfers, getting around via wheelchair or ambulation, and stairs. The potential score that can be attributed to any particular item varies: 0–1 points in relation to grooming and bathing, 0–2 available in relation to sphincter control and most other items, and 0–3 in relation to mobility and transfers. For example, in grooming, with its range from 0 to 2, 0 signifies "needs help" and 1 indicates independence (implements can be provided). In feeding, with its range from 0 to 3, 0 signifies inability; 1 indicates that the person needs help cutting, spreading butter; and 2 indicates independence. In general, a middle score indicates that the patient supplies more than 50% of the effort. Within the item of mobility, with its range from 0 to 3, 0 indicates immobility; 1 indicates wheelchair independence, including corners; 2 indicates that the individual walks with the help of one person (verbal or physical); and 3 signifies independence (may use any aid). In general, the use of aids is allowed in being "independent."

The scale can be insensitive to the graded differences that can occur in the context of a rehabilitation program. The rationale for the various weights given to certain items and the distribution of weights given for any combination that go to make up the total are unclear. Furthermore, very major differences are sometimes found in outcome of community living depending on the kind and degree of support necessary. The scores do not reflect these distinctions. For example, a caregiver may be able to provide supervision when he or she is unable, because of frailty, to provide physical support. Furthermore, even when physical support is necessary, degrees of such may be possible.

Functional Independence Measure

The FIM is similar to other forms of basic measures of daily living as exemplified by most inpatient rehabilitation programs. Its validation is described earlier in this chapter in relation to the general issues of disability. Its use is widespread, particularly in the United States. Training is available for certification in its scoring. It can be used to compare programs in terms of change during the course of inpatient rehabilitation and to predict those who might benefit from admission to such programs. It has also found use to measure gradation in change during such programs. The difference in scale scores frequently reflects the changes found during the weekly intervals that are normally used to assess progress. It is not a true interval scale in that an equivalent difference does not necessarily exist between each of the scale scores. However, techniques have been used that can transform the scores from an ordinal to an interval scale.[72]

The FIM contains 18 items: 13 dealing with sphincter control, self-care, and mobility, forming a motor subscale, and 5 items dealing with social interaction and communication, forming a cognitive subscale. Unlike the BI, each item is scored the same, ranging from 1 to 7, with the higher scores indicating a diminution in the burden of care. A score from 0 to 4 reflects the need for physical assistance, with 1–2 defined as complete dependence, 3 indicating moderate assistance with the patient providing 50% of the effort, 4 indicating minimal assistance with the patient providing 75% of the effort, 5 indicating need for supervision, 6 indicating independence with the use of aids, and 7 indicating independence. Within the range of need for physical assistance, a major difference can exist in the viability of community living when one reaches a 4, which reflects the need for only minimal assistance. The patient is then able to carry out 75% of tasks with perhaps only physical contact guidance required. This is particularly important in relation to the transfer item. This level of physical assistance has been found to be consistent with the capability of many caregivers. Need for greater degree of physical assistance has generally not been consistent with satisfactory caregiving by family members over an extended time.

As with the BI, the FIM samples only a basic set of items and fails to sample more complex items that are exemplars of more truly independent community living. *Extended ADL*, rather than so-called instrumental, is the term recommended to describe the broader set of skills such as shopping and use of transportation that would permit a person to carry on his or her life without the need for outside support.[73]

Frenchay Activities Index

The Frenchay activities index (FAI) has been recommended as a scorable measure that reflects these more extensive activities complementing the BI.[74] It can also serve as a basis for a global score of disability.[65] A summary of both basic and extended scales is encompassed within the functional level, ranging from I to V, in addition to the impairment score described above.

The FAI contains 15 items concerning activities within and outside the home. It consists of a summary score (15–60) and subscale scores for domestic, leisure and work, and outdoor activities. Each item ranges from 0 to 3, with the higher score reflecting a greater frequency of activity. The frequency varies depending on the character of the task. For example, items that deal with eating, such as food preparation, are assessed as follows: 0 indicates never, 1 indicates less than once a week, 2 indicates 1–2 times a week, and 3 indicates most days. Items such as washing clothes, housework, shopping, walking outside for more than 15 minutes, and driving or going on a bus are assessed in the longer time frame of 3 months: 0 indicates never, 1 indicates 1–2 times, 2 indicates 3–12 times, and 3 indicates at least once a week. Travel outings and reading books are assessed within a time frame of 6 months with a similar range of scores. Gainful employment ranges from none to more than 30 hours a week, with intermediate scores for intermediate degrees.

Measurement of a more extended set of activities is a highly welcome broader appreciation of potential function after stroke. The FAI is representative of the limitations of any such scale. Although designed specifically for persons with stroke, it reflects the characteristics of life in Britain, where it was developed. Given the wide range of settings and interests, no scale can sample the equivalent variety of possible activities that a substantial number of persons may choose to do. Even the basic set of ADL does not necessarily reflect the variety of persons who are being served. For example, dressing, which forms an important set of components in the personal ADL scores and an important part of the effort expended within an inpatient rehabilitation program, may not be a priority for all. If one wishes to carry out other activities outside the house such as return to gainful work, it may be inappropriate to spend one's energy trying to become fully independent in this area.

In clinical practice and also in research studies, one must ultimately measure the effects of treatment in the amelioration of specific problems that are often idiosyncratic to the person. Single-case research design can be used.[75] One defines the initial status of the activity over a baseline period before treatment and then assesses the effects in relation to some criterion. The technical aspects of this approach are described in Chapter 3. Still another methodologic issue is the impact of outcome measurement on the system being measured. Regardless of the measure being used, the goal must ultimately be not only knowledge of what outcome was achieved but also how to improve results. The process of data collection, data analysis, and feedback is in itself an important aspect. The use of single-case design may make it possible to incorporate within standard clinical practice an awareness of quality improvement.[61]

Measurement of Degree of Handicap and Quality of Life

The issues during the continuing care phase of the person's life after stroke extend beyond the family into re-establishing life in the wider community. The term *handicap* describes the degree to which the person fails to function in his or her social role as a result of impairment and subsequent disability. The WHO definition is that a handicap exists when individuals with disability are unable to fulfill one or more of the roles considered normal for their age, gender, and culture. The components of this multidimensional life measure incorporate issues of physical independence, mobility, orientation, social integration, occupation, and economic self-sufficiency. A scale proposed by WHO assigns a score of 0–8 in each of these areas, with the higher score reflecting greater severity of handicap.

Even more global has been the concept of QOL, which encompasses the full range of disease effects. These include elements of physical health, reflecting the disease process and the resultant impairments; functional health, reflecting the disabilities that result from those impairments; social health, reflecting the handicaps; and psychological health, reflecting the person's response to those other aspects.[76] These elements can include depression and anxiety as major problems that affect performance after stroke. Technical issues include the fact that the source of data is mainly self-report via questionnaires. For persons with cognitive or language impairment, the reports must generally come from caregivers, with the consequent question as to the accuracy of the report. Another aspect is development of utility values by which QOL can be measured. The issue here is the identity of the persons who establish the values. It is an elusive concept and highly dependent on the person who must ultimately define it. QOL is nevertheless the sense of well-being in response to the entire spectrum of effects of the stroke. It thus identifies an important measure of outcome. Discussion here is limited to those measures that have been used for persons with stroke. Multiple measures are frequently necessary given the multidimensional quality of the outcome.

Sickness Impact Profile

The sickness impact profile is a widely accepted generic measure that contains 136 items divided into 12 subscales.[77] It was designed to be an objective measure, sensitive to even minor changes in health status and for use in evaluation and program planning across types and severity of illness and across demographic and cultural subgroups. It has been shown to be applicable to persons with stroke.[78] It has been shortened to 30 items and made more relevant to persons with stroke in what is called the *stroke-adapted sickness impact profile 30*.[79]

Eight subscales are retained from the original version, with items and scales selected on the basis of applicability to a sample of elderly persons 6

months after stroke. In this initial study of convergent validity, persons with communication problems were excluded. The subscales contain a varying number of items. The body care and movement subscale with five items includes as an example, "I get in and out of bed or chairs by grasping someone for support or using a cane or walker." The social interaction subscale also contains five items, such as "I am doing fewer social activities with groups of persons." The mobility subscale includes three items, such as "I stay home most of the time." The ambulation scale also contains three items, such as "I get around only by using a walker, crutches, cane, walls, or furniture." Alertness behavior (with three items) contains "I am confused and start several actions at a time." The next subscales each contain four items: Communication includes items such as "I have difficulty speaking, for example, get stuck, stammer, slur my words." Emotional behavior contains items such as "I say how bad or useless I am, for example, that I am a burden to others" or "I get sudden frights." Household management incorporates "I am not doing any of the shopping I usually do or house cleaning or clothes washing or maintenance work."

Health Status Questionnaire SF-36

The health status questionnaire is a modification of the SF-36 with the addition of a depression screen. The SF-36 is a short form of the health status measure derived from the medical outcomes project developed by Rand Corporation.[80] A generic measure, its validity was assessed in a group of 1-year stroke survivors.[81] Scores range up to 100, with higher scores indicating better health state. It comprises eight health scales: physical functioning (10 items), role limitations–physical (4 items), bodily pain (2 items), general health (5 items), vitality (4 items), social functioning (2 items), role limitation–emotional (3 items), and mental health (5 items).

The score to be assigned to each of the scales varies depending on the number of items and also the range of scores that are included. For example, the potential score derived from the physical functioning scale is 30 because each item can be scored on a scale from 1 to 3; the potential of the role limitation–physical scale is 8 because each item can be scored on a scale of yes or no only. In general, the questions are posed so that one can give a subjective answer and in relation to the past week. The two core dimensions of physical and mental health can be derived from the various subscales. Relatively poor correlation was found with other measures of social functioning; correlation was better with physical and mental health measures. In light of these findings, recommendations include the use of a supplemental measure of social functioning. The subjective nature of the questions makes problematic the use of proxies for persons with cognitive and language impairment.[82]

EuroQoL

The EuroQoL is a generic instrument for the assessment of health-related QOL. It exemplifies the use of health utility values. In this instance, the values had been assigned by a group of persons who were free of stroke. It can thus be used in studies that compare allocation of resources to various treatments and disease states. Concurrent validity for persons after stroke (median of 72 weeks) has been established in relation to other standard instruments in the various domains sampled, and it also appears to discriminate between functional outcomes in various stroke syndromes.[83] Five dimensions are assessed: mobility, self-care, social (usual activities), and pain and psychological (anxiety and depression), along with a visual analogue scale that assesses global function. Each domain contains a single item with a three-point scale that ranges, for example in the mobility area, from "no problem in walking about," to "some problems in walking about," to "I am confined in bed." Each possible answer has a utility established, and thus an overall weighted score can be generated. Its test-retest reliability is poor and similar to that of the SF-36.[84] Its simplicity and brevity in comparison to the SF-36 can increase the likelihood of a response when it is used in large-scale studies. Mobility correlates best with social functioning and least with psychological outcome. This reflects findings with other QOL measures, such as a visual analogue scale in which improvement in physical functioning did not necessarily lead to improved perception of QOL because of ongoing psychological difficulty.[85]

The significance of the source of health utility measures is emphasized when one assesses the values derived from a group of chronically ill disabled persons compared with those of people who are not disabled. Research on QOL most often has focused on the extent to which people experience attainment of various states that are commonly regarded as desirable, such as health or good social relations. However, because most people have different views of what is important in life, a fair picture of how they evaluate their life situation is only obtained when the subjective evaluation of both the importance and the degree of attainment of the different areas of life is considered. Satisfaction with life can be viewed as a function of the distance between the subjective importance of life values and perceived attainment. The smaller the gap, the greater is the satisfaction with life.[86] Disabled persons, with the largest group represented by those with MS, gave lower importance ratings to functions related to health and mobility. The attainment levels in those same areas were also markedly lower. It appears that disabled persons may adjust to their life situation by de-emphasizing the importance of the physical functions affected by the disability.

The approach of determining utility values from the specific population that might be called on to make decisions is an important new development for assessment of QOL issues. For example, a group of persons referred for ultrasound evaluation of their carotid arteries, and thus at risk for stroke and potential candidates for surgical treatment of their carotid stenosis, were asked to assess their degree of aversion to a set of scenarios. Several degrees of impairment in motor, language, and cognitive areas as well as death and state of perfect health were described.[87] It is interesting that aversion to severe motor impairment was greater than to general confusion, global aphasia, and death. The values assigned to the different scenarios might well reflect the concerns of this elderly (average age, 73 years) urban population, who are likely to rely heavily on mobility to preserve their autonomy.

An example of another population is that of relatively young persons who were diagnosed as having an arteriovenous malformation (AVM) and who thus would be candidates for the use of surgery versus radiation therapy for treatment.[88] Some, but not all, had already experienced a stroke due to their AVM. Once again, scenarios were provided, in this instance of a major stroke and minor stroke as well as current life situation. A gambling technique was used in which one could choose to remain in the present state for the remainder of one's life or to gamble, which either results in perfect health or immediate death. Considerable individual variation existed in the utilities assigned. It was suggested that this technique could be used for tailoring medical decision making to individual preferences.

Ultimately, the evaluation of outcomes provides a technique by which individuals can contribute to their own management. When a group of stroke survivors were asked about their definition of satisfactory QOL after stroke, their answers clustered in three major areas: (1) opportunities provided in their environment, such as accessibility, exercise opportunities, and ability to travel and carry out their other interests; (2) opportunity to do meaningful work whether paid or voluntary; and (3) being treated as an intelligent person, to be able to make one's own decisions, and being allowed to think for oneself and do for oneself. It is this last aspect that may be the most important. The process is crucial. The very fact that the patient is asked about his or her goals and priorities is the key. Being asked rather than told, being encouraged to speak for oneself rather than being spoken for, and re-establishing a sense of control over one's life are the outcomes to be sought.

References

1. Bonita R, Solomon N, Broad JB. Prevalence of stroke and stroke related disability: estimates from the Auckland stroke studies. Stroke 1997;28:1898.
2. Taylor TN, Davis PH, Torner JC, et al. Lifetime costs of stroke in the United States. Stroke 1996;27:1459.
3. Broderick J, Blott T, Kothari R, et al. The Greater Cincinnati/Northern Kentucky stroke study. Stroke 1998;29:415.
4. Gorelick PB. Cerebrovascular disease in African Americans. Stroke 1998;29:2656.
5. National Center for Health Statistics. Monthly Vital Statistics: Report 1995;(suppl 2):45.
6. Robins M, Baum HM. Incidence. Stroke 1981;1(suppl 12):145.
7. Foulkes MA, Wolf PA, Price TR, et al. The stroke data bank: design, methods and baseline characteristics. Stroke 1988;19:547.
8. Hahn RA, Teutsch SM, Rothenberg RB. Excess deaths from nine chronic diseases in the United States. JAMA 1990;264:2654.
9. Sacco RL, Wolf PA, Kannel WB, et al. Survival and recurrence following stroke: the Framingham Study. Stroke 1982;13:290.
10. Pickle LW, Mungiole M, Gillum RF. Geographic variation in the mortality of blacks and whites in the United States. Stroke 1997;28:1639.
11. Goldstein M. The decade of the brain: challenge and opportunities in stroke research. Stroke 1990;21:373.
12. Burn J, Dennis M, Bamford J, et al. Long-term risk of recurrent stroke after a first-ever stroke. Stroke 1994;25:333.
13. Wolf PA, D'Agostino RB, Belanger AJ, et al. Probability of stroke: a risk profile from the Framingham Study. Stroke 1991;22:312.
14. Gorelick P. Stroke prevention. Arch Neurol 1995;52:347.
15. Miller NH, Hill M, Kottke T, et al. The multi-level compliance challenge: recommendation for a call to action. Circulation 1997;95:1085.
16. Matcher DB, Duncan PW. Cost of stroke. Stroke Clinical Updates (NSA) 1994;5:9.
17. Dennis M, O'Rourke S, Lewis S, et al. A quantitative study of the emotional outcome of people caring for stroke survivors. Stroke 1998;29:1867.
18. Schneider EL, Guralnick JM. The aging of America: impact on health care costs. JAMA 1990;263:2335.
19. Caplan LR. Neurological Management Plan. In MN Ozer, RS Materson, LR Caplan (eds), Management of Persons with Stroke. St. Louis: Mosby–Year Book, 1994;63–89.
20. Silvestri M, Cupini LM, Placidi F, et al. Bilateral hemispheric activation in the early recovery of motor functions after stroke. Stroke 1998;29:1305.
21. Goldstein LB. Potential effects of common drugs on stroke recovery. Arch Neurol 1998;55:454.
22. Walker-Batson D, Smith P, Curtis MA, et al. Amphetamine paired with physical therapy accelerates motor recovery after stroke. Stroke 1995;26:2254.
23. Katz DI. The Neurologic Rehabilitation Model in Clinical Practice. In VM Mills, JW Cassidy, DI Katz (eds), Neurologic Rehabilitation: a Guide to Diagnosis, Prognosis and Treatment Planning. Malden, MA: Blackwell Science, 1997;1–27.
24. Kittner SJ, Stern BJ, Wozniak M, et al. Cerebral infarction in young adults: the Baltimore-Washington cooperative young stroke study. Neurology 1998;50:890.
25. Gillum RF. Epidemiology of stroke in Hispanic Americans. Stroke 1995;26:1707.
26. Sacco RL, Hauser WA, Mohr JP. Hospitalized stroke in blacks and Hispanics in northern Manhattan. Stroke 1992;22:1491.
27. Sacco RL, Kargman DF, Gu Q, et al. Race-ethnicity and determinants of intracranial atherosclerotic cerebral infarctions: the Northern Manhattan Study. Stroke 1995; 26:14.
28. Feldman E, Daneault N, Kwan E, et al. Chinese-white differences in the distribution of occlusive cerebrovascular disease. Neurology 1990;40:1541.
29. Hoffmann M, Sacco RL, Mohr JP, et al. Higher cortical function deficits among acute stroke patients: the Stroke Data Bank experience. J Stroke Cerebrovasc Dis 1997;6:114.
30. Macciocchi SN, Diamond PT, Alves WM, et al. Ischemic stroke: relation of age, lesion location and initial neurologic deficit to functional outcome. Arch Phys Med Rehabil 1998;79:1255.
31. Cifu DX, Lorish TR. Stroke rehabilitation. Stroke outcome. Arch Phys Med Rehabil 1994;75(suppl):56.

32. Reding MJ, Potes E. Rehabilitation outcome following initial hemispheric stroke: life table approach. Stroke 1988;19:1354.

33. Gan R, Sacco RL, Kargman DE, et al. Testing the validity of the lacunar hypothesis: the Northern Manhattan Stroke Study. Neurology 1997;48:1204.

34. Miyai I, Blau AD, Reding M, et al. Patients with stroke confined to basal ganglia have diminished response to rehabilitation efforts. Neurology 1997;48:95.

35. Bohannon RW. Measurement and treatment of paresis in the geriatric patient. Top Geriatr Rehabil 1991;7:15.

36. Ozer MN. Central Nervous System. In SL Demeter, GBJ Andersson, GM Smith (eds), Disability Evaluation. St. Louis: Mosby, 1996;452–463.

37. Brott T, Adams HP, Olinger LP, et al. Measurements of acute cerebral infarction: a clinical examination scale. Stroke 1989;20:864.

38. Heinemann AW, Harvey RL, McGuire JR, et al. Measurement properties of the NIH stroke scale during acute rehabilitation. Stroke 1997;28:1174.

39. Lyketsos CG, Treisman GJ, Lipsey JR, et al. Does stroke cause depression? J Neuropsych Clin Neurosci 1998;10:103.

40. Prescott RJ, Garraway WM, Akhtar AJ. Predicting functional outcome following acute stroke using a standard clinical examination. Stroke 1982;13:641.

41. Lichtman CD, Dietz M, Reding MJ. Clinical examination is more predictive of ambulation recovery than CT location following subcortical ischemic stroke. J Neurorehab 1994;8:55.

42. Chae J, Johnston M, Kim H, et al. Admission motor impairment as a predictor of physical disability after stroke rehabilitation. Am J Phys Med Rehabil 1995;74:218.

43. Perry J, Garrett M, Gronley JK, et al. Classification of walking handicap in the stroke population. Stroke 1995; 26:982.

44. Roth EJ, Heinemann AW, Lovell LL, et al. Impairment and disability: their relation during stroke rehabilitation. Arch Phys Med Rehabil 1998;79:329.

45. Stineman MG, Goin JE, Granger CV, et al. Discharge motor FIM-functional related groups. Arch Phys Med Rehabil 1997;78:980.

46. Stineman MG, Jette A, Fiedler R, et al. Impairment-specific dimensions within the functional independence measure. Arch Phys Med Rehabil 1997;78:636.

47. Mauthe NH, Haaf DC, Hayn P, et al. Predicting discharge destination of stroke patients using a mathematical model based on six items from the functional independence measure. Arch Phys Med Rehabil 1996;77:10.

48. Alexander MP. Stroke rehabilitation outcome: a potential use of predictive variables to establish levels of care. Stroke 1994;25:128.

49. Stineman MG, Fiedler RC, Granger CV, et al. Functional task benchmarks for stroke rehabiitation. Arch Phys Med Rehabil 1998;79:497.

50. Panel. Post-stroke Rehabilitation: Clinical Practice Guideline No. 16. Rockville, MD: Agency for Health Care Policy and Research, 1995.

51. Retchin SM, Brown RS, Shu-Chuan JY, et al. Outcomes of stroke patients in Medicare fee-for-service and managed care. JAMA 1997;278:119.

52. Kane RL, Chen Q, Blewett LA, et al. Do rehabilitative nursing homes improve the outcomes of care? J Am Geriatr Soc 1996;44:545.

53. Kramer AM, Steiner JF, Schlenker RE, et al. Outcomes and costs after hip fractures and stroke: a comparison of rehabilitation settings. JAMA 1997;277:396.

54. Samsa GT, Cohen SJ, Goldstein LB, et al. Knowledge of risk among patients at increased risk of stroke. Stroke 1997;28:916.

55. Wagner EH. Managed care and chronic illness: health service research needs. Health Serv Res 1997;32:702.

56. Ozer MN. Ensuring Continuity of Medical Care. In MN Ozer, RS Materson, LR Caplan (eds), Management of Persons with Stroke. St. Louis: Mosby–Year Book, 1994;451–454.

57. Ozer MN. Patient participation in the management of stroke rehabilitation. Top Stroke Rehabil 1999;6:43.

58. Glass TA, Matcher DB, Belyea M, et al. Impact of social support on outcome in first stroke. Stroke 1993;24:64.

59. Scholte WJM, deHaan RJ, Rijinders PT, et al. The burden of caregiving in partners of long term stroke survivors. Stroke 1998;29:1605.

60. Evans RL, Matlock A-L, Bishop DS, et al. Family intervention after stroke: does counseling or education help? Stroke 1988;19:1243.

61. Berwick DM. Harvesting knowledge from improvement. JAMA 1996;275:877.

62. Stroke Group. Thrombolytic therapy for acute ischemic stroke. Summary statement. Neurology 1996;47:835.

63. Muir KW, Grosset DG, Lees KR. Interconversion of stroke scales: implications for therapeutic trials. Stroke 1994;25:1366.

64. Muir KJ, Weir CJ, Murray GD, et al. Comparison of neurological scales and scoring systems for acute stroke prognosis. Stroke 1996;27:1817.

65. Kelly-Hayes M, Roberson JT, Broderick JP, et al. The American Heart Association stroke outcome classification. Stroke 1998;29:1274.

66. Fugl-Meyer AR, Jaasko L, Leyman I, et al. The post-stroke hemiplegic patient. 1. A method for evaluation of physical performance. Scand J Rehabil Med 1975;7:13.

67. Twichell TE. The restoration of motor function following hemiplegia in man. Brain 1951;74:443.

68. Demeurisse G, Demol O, Robaye E. Motor evaluation in vascular hemiplegia. Eur Neurol 1980;19:382.

69. Collin C, Wade DT. Assessing motor impairment after stroke: a pilot reliability study. J Neurol Neurosurg Psychiatry 1990;53:576.

70. Carr JH, Shepherd RB, Nordholm L, et al. Investigation of a new motor assessment scale for stroke patients. Phys Ther 1985;65:175.

71. Collin C, Wade DT, Dav S, et al. The Barthel index: a reliability study. Int Disabil Stud 1988;10:61.

72. Heinemann AW, Linacre JM, Wright BD, et al. Relationships between impairment and physical disability. Arch Phys Med Rehabil 1993;74:566.

73. Wade DT. Measurement in Neurologic Rehabilitation. Oxford, UK: Oxford University Press, 1992;85.

74. Pederson PM, Jorgensen HS, Nakayama H, et al. Comprehensive assessment of activities of daily living in stroke:

the Copenhagen Stroke Study. Arch Phys Med Rehabil 1997;78:161.

75. Wagenaar RC. Functonal recovery after stroke. J Rehabil Sci 1991;4:13.

76. deHaan R, Aaronson N, Limburg M, et al. Measuring quality of life in stroke. Stroke 1993;24:320.

77. Bergner M, Bobbitt RA, Carter WB, et al. The sickness impact profile: development and final revision of a health status measure. Med Care 1981;19:787.

78. deHaan RJ, Limburg M, Van der Meulen JM, et al. Quality of life after stroke: impact of stroke type and lesion location. Stroke 1995;26:402.

79. Van Straten A, deHaan RJ, Limburg M, et al. A stroke adapted 30-item version of the sickness impact profile to assess quality of life (SA-SIP30). Stroke 1997;28:2155.

80. Ware JE, Sherbourne CD. The MOS 36 item short form health survey SF-36. I. Conceptual framework and item selection. Med Care 1992;30:473.

81. Anderson C, Laubscher S, Burn R. Validation of the short form 36 (SF-36) health survey questionnaire among stroke patients. Stroke 1996;27:1812.

82. Segal ME, Schall RR. Determining functional/health status and its relation to disability in stroke survivors. Stroke 1994;25:2391.

83. Dornan PJ, Slattery J, Farrell B, et al. Randomized comparison of the EuroQoL and SF-36 after stroke. BMJ 1997;315:461.

84. Dornan PJ, Slattery J, Farrell B, et al. Qualitative comparison of the reliability of health status assessments with the EuroQoL and SF-36 questionnaires after stroke. Stroke 1998;29:63.

85. Ahlsio B, Britton M, Murray V, et al. Disablement and quality of life after stroke. Stroke 1984;15:886.

86. Montgomery H, Persson L-A, Ryden A. Importance and attainment of life values among disabled and non-disabled people. Scand J Rehabil Med 1996;28:233.

87. Solomon NA, Glick HA, Russo CJ., et al. Patient preferences for stroke outcomes. Stroke 1994;25:1721.

88. Shin AY, Porter PJ, Wallace MC, et al. Quality of life of stroke in younger individuals: utility assessment in patients with arteriovenous malformation. Stroke 1997; 28:2395.

Chapter 5

Management of Persons with Spinal Cord Injury

Pamela H. Ballard

Nature of the Problem

Extent of the Problem

Incidence and Prevalence

SCI has many causes, including trauma, tumors, vascular disorders, developmental disorders, and infections. This chapter focuses on trauma as the largest single cause of SCI. The annual incidence of traumatic SCI in the United States is between 30 and 50 cases per 1 million population.[1] It is estimated that 10,000 new cases occur each year. Approximately 200,000 people in the United States are living with SCI. These statistics are estimates derived from multiple studies.

The National Spinal Cord Injury Database was developed in 1973. It is comprised of data from approximately 15% of new SCI cases in the United States.[2] Data were collected from up to 24 federally funded SCI Model Care Systems, which represent information on nearly 19,000 individuals with traumatic SCI as of September 1998. This database provides a major source for statistical information about people with SCI who were admitted to participating centers (currently 18 centers).[1,2]

Over the last 30 years, significant advances have been made in the management of SCIs and the coordination of emergency, acute, and rehabilitative care. Data collected from the SCI Model Systems reveal that the overall extent of neurologic injury in persons with spinal fracture or insult decreased by

24% from 1972–1992.[1] Time between injury and admission into the specialized SCI Model Systems has also decreased. Factors that contribute to these changes include injury prevention activities, such as safer automobiles, mandatory seat belt laws, posted diving precautions, and coordinated emergency medical systems within the model system. In addition, the length of stay in acute care units for patients with SCI dramatically decreased from an average of 25 days to 15 days from 1974 to 1996. This appears to be related to the facilitation of appropriate medical and surgical stabilization and the integration of rehabilitation into the acute care process. Mortality during initial hospitalization decreased as well, from 13% to 5% for patients who were treated in the model system.[1,3]

Demographics

According to Model Systems statistics, people with SCI are generally young (between 16 and 30 years of age), with 19 years the most frequent age of injury. SCI occurs more frequently in men (82%) than women (18%), representing a greater than 4 to 1 male to female ratio. The most common causes of SCI are motor vehicle accidents, followed by violence, falls, sports, and other causes. In some urban settings, violence is the leading cause of SCI. Acts of violence and sports are less contributory factors with an increase in age. After age 45, falls become the leading cause of injury. Over one-half of the people who experience SCI are single at the time of injury. Individuals with SCI have a reduced likelihood of getting married or remaining married after injury compared with those in the uninjured population. More than 60% of persons are employed at the time of their injury. The employment status appears higher in paraplegic (35%) than in tetraplegic persons (23%) by 10 years after injury.[1,2]

Since 1988, a larger number of injuries have been incomplete than complete, 55% versus 45%, respectively.[1] Complete injury does not imply that the spinal cord has been severed. *Complete injury* refers to the loss of motor or sensory function below the level of the injury. Incomplete injury describes a partial loss of sensory or motor function, or both, below the injury. The majority of injuries result in tetraplegia. The proportion of tetraplegic injuries increases significantly after age 45, such that two-thirds of all injuries after age 60 years and almost 90% of all injuries after age 75 years result in tetraplegia.[1,2]

The alarming growth of SCI due to violence is particularly evident in some urban areas, where violence is often the number one cause of SCI. Minority teens and young adults are at especially high risk. Acts of violence contribute to 42.5% of all SCI injuries among blacks and 37.4% of all SCI among Hispanics compared with 7.1% of all SCI among whites since 1973. These percentages among blacks and Hispanics have risen since 1990.[1] This increase parallels a disproportionately high homicide rate among blacks compared with whites in the general population. Acts of violence or falls were both the second leading cause of SCI among Asians.[1] However, some studies have suggested that lower socioeconomic status plays a more significant role than race or ethnicity in contributing to violence-related injury.

Alcohol or drug abuse, or both, has also been shown to be a contributing factor in approximately 50% of SCIs that result from violence.[4] These injuries often occur as a result of a failed drug deal or robbery attempt with associated assault. Some urban neighborhoods are prone to drive-by shootings and robberies in which a bystander may be at risk for injury. In addition, these individuals tend to be younger and less educated and are frequently unemployed or have lower-quality occupations.[5] These premorbid characteristics and lifestyles must be considered in the development of a rehabilitation program.

Morbidity and Mortality

Acute and long-term survival rates have improved significantly in the last 50 years for people with SCI due to improved medical care.[6] However, life expectancy remains below normal for most of this group. Elderly patients with complete tetraplegia continue to have a poor prognosis. In contrast, life expectancy has improved and approaches normal life expectancy in functionally motor-incomplete injury patients with normal bladder function.[7] For example, for people who survive at least 1 year after injury, with functional motor strength at any neurologic level and with injury at age 20 years, the life expectancy is 51.1 years, compared with 56.8 years with no SCI.[2]

Mortality is much higher during the first year than in the succeeding years. This is especially true in patients with severe SCI. According to the SCI Model Systems data, mortality was 3.8% during the first year after injury, 1.6% during the second year, and approximately 1.2% per year over the next 10 years.[6] Prognostic factors related to survival include injury severity (i.e., neurologic level), degree of completeness, ventilatory dependency, and age. Psychological factors such as subjective or overall QOL, decreased activity, dependency, and unemployment have been found to be significant predictors of mortality.[8] The overall frequency of death decreases with time after injury, especially beyond 1 year.

The leading cause of death among persons with SCI initially was related to complications of the urinary tract with eventual renal failure. With diligent management of urinary tract complications, those statistics have improved. Currently, the leading cause of death is pneumonia and other complications related to the respiratory system, including pulmonary emboli in all neurologic levels.[6,7] This is particularly evident in persons with tetraplegia. Death due to pneumonia, however, is evident in all age groups and all postinjury periods. The second and third overall leading causes of death are nonischemic heart disease and septicemia, respectively. Among paraplegics, the leading causes of death include septicemia, suicide, heart disease, and cancer. As people with SCI age and medical treatment improves, it is anticipated that mortality due to these secondary complications will decrease and mortality will be secondary to unrelated medical illnesses such as cancer and cardiovascular disease.[6,7]

Aging Effects

An increasing number of aging individuals have SCI, and it is estimated that 40% of SCI survivors in the United States are older than 45 years and that one-fourth have lived more than 20 years with the disability.[9] Aging with SCI is a dynamic process with concomitant increases in morbidity.[10] Upper extremity pain syndromes develop as a result of arthritis and tendonitis, as well as overuse injuries due to prolonged reliance on the arms to compensate for varying degrees of paralysis. Close monitoring of the cardiac and pulmonary systems is required because of patient immobility and potential underlying restrictive lung disease. Patients with SCI have an increased risk for fractures due to osteoporosis and declining functional skills. Psychological issues, including depression, may occur with aging, along with social and vocational issues.[9,11]

Menter et al.[11] proposed three major dimensions to be considered when evaluating the impact of aging in people with SCI. These include (1) the possibly decreased ability to adapt to injury when the individual is older, (2) potentially accelerated aging after SCI due to increased demands on the body and decreased adaptability, and (3) the potential altering of the aging process according to completeness and type of injury (tetraplegia versus paraplegia). Individuals older than 45 years with SCI have an increased prevalence for premorbid conditions, such as diabetes mellitus, obesity, cardiac disease, and arthritis, when compared with a younger population. They also have decreased functional status, an increase in nursing home discharges, and an increase in the prevalence of pneumonia, pulmonary embolism (PE), renal stones, gastrointestinal hemorrhage, and ventilator use.[11,12]

A study by Gerhart et al.[9] of 279 individuals with chronic SCI (over 20 years) showed that almost one-fourth reported the need for increased assistance over the years. The major reported area of assistance, at 45%, was in performing transfers. Those who required increased assistance were older tetraplegic individuals, and the decline in function occurred earlier than in the nondisabled population. Multifactorial reasons were cited for this functional decline, including fatigue, weakness, weight gain, altered posture, and shoulder pain. These patients had an increased need for attendant care, and their perceived QOL appeared to be lower than that of those who did not require more assistance.

The aging individual with SCI was also reported to develop acquired scoliosis with each 5-year postinjury interval. An increase in pressure sores that subsequently required surgical closure also contributed to increased costs. Paraplegics reported more complications, such as urinary tract infections (UTIs), more frequent and longer rehospitalizations, and twice as much spasticity compared with tetraplegics. Thus, SCI in aging individuals is a complex phenomenon associated with increased physiologic decline, increased disability and handicap, increased costs, and probably an increased burden of care to the caregiver. Interventions during this time period could possibly delay or prevent these secondary conditions.[11]

Economic Impact

The economic impact of SCI on the individual and society is significant. This impact can be measured in terms of direct costs, reflecting charges incurred by the patient as a result of the injury, and in terms of indirect costs related to loss of earning and productivity. Direct costs are rising rapidly due to longer life expectancy and improved medical technology. The indirect costs of SCI are high and often exceed direct costs because SCI primarily affects a younger population. Significant variations exist, however, and these are based on severity of injury, education, and premorbid employment history.[13]

Most studies have not adequately addressed the issue of actual total costs for the individual with SCI or for society. Multiple variables exist, and it is often difficult, time consuming, and expensive to collect information. The SCI Model Systems initiated a collaborative study of people initially treated at model systems, and direct costs were based on actual charges.[13] Individuals were categorized into four neurologic groups because charges varied significantly according to severity of injury. Mean charges in 1992 during the first year were $417,067 in patients with high-level C1–C4 tetraplegia, $269,324 in those with low C5–C8 tetraplegia, and $152,396 in paraplegia, compared with $122,914 in persons with incomplete motor function at any neurologic level. Considerable variation was noted within each group. Average yearly expenses for each subsequent year ranged from $8,614 to $74,707, depending on level of injury.

Although the incidence of SCI secondary to motor vehicle accidents and sports has diminished, the incidence due to violence has increased. The treatment of residual disability in persons who are subject to violence is particularly problematic. With improved care, the prevalence of persons living with SCI has remained high. Increased longevity has led to medical illness secondary to the aging process, which complicates initial adaptation to the functional disabilities caused by SCI. Despite the relatively low incidence of SCI, its high prevalence and the usually young age of persons injured have led to a high burden of care. This is due not only to the indirect costs of lost earnings but also to the ongoing direct costs within the health care system for secondary medical illness. The management of persons with SCI must be responsive to these issues.

Nature of the Disease

Primary and Secondary Injury

Typically, SCI is caused by abrupt disruption of the spinal cord or its vascular supply by trauma. The injury can be of two types: primary or secondary. The mechanism of primary injury involves compression, laceration, contusion, or stretch injury of the cord. Mechanical disruption of axons occurs at the site of injury, ischemia is present that results in local infarction and central microhemorrhages, and edema within the spinal cord impairs the transmission of nerve impulses. Large myelinated axons appear to be more susceptible to injury. The ability to propagate nerve action potentials is impaired due to damage to the nodes of Ranvier that are interspersed among the myelinated segments of an axon. The majority of the damage occurs in the central or gray matter of the cord, with the rim of white matter preserved.[14,15]

Secondary injury, which occurs within 24–72 hours after initial injury, can further damage or compromise remaining axons.[14] This involves multiple pathophysiologic changes. Post-traumatic spinal cord ischemia occurs, along with neuronal electrolyte shifts with an increase in intracellular Ca^{2+} and Na^+ and loss of intracellular K^+. This gives rise to impaired metabolic activity and release of oxygen free radicals that cause further tissue damage and necrosis by reacting with cellular proteins and lipids. Inflammation and toxic extracellular accumulation of endogenous neurotransmitters such as glutamate occur. Demyelination of spinal cord axons occurs as a result of primary and secondary injury. Impaired conduction of nerve action potentials contributes to neurologic deficits. The recovery process is prolonged due to incomplete remyelination.[14,15]

Extensive experimentation and therapeutic trials of methods to counteract these primary and secondary mechanisms have been performed and are ongoing.[14,15] Clinical trials aimed at treatment that can improve nerve conduction of axons and stimulate remyelination within the spinal cord in persons with chronic SCI are under way. A drug called *4-aminopyridine* has been found to increase the excitability of demyelinated axons and improve the ability of the axon to conduct the nerve action potential. Research is also focused on potential factors that may stimulate growth and development of oligodendroglia cells within the spinal cord and the use of N-methyl-D-aspartate (NMDA) and non-NMDA receptor antagonists to prevent intracellular accumulation of Ca^{2+} in neuronal or glial cells.[14,15]

A major breakthrough in the treatment of acute SCI occurred as a result of the findings of the National Acute Spinal Cord Injury Studies (NASCIS 2) in 1990 by Bracken et al.[16] In a multicenter randomized control study, the efficacy of three drugs, methylprednisolone, naloxone, and tirilizad mesylate, were evaluated. Methylprednisolone given as a bolus (30 mg/kg body weight), followed by infusion (5.4 mg/kg/hour for 23 hours within 8 hours after injury), was found to be effective.[16] Significant improvement in motor and sensory recovery was noted in those patients who were thought to have complete SCI as well as in those with incomplete injuries. A third NASCIS randomized controlled trial was completed in May 1997 that compared the efficacy of methylprednisolone given for 24 hours and 48 hours and a bolus of methylprednisolone followed by tirilizad mesylate given for 48 hours.[17] The study showed that patients who were treated with 48 hours of methylprednisolone showed one full neurologic grade improvement in 6 months than the group

Figure 5-1. Lamination of the spinal cord tracts. C = cervical; T = thoracic; L = lumbar; S = sacral. (Reprinted with permission from W Haymaker. Bing's Local Diagnosis in Neurological Diseases. St. Louis: Mosby, 1956.)

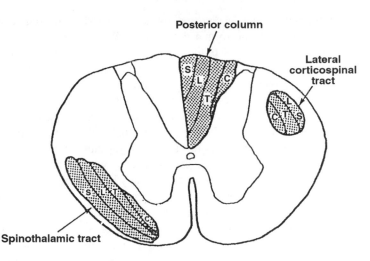

that received the 24-hour regimen. The 48-hour tirilizad treatment group showed motor recovery similar to that of the 24-hour methylprednisolone group. The authors concluded that methylprednisolone treatment initiated within 3 hours of injury should be maintained for a 24-hour regimen and that treatment initiated within 3–8 hours should be maintained for 48 hours.[17]

Anatomic Considerations

The residual effects of SCI are greatly influenced by the anatomy of the spinal cord such that "anatomy is destiny" (Figure 5-1). The spinal cord emerges from below the foramen magnum and ends at the lower part of the first lumbar vertebrae. The L4–L5 segmental level of the spinal cord is located at the T11–T12 vertebral interspace. The S2 cord level is located at the T12–L1 interspace and the S4 level at the L1 interspace. When a highly mobile vertebral segment joins a less mobile segment, injuries tend to occur. This is observed in the lower cervical region and in the thoracolumbar junction.[18,19]

In the cervical spine, the spinal cord takes up approximately one-third of the space enclosed by the arch of the atlas (C1). Below that region, 50% of the spinal canal is occupied by the cord. At the C5 level, the cord is at its largest width due to cervical enlargement. With neck extension, limited room is available within the subarachnoid space. Subsequently, the elderly, who have a tendency for disk bulging and spondylitic ridges anteriorly and buckling of the ligamentum flavum posteri-

orly, are at high risk for cord compromise with neck extension.[18,19]

In the thoracic cord, the incidence of complete lesions is higher. This appears to be due to the relative narrowness of the thoracic canal between T1 and T10. Between segments T10 and T12, the cord is the largest, and less free space is available. In addition, the blood supply in the thoracic region is tenuous and can lead to perfusion problems, particularly at T5 and L1. The central gray matter and the ventral aspect of the posterior columns can also be compromised due to the character of the blood supply in the spinal cord. Ischemic injury to the central region of the cord results in relative sparing of the sacral motor and sensory function. This reflects lamination of the corticospinal and spinothalamic tracts with the caudal portion most lateral. The anterior aspect of the spinal cord is particularly vulnerable with one anterior spinal artery compared with the pair of posterior spinal arteries that tend to protect the posterior portion.[18,19]

The canal is quite large in the lumbar region. The spinal cord ends at the L1–L2 vertebral level, and because the canal contains only the roots of the cauda equina, a modest amount of free space is available. Subsequently, a large displacement of vertebral bodies is required to cause neurologic impairment at this segment.

Gunshot Wounds

The incidence of gunshot wounds to the spine has increased steadily, and the majority of these wounds result in SCI. In a prospective study of 135 patients with SCI due to gunshot wounds, Waters et al.[20] found that in 42% of the cases the bullet traversed the cord and in 30% the bullet or major fragment remained in the canal. In approximately 27% of the cases, the bullet did not enter or traverse the cord and the injury was sustained from the concussive effects of the impact of the bullet.[20]

Studies have shown that most civilian gunshot wounds are from low-velocity weapons with medium-caliber bullets. A prospective study by the Rancho Los Amigos Medical Center found that twice as many patients were shot in the back as in the front and that left-sided entry was more common than right. These injuries usually resulted in paraplegia because of the location of spinal injury, with thoracic injury most common (50%), thoracolumbar injury next (30%), and cervical injury least common (20%).[21]

Most gunshot wounds to the spine are thought to be stable. If one pedicle and facet remain intact, instability is unlikely. However, early surgical stabilization with posterior fusion is indicated if instability is suspected to facilitate rehabilitation and early mobilization. The SCI Model Systems data revealed that 91% of patients with injuries due to gunshot wounds were treated nonoperatively. Symptomatic treatment such as analgesic administration or orthosis is often required. Patients with a retained bullet or fragment should be monitored for neurologic symptoms or neurologic loss.[22]

Generally, bullet removal is not recommended unless the neurologic status deteriorates. Retained bullets rarely have been shown to cause lead toxicity, delayed infection, or late neurologic decline that would warrant prophylactic removal. Incidence of pain after injury also has not been significantly altered by removal of the bullet. However, in a multicenter study by the National Model Spinal Cord Injury Systems, surgical removal of bullets from the thoracolumbar spine (T12–L4) statistically improved motor recovery in both complete and incomplete injuries. No significant improvement in recovery was noted in thoracic cord lesions (T1–T11).[23]

Anatomic differences in the spinal cord appear to contribute to different effects when a bullet is removed from the thoracic cord versus the thoracolumbar region. Above T12 in the thoracic spine, nerve roots exit the spinal canal just below the level from which they branch from the spinal cord, and thus a bullet at this level can only compress nerve roots that emanate from one neurologic level and the spinal cord.[21] The lumbar and sacral roots that arise from the conus may descend multiple levels before exiting. Subsequently, a bullet or fragment located in the spinal canal at or below T12 can lead to multiple nerve root compression and contribute to a greater effect on motor function. In addition, injury of peripheral nerves in the cauda equina has a greater chance for recovery than does injury within the spinal cord itself.

Spinal injury secondary to firearms has been found to result in less spine instability or fracture that would require surgical stabilization or the need for an orthosis. Compared with injury secondary to motor vehicle accidents, injuries secondary to firearms generally require a shorter length of stay to achieve the same outcome because of the difference in concomitant injury and a tendency toward less residual deficit, with more paraplegic patients seen.[24]

Nature of the Impairments

The ability to accurately classify the degree of motor and sensory loss ultimately affects functional outcome and the efficacy of medical management. An individual with SCI displays different types of problems based on the degree of impairment. The longitudinal level of injury and the extent of the injury in the transverse plane (incomplete versus complete) are the two variables. The currently recognized system to describe the level and extent of injury is based on the International Standards for Neurological and Functional Classification of Spinal Cord Injury. A systematic motor and sensory examination is performed. The new term, *tetraplegia*, has replaced *quadriplegia* and refers to an injury to the cervical area of the spinal cord. The term *paraplegia* refers to injury that involves the thoracic, lumbar, or sacral region of the spinal cord and includes the conus medullaris and the cauda equina. The terms *quadriparesis* and *paraparesis* are no longer used.

The American Spinal Injury Association (ASIA) impairment scale has replaced the Frankel classification grade in defining the extent of the injury (Table 5-1). A person with SCI is classified by grades that range from A, which refers to motor

Table 5-1. American Spinal Injury Association Impairment Scale

A	Complete: No motor or sensory function is preserved in the sacral segments S4–S5.
B	Incomplete: Sensory but not motor function is preserved below the neurologic level and includes the sacral segments S4–S5.
C	Incomplete: Motor function is preserved below the neurologic level, and more than half of the key muscles below the neurologic level have a muscle grade less than 3.
D	Incomplete: Motor function is preserved below the neurologic level, and at least half of the key muscles below the neurologic level have a muscle grade of 3 or more.
E	Normal: Motor and sensory function is normal.

Source: Reprinted with permission from F Maynard Jr. International Standards for Neurological and Functional Classification of Spinal Cord Injury. Chicago: American Spinal Injury Association, 1996;18–19.

Table 5-2. Key Muscles for Motor Level Classification

C5	Elbow flexors
C6	Wrist extensors
C7	Elbow extensors
C8	Finger flexors (distal phalanx of the middle finger)
T1	Finger abductors (little finger)
T2–L1	No testable myotome and sensory levels are used to determine level
L2	Hip flexors
L3	Knee extensors
L4	Ankle dorsiflexors
L5	Long toe extensors
S1	Ankle plantar flexors

Source: Reprinted with permission from F Maynard Jr. International Standards for Neurological and Functional Classification of Spinal Cord Injury. Chicago: American Spinal Injury Association, 1996;14.

and sensory complete SCI, to E, which refers to complete recovery.[25]

Neurologic Level of Injury

The *neurologic level of injury* is defined as the most caudal neural segment with normal sensory and motor function on each side of the body; however, as many as four levels can be recorded if the neurologic level is asymmetric. Both sensory and motor levels are described on both sides of the body to provide a more accurate description. Muscles are given a motor grade based on the 0–5 scale and tested in the supine position. A muscle with a grade of 3/5 is considered to have intact innervation provided that the most rostral muscle has 5/5 strength. Five key muscles are located in each upper extremity for levels C5–T1 and five key muscles in each lower extremity for L2–S1 (Table 5-2). A motor index score is derived by adding the muscle scores of each key muscle. The maximum total score possible is 100.[25]

Twenty-eight key dermatomes are used for sensory testing. Each dermatome is tested for light touch and pinprick–dull touch and based on a three-point scale, with 0 indicating absent, 1 indicating impaired, and 2 indicating intact. Facial sensation is used as the control area for comparison. A score of 0 is given if the person is unable to distinguish between sharp and dull. If the person can distinguish between sharp and dull and the pinprick is not perceived as sharp as on the face, a score of 1 is given. A sensory index score is obtained by adding the scores derived from each dermatome for a total of 112 points for light touch and pinprick (Table 5-3). It is important to assess position sense and deep pressure, although these are not included in the sensory index score. Another important clinical term is *zone of partial preservation*. This refers to partially innervated dermatomes and myotomes caudal to the neurologic level. The term is referenced only in a complete injury.[25]

Incomplete Syndromes

Determination of complete versus incomplete SCI is currently based on the sacral sparing definition.[26] A rectal examination is essential to determine whether motor function or sensory preservation is present at the anal mucocutaneous junction, as well as deep anal sensation. *Complete injury* describes absence of sensation and motor function in the lower sacral segment. *Incomplete SCI* describes the presence of partial sensation or motor function below the neurologic level and includes the lower sacral segment.[25] The presence of sacral sparing implies some continuity of long tracts within the

Table 5-3. Key Sensory Points for Sensory Level Classification

C2	Occipital protuberance
C3	Supraclavicular fossa
C4	Top of the acromioclavicular joint
C5	Lateral side of the antecubital fossa
C6	Thumb
C7	Middle finger
C8	Little finger
T1	Medial side of the antecubital fossa
T2	Apex of the axilla
T3	Third IS
T4	Fourth IS (nipple line)
T5	Fifth IS (midway between T4 and T6)
T6	Sixth IS (level of xiphisternum)
T7	Seventh IS (midway between T6 and T8)
T8	Eighth IS (midway between T7 and T9)
T9	Ninth IS (midway between T8 and T10)
T10	Tenth IS (umbilicus)
T11	Eleventh IS (midway between T10 and T12)
T12	Inguinal ligament at midpoint
L1	Half the distance between T12 and L2
L2	Midanterior thigh
L3	Medial femoral condyle
L4	Medial malleolus
L5	Dorsum of the foot at the third metatarsophalangeal joint
S1	Lateral heel
S2	Popliteal fossa in the midline
S3	Ischial tuberosity
S4-5	Perianal area (taken as one level)

IS = intercostal space.
Source: Reprinted with permission from F Maynard Jr. International Standards for Neurological and Functional Classification of Spinal Cord Injury. Chicago: American Spinal Injury Association, 1996;9–12.

Table 5-4. Clinical Syndromes

Central cord syndrome	A lesion, occurring almost exclusively in the cervical region, that produces sacral sensory sparing and greater weakness in the upper limbs than in the lower limbs.
Brown-Séquard's syndrome	A lesion that produces relatively greater ipsilateral proprioceptive and motor loss and contralateral loss of sensitivity to pain and temperature.
Anterior cord syndrome	A lesion that produces variable loss of motor function and of sensitivity to pain and temperature while preserving proprioception.
Conus medullaris syndrome	Injury of the sacral cord (conus) and lumbar nerve roots within the neural canal, which usually results in an areflexic bladder, bowel, and lower limbs. Sacral segments occasionally show preserved reflexes, e.g., bulbocavernosus and micturition reflexes.
Cauda equina syndrome	Injury to the lumbosacral nerve roots within the neural canal resulting in areflexic bladder, bowel, and lower limbs.

Source: Reprinted with permission from F Maynard Jr, International Standards for Neurological and Functional Classification of Spinal Cord Injury. Chicago: American Spinal Injury Association, 1996;19.

spinal cord. Sparing of the sacral fibers is likely due to their peripheral location in the spinal cord. It is unlikely that a patient's injury would change from complete to incomplete if classified under this definition.[26]

Neuroanatomic syndromes of the spinal cord are also defined in this classification system (Table 5-4). These include the central cord, Brown-Séquard's, anterior cord, conus medullaris, and cauda equina.[25,27]

The central cord syndrome is the most common incomplete syndrome. It involves a lesion in the medial white matter and the central gray matter of

the cervical spinal cord. Clinically, greater arm than leg weakness is noted. Sacral sparing with bowel and bladder control is attributed to the lateral position of the corticospinal and spinothalamic tracts in the spinal cord (see Figure 5-1). A frequent mechanism of injury involves hyperextension of the degenerative spine.[25,27]

Brown-Séquard's syndrome describes a lesion that involves hemisection of the spinal cord. It results in ipsilateral motor and proprioception loss and contralateral loss of pain and temperature sensation. The mechanism of injury classically involves stabbing or gunshot wounds as a result of local trauma, which is seen in a small number of all traumatic SCIs. A "Brown-Séquard plus" syndrome is more typically seen with relative ipsilateral hemiplegia and contralateral hemianalgesia. The cause of injury is variable.[28]

Anterior cord syndrome develops as a result of a lesion in the anterior two-thirds of the spinal cord. A variable loss of motor function and temperature sensation and pain occur. Proprioception is preserved due to sparing of posterior columns, which is attributed to the dual blood supply of the posterior spinal arteries.

The *conus medullaris syndrome* describes an injury to the sacral cord, that is, the conus and the lumbar roots that travel within the spinal canal. Lesions here usually result in an areflexic bowel and bladder and flaccid paralysis. Some preservation of sacral reflexes may be seen, such as bulbocavernosus and micturition reflexes. The *cauda equina syndrome* refers to an injury of the lumbosacral nerve roots located within the neural canal. This results in an areflexic bowel, bladder, and lower extremities.

Prognoses

Functional prognostication after SCI requires an understanding of the spinal cord syndromes and is based on results of the neurologic examination. The timing of the initial examination is important so that the evaluation on the day of the injury helps to establish a baseline and to determine the extent of primary and secondary injuries. However, it is not as accurate for prognosis.[29] Recovery in the zone of injury proceeds differently from that below the level of injury and may continue for an extended period. Ultimate recovery is also influenced by the level of injury, completeness of the injury, and the initial strength of the muscle in question.

A multicenter study by Ditunno et al. in 1992[30] found that C4, C5, and C6 motor-complete tetraplegic patients with some motor power in the zone of partial preservation recovered earlier, with a plateau within 1 year of injury. Subjects with no initial motor power may not plateau until 2 years or more. This supports the need for ongoing re-evaluations to reassess changes in motor function to determine the need for further therapeutic intervention or equipment modifications.

Three windows of motor recovery in the zone of injury have been postulated. *Neuropraxic resolution* refers to resolving the neuropraxic block at the level of the injury and occurs within the first few months after injury. This is considered actual return of function of original motor units. Peripheral sprouting of intact nerves to denervated mus-

cle and hypertrophy of functioning muscle occur in 2–6 months. During this phase, muscles are subject to earlier fatigue and overwork weakness. Axonal regeneration may play a role beyond 12 months.[27]

Recovery below the zone of injury in individuals with motor and sensory complete SCI carries a poor prognosis of functional recovery overall.[27,28] Conversion from complete to incomplete ranges from 0 to 9%. However, unreliable motor and sensory examinations can lead to misdiagnosis. Data from the SCI Model Systems report that up to 11% of Frankel grade A patients gain one classification grade of function. However, fewer than 3% gain to grade C or D.[28] Those classified initially as complete usually remain complete.

The presence of motor function below the injury, that is, motor-incomplete SCI, suggests a better prognosis. Rapid recovery is associated with good prognosis. The faster rate of recovery in tetraplegia tends to occur within the first 3 months, and most upper extremity recovery takes place within 6 months.[28] Recovery may continue for up to 2 years at a slower rate. Brown-Séquard's syndrome has the best prognosis of the motor-incomplete syndromes. Recovery occurs from 1 to 6 months after injury. Function of the ipsilateral lower extremity recovers more slowly than that of the leg contralateral to the injury. However, if lower extremity strength is greater than that of the upper extremities, the prognosis for ambulation is better. The proximal extensors on the side of injury recover before the distal flexors. Recovery of bowel and bladder function is favorable. This recovery pattern is also seen in Brown-Séquard plus syndrome.[28]

The central cord syndrome carries an overall good prognosis. The typical pattern of recovery is lower extremity motor power, bladder function, proximal upper extremity motor power, and intrinsic hand function, and sensation recovery is variable. A more favorable outcome occurs in younger patients (younger than 50 years). The recovery of ambulation in younger individuals with central cord syndrome is reported to be 50% or greater.[31] The ability to ambulate is also affected by the residual weakness in the upper extremities, which prevents the use of assistive devices. The sparing of pain sensation in the sacral area suggests a good prognosis with bowel and bladder function recovery. In 1990, Penrod et al.[31] proposed possible differences between age groups due to concurrent morbidity, effect of spondylosis, effect of arteriosclerosis, and effect of different disease processes. Anterior cord syndrome has a poor prognosis for any functional return, with only a 10–20% recovery rate that is accompanied by significantly impaired muscle strength and coordination. Conus medullaris syndrome shows minimal improvement, and some motor return of function is seen in the cauda equina syndrome.[19,27]

Individuals with sensory-incomplete SCI who have intact pinprick have been shown to ambulate in 66–88% of cases.[32] The extent and type of sacral sparing appear to be important. Preserved pinprick in the S2–S4 dermatome is a good prognostic indicator, suggesting intact spinothalamic tract function and possible sparing of nearby corticospinal tracts.[28,32] The retrospective study by Crozier et al. in 1991[32] revealed that 88% of patients with preserved pinprick ambulated and that only 11% of patients without preserved pinprick ambulated. Those with light touch only below the level of injury had a poor prognosis for ambulation.

The level and transverse extent of the injury determine to a significant degree the severity of impairment, yet the functional consequences of the impairments in the life of the person are a function not only of the impairments but also of the person in whom they occur. The major opportunities are to learn to use compensatory techniques to minimize the degree of illness and to otherwise limit the degree of disability.

Nature of the Disabilities

Disability is a functional consequence of an impairment. Functional potential or ability of an individual to compensate for the impairment by reducing disability depends on the severity of the impairment (i.e., level and completeness of injury). It is also greatly influenced by the age of the patient, comorbidities, motivation, physical limitations, and availability of assistive devices and resources. The functional prognosis triad model is helpful in clarifying the key issues: (1) motor power, referring to what a person may do; (2) functional capacity, which refers to what a person can do; and (3) performance, which is what a person actually does.[27]

Mobility and Activities of Daily Living

Generally, a given neurologic level has functional expectations. Table 5-5 describes functional expectations in mobility and ADL.

In summary, a patient with a lesion above C4 is respiratory dependent and requires a power wheelchair. A C4 level patient can potentially breathe without a ventilator; however, he or she remains dependent in all mobility and ADL and uses a power-driven wheelchair. At the C5 level, the individual can propel a power wheelchair and perform partial upper extremity ADL using adapted equipment. A person with C6 level function may achieve independence with ADL and mobility. The person with C7 level function gains full independence and can propel a manual wheelchair for community distances.

Patients with C8–T10 level injuries are independent in all ADL and mobility at the wheelchair level. Individuals with a T11 or T12 level injury may achieve additional independence with standing, using long leg braces, and the potential for ambulation with braces is more likely with the assistance of functional electrical stimulation to the lower extremities. Household ambulation potential increases significantly with the presence of active hip flexion with L2 function. Patients with L3–S1 injuries can become community ambulators with variable types of leg braces, and those with S2–S5 level injuries can ambulate, possibly without a brace.[33]

In addition to issues of mobility and ADL, illness due to medical problems is a major treatable cause of disability after SCI. Serious medical complications, significant morbidity, and eventual death can occur if the illnesses are ignored and untreated. A major goal of rehabilitation is to learn how to reduce disability due to illness by learning how to anticipate and recognize potential medical complications given impaired sensory input and motor control. The patient is taught compensatory strategies to prevent or minimize illness. A brief overall review of some of the more commonly recurring and often preventable medical illnesses is presented in the next section.

Depression

Underlying the ability to make the adaptations necessary to maintain health as well as deal with mobil-

Table 5-5. Functional Expectations Based on Neurologic Level

Neurologic Level	Sensory	Motor	Test	Goals
C1–C3	Neck	Cervical flexors and extensors	Trapezius Shoulder shrug	Respiratory dependent Blink or head control powers wheelchair Environmental control unit Computer Mouth stick
C4	Shoulder mantle	Deltoid diaphragm	Shoulder abduction Breathing	Dependent Electric wheelchair with chin control
C5	Lateral arm and thumb	Biceps	Elbow flexion	Partially independent with adaptive equipment Electric wheelchair with arm control
C6	Index, long fingers	Wrist extensors	Wrist extension	Independent with equipment Driving hand controls Manual wheelchair with pegs
C7	Index, long fingers	Triceps Wrist flexor Finger extensors	Elbow extension Finger extension	Independent transfers and ADLs Standard manual wheelchair
C8	Fifth finger	Finger flexors Interosseus	Flex fingers Spread fingers	Independent ADLs without splints Independent transfers
T1–L10	Chest to umbilicus	Intercostals Spine extensors	Normal upper extremity	Independent in all skills for living
T11–L12	Inguinal ligament	Rectus abdominis	Elevate trunk	Independent stand in long leg braces
L1–L2	Anterior and medial thigh	Iliopsoas adductors	Hip flexion	Ambulation with long leg braces in household
L3–L4	Medial calf	Quadriceps Hamstrings	Knee extension	Community ambulation with long leg (possibly short leg) braces
L4–L5	Dorsal foot	Anterior tibial	Dorsiflexion of foot	Community ambulation with short leg braces
L5–S1	Lateral foot	Gastrocnemius Toe flexors	Plantar flexion of foot	Community ambulation with short leg braces
S2–S5	Perianal region	Gluteus Sphincters	Hip extension Anal tone	Community ambulation, possibly without braces

ADLs = activities of daily living.
Source: Reprinted with permission from D Apple Jr. Spinal Cord Injury Rehabilitation. In RH Rothman (ed), The Spine (3rd ed). Philadelphia: Saunders, 1992;1244.

ity and ADL is the degree to which the person is willing to learn new ways of living. The ability to make often profound changes is significantly affected by psychosocial issues. Individuals with SCI require major psychological adjustments after the injury. The process of readaptation involves feelings of denial, grief, anger, depression, and eventual coping. Patients often mourn the loss of the physically active person they were before the injury. The individual may stop anywhere along any of these stages, which may have an impact on the rehabilitation process and the ability to achieve independence in functional status. Direct and indirect self-destructive behavior contributes to increased illness, morbidity, and mortality. A high rate of suicide among individuals with SCI has been noted in complete paraplegics within 5 years of injury[7] and among marginally disabled paraplegic patients when compared with even far more functionally impaired complete tetraplegic patients.[34] Often, the underlying issue is related to depression.

The complexity of the psychosocial issues and their impact on subsequent function are illustrated by the following case: A 20-year-old man with T12 paraplegia for 1 year presented to an acute care hospital with multiple pressure ulcers and signs and symptoms of sepsis. He gave a history of prior completion of a 6-week inpatient rehabilitation program with independence at a wheelchair level for mobility and daily living skills. He had minimal outpatient medical and rehabilitation follow-up because of financial and transportation issues. He lives with his grandmother in a wheelchair-inaccessible home with bathroom and bedroom on the second floor with 13 steps. He negotiated the stairs using a "bumping" technique and, over time, noted bilateral ischial pressure ulcers that were draining and foul smelling. He became essentially bed confined in attempts to heal the wounds. He reported feeling isolated and hopeless. He admitted to increased alcohol use due to feeling "down." He ate one meal per day in hopes of decreasing his need to perform the bowel program, with digital stimulation and suppositories one to two times a week. He experienced frequent UTIs and often limited fluid intake in an attempt to limit the need to catheterize. Before his injury, he was unemployed and had completed the eleventh grade. He had no active school or vocational interests or pursuits before or after his injury.

Despite adequate mobility, the patient was nevertheless bed-bound because of medical illness caused by skin ulcers as well as UTI. To be successful, his preparation for a life after SCI could not be limited to being instructed in methods for assuring mobility. It is clear that adequate follow-up and management of psychosocial issues were essential for an adequate treatment plan.

Significant depression after SCI is not universal. The SCI in itself does not change a person's basic personality, so that one who was successful in dealing with problems or life events before the injury will do so even after the injury. It is important to be able to identify those patients who are at higher risk for depression. Some of those risk factors include history of depression, positive family history of depression with suicide attempts, chronic pain, age of less than 40 years at onset, female gender, inadequate social support, multiple life stressors, and concurrent medical or substance abuse.[35] Accompanying symptoms may be insomnia or hypersomnia, loss of interest, hopelessness and guilt, fatigue and loss of energy, and impaired appetite.[35] Psychological or pharmacologic intervention, or both, are indicated in individuals with significant symptomatology.

Psychological adjustment after the SCI is particularly difficult among urban youth. Typically, they are very self-conscious of their image and of being accepted. These individuals may refuse to return to school for fear of rejection from peers and concern over social stigma. Some fear being targeted for further violence due to limitations in mobility. Others may return to illicit drug activity or substance abuse for financial reasons or as an attempt to relieve pain or psychological distress. Altered self-esteem affects the ability to cope with daily life pressures and peer relations. The combination of these and other social factors frequently impedes the ability to engage in the rehabilitation process. Supportive family and friends are the key ingredients to successful patient participation and progress in the rehabilitation process, especially in transitioning to home. For many urban poor families, participation may be difficult and often impossible due to the inability to obtain leave from work, lack of transportation, and child care limitations. Families are often unable to provide the ongoing emotional support and financial assistance needed. Feelings of abandonment are frequently expressed. In addition, patients and families are often unprepared to navigate the health care system or social services to obtain appropriate care.

Community reintegration is also hampered by returning to the fairly hostile environments that initially contributed to the violence associated with the SCI. Architectural barriers are a major issue in inner-city housing that leads to individuals being virtually confined to the home. This contributes further to feelings of isolation and social rejection. Day-to-day survival issues, such as lack of food, clothing, and money as well as limited education, vocational opportunities, and financial resources, further add to the challenges of a successful return to the community.

Weitzenkamp et al.[36] found that spouses who provide supportive care display more depressive symptoms, such as increased physical and emotional stress, fatigue, burnout, and low self-esteem, than do noncaregiving spouses. It is unclear whether the stress and depression reported by the spouse are secondary to being the caregiver or related to having a dependent spouse. Caregiving spouse issues are multiple and may include financial concerns about loss of income by the wage earner, change in family role, and feelings of inadequacy or being overwhelmed by managing the medical care.

A major goal of rehabilitation must be to assist the patient during the psychological adjustment after injury and facilitate as much independence as possible, which will ultimately decrease the caregiver burden. This assistance helps to develop positive coping skills and allows the person to capitalize on his or her strengths and to maximize remaining functional abilities. Support of family and friends is also crucial and can assist the person with SCI in adapting during the rehabilitation phase and in managing his or her life. Periodic follow-up with health professionals to assess overall well-being and psychological status is indicated, given the higher risk for suicide among individuals with SCI.

Respiratory Complications

Pneumonia and other related pulmonary complications are the most common causes of death.[37] Respiratory system complications are especially common in patients with high-level tetraplegia, such as C1–C4. Upper respiratory infection, tracheitis, and bronchitis lead to significant morbidity, and aspiration and ventilatory failure are frequently seen in the acute phase of injury. Several factors can contribute to the increased risk of pulmonary dysfunction. In tetraplegics, a major factor is weakened diaphragm muscles and partially innervated phrenic nerves, as well as paralysis of the chest and abdominal muscles, which inhibits the ability to perform an effective cough. This significantly reduces maximal respiratory vital capacity and tidal volume in tetraplegics and in higher-level paraplegic patients, which can further compromise the respiratory system. Development of mucous plugs also impairs gas exchange. Other contributing factors include immobility, medication with sedation effects, and potential for nighttime desaturation. A higher incidence of pneumonia, aspiration, atelectasis, and ventilatory failure is seen in older age groups (older than 60 years) and in higher, neurologically complete injuries.[37]

Comprehensive prophylactic respiratory therapy program measures are instituted to decrease potential mortality and morbidity from pulmonary complications. The program includes components such as frequent turning (every 2 hours), vigorous pulmonary toileting (including postural drainage), chest physical therapy, nebulization treatment, assisted coughing, strengthening exercises for the diaphragm and other accessory muscles, and incentive spirometry and bronchodilators. It has been helpful to translate such preventive programs into clear objectives that are measurable by patient as well as staff. One such objective measurement that lends itself to ongoing patient participation in monitoring is the tidal volume with the use of incentive spirometry. The degree of oxygen saturation is another measure that can be easily communicated to the patient.

Long-term pulmonary management is important as a person with SCI ages. Risk factors for recurrent or chronic pulmonary conditions include complete higher-level injuries, spasticity involving the chest and abdominal walls, skeletal deformities of the spine that may impair the ability to cough, obesity, and smoking.[37]

Cardiovascular Complications

Cardiovascular complications such as deep vein thrombosis (DVT), PE, and autonomic dysreflexia contribute to significant complications in acute and chronic phases of SCI. Thromboembolic disease frequently develops during the acute phase of SCI, especially within the first 2 weeks, with a lower occurrence rate seen in patients with chronic SCI. It is influenced by immobility, hypercoagulable state, and decreased venous return and is seen more frequently in patients with complete motor paralysis. Clinical signs of DVT are apparent in approximately 16.3% of persons with SCI according to SCI Model Systems reports.[37] A high index of suspicion must be maintained. Common signs may include fever, tachycardia, discrepancy in thigh girth measurement, autonomic dysreflexia, increased warmth, and erythema. Objective evidence of DVT is detected with a Doppler ultrasound of the lower extremities. If tests are negative or indeterminate, confirmation is obtained via venogram of the lower extremities. Prophylactic treatment is recommended for the first 2 weeks with compression hose or pneumatic devices applied to the legs. Indications for placement of a vena cava filter include failed anticoagulation prophylaxis, contraindication to anticoagulation, high cervical lesions, or poor cardiopulmonary reserve.[38] Filter placement does not substitute for anticoagulation prophylaxis. Early mobilization of patients and passive range of motion are crucial. Within 72 hours of injury, anticoagulation prophylaxis with low-molecular-weight heparin or an unfractional heparin fixed or adjusted dose is initiated unless contraindicated. Anticoagulation is continued until discharge from the hospital in ASIA D motor-incomplete patients, up to 8 weeks in ASIA C patients, at least 8 weeks in motor-complete patients, and 12 weeks for those who are motor complete with additional risk.[38]

PE is a serious potential complication of DVT. It is the leading cause of death in SCI patients, and the incidence is approximately 5% in acute SCI. Frequency of death as a result of PE is reduced as the time advances after injury, so that it represents 2.5% of deaths after the fifth postinjury year.[39] Signs and symptoms of pleuritic chest pain, hemoptysis, and dyspnea may be masked in SCI patients, and these signs may be present with autonomic dysreflexia or tachycardia. A high index of suspicion is required, and diagnosis should be confirmed with a ventilation-perfusion scan or a pulmonary angiogram. Treatment involves full anticoagulation therapy with intravenous heparin and warfarin (Coumadin) for at least 3 months in the case of a DVT and 6 months for PE.[37] Alternative treatment with low-molecular-weight heparin in persons with SCI must be further evaluated as to safety and effectiveness as a traditional treatment.

Autonomic Dysreflexia. Autonomic dysreflexia is a potentially life-threatening condition that may develop after spinal shock has resolved and reflex activity has returned. It is particularly important that caregivers and patients become aware of its characteristics and treatment. It is a phenomenon triggered by noxious stimuli below the level of injury that results in unopposed sympathetic hyperactivity leading to severe hypertension. Autonomic dysreflexia occurs in individuals with injuries at or above the T6 level, which is above the major sympathetic outflow. The incidence varies from 15% to 85% of tetraplegic patients, who are at greatest risk.[37,40]

The pathophysiology of autonomic dysreflexia is somewhat complex. The major splanchnic out-

flow is located between T6 and L2. Sensory nerve impulses below the level of injury travel to the spinal cord and ascend in the posterior column and spinothalamic tracts. Subsequently, these impulses stimulate the intermediolateral gray matter sympathetic neurons. The inhibitory sympathetic impulses that arise above T6 are unable to transmit impulses because they are blocked by the injury. The sympathetic outflow, T6–L2, below the injury level remains unopposed. The release of neurotransmitters, such as norepinephrine, dopamine, and others, may result in skin pallor, sweating, and severe arterial vasoconstriction, leading to an abrupt hypertensive state and concomitant headache.[40]

The hypertension is detected by carotid and aortic baroreceptors. Compensatory vasomotor brain stem reflexes are, however, unsuccessful in lowering the blood pressure. Bradycardia develops as a result of increases in vagal (cranial nerve X) parasympathetic stimulation; however, severe vasoconstriction cannot be halted because any increase in sympathetic inhibitory output is unable to travel below the injury level. Subsequently, profuse sweating, skin flushing, and vasodilatation occur above the level of the lesion.[40] An increase of just 20–40 mm Hg above the usual state without other symptoms may be a significant sign. Other reported symptoms are pounding headache, blurred vision, nasal stuffiness, pupil dilation, cardiac arrhythmias, or spots in a patient's visual fields.

Treatment of an acute episode of autonomic dysreflexia is a medical emergency for those with SCI. At the first indication of signs or symptoms, initial treatment should be to place the patient in a sitting position and loosen clothing and devices. The patient should be quickly screened head to toe to localize and eliminate the source of noxious stimuli. Special attention is focused on the anogenital region to assess for bladder and bowel distention or retention. Resumption of normal blood pressure and pulse occurs quickly if the primary cause of autonomic dysreflexia, such as unkinking a Foley catheter with immediate urinary flow, is found and eradicated. If the source is not found and blood pressure is above 150 mm Hg systolic, treatment with a short-acting antihypertensive agent, such as nifedipine or nitrate, is indicated.

It is important to institute prophylactic measures, such as diligent management of multiple organ systems that can contribute to this condition, to prevent recurrent episodes. Autonomic dysreflexia has many potential causes; more frequent etiologies include distention of the bladder, UTI, bladder or kidney stones, detrusor sphincter dyssynergia, urodynamics, and cystoscopy. Other causes of noxious stimuli below the level of injury, such as bowel distention or impaction, pressure sores, ingrown toenails, pain, DVT-PE, gastritis, and pregnancy (especially labor and delivery), can contribute to this phenomenon. The patient and family should be instructed as to the potential causes of autonomic dysreflexia and appropriate preventive measures.

Orthostatic Hypotension. Orthostatic hypotension commonly occurs in higher-level SCI. Pooling of blood in distal extremities, loss of sympathetic tone with impaired vasoconstriction, and absence of muscle contraction contribute to its occurrence, especially with quick changes from a supine position. The dependent position of the extremity along with the lack of compressive muscle forces contribute to the problem. Prompt treatment involves placing the patient in a reclining position and elevating the legs. Prophylactic treatment may involve lower extremity elastic stockings, an abdominal binder, prolonged leg elevation, gradual transition to a sitting position, and liberalization of salt intake; medications such as ephedrine sulfate or fluorinated corticosteroids can also be used.[37]

Dependent edema occurs frequently and is usually bilateral. The prolonged dependent position of a lower extremity, along with a lack of compressive muscle forces, contributes to the condition. Unilateral swelling suggests DVT or heterotopic ossification that requires further workup. Primary treatment involves elevation and elastic stockings.

Pressure Ulcers

Pressure ulceration is a frequent complication of SCI patients, with the key factors including a combination of pressure, shear, and friction. Secondary factors include sensory loss, infection, hypoproteinemia, anemia, impaired mobility, advanced age, impaired mental status, and fecal and urinary incontinence. Other associated factors reportedly include poor nutrition, complete lesions, acute illness, or cigarette smoking.[40] Psychological adjustment has been linked with development of pressure ulcers. Clinically, pressure ulcers are often seen in those patients who do not follow diligent skin-monitoring techniques because of depression or lack of motivation, inadequate caregiver support, or alcohol or substance abuse.

Pressure ulcers occur most commonly after prolonged pressure that exceeds mean capillary pressure, over bony prominences. The initial damage occurs in deep muscle with progression toward the skin.[41] According to SCI Model Systems data, the most common sites of ulcer development were the sacrum (37.4%), the heel (15.9%), and the ischium (9.2%).[42] Two years after injury, however, distribution had shifted due to increased time in a sitting position, with 24.3% occurring at the ischium, 20.3% at the sacrum, 12.5% at the trochanter, and 10.9% at the heel.[42]

The essential treatment must be prevention. The need for a comprehensive approach to the management of skin ulcers is illustrated by the following case: A man with C6 tetraplegia secondary to a motor vehicle accident remained withdrawn during his entire rehabilitation stay. He reported no need to participate because of his belief in eventual divine healing. During his stay, sacral pressure ulcers developed, and he resisted all attempts to learn how to perform dressing changes or direct his caregiver in treatment or skin management techniques. He required significant assistance for mobility and ADL even at discharge. The wound eventually healed with his wife's diligent treatment. Depressed affect was evident; however, he refused all antidepressant pharmacologic treatment or counseling within the spinal cord support group or individual treatment. A recurrent pressure ulcer developed while he was an outpatient. It took almost 1 year for the patient to develop a sense of empowerment and return to activities within the community, including the resumption of ministerial duties.

Management of existing pressure sores involves frequent pressure relief with avoidance of shear, prevention of excessively dry conditions, and maximization of nutrition. To prevent dehydration, 1 liter or more of water a day is recommended. Major caloric intake should be from carbohydrates and 1.5–2.0 g protein/kg of body weight. Zinc and iron supplementation is recommended only if levels are found to be deficient. Vitamin C, 1 g per day in divided doses, has been found to improve healing of pressure ulcers.[41] The patient should also be evaluated and treated for underlying medical conditions that may aggravate the healing process.

Initially, the nursing staff is responsible for proper skin protection management. A frequent turning schedule every 2 hours in bed and proper bed positioning are instituted. It is imperative to inspect the skin, and if hyperemia is noted for longer than 30 minutes, an increase in frequency of turning is implemented.

Once the patient is sitting on his or her own, prevention is heavily dependent on whether the individual becomes a participant in his or her own management. The patient must have some ability to monitor the status of the skin. A mirror can enable the patient to check him- or herself after sitting. Early mobilization into a wheelchair decreases the risk of pressure ulcers being caused by lying in bed. Sitting programs are limited initially to 30- to 60-minute intervals, depending on the presence of persistent hyperemia. Reducing the likelihood of breakdown requires pressure relief to permit venous return of waste products. In the absence of sensory input such as burning pain, the usual method is to use a clock to indicate the need for pressure relief. Pressure-relieving seating systems and mattresses are used as well as protective boots to prevent pressure ulcers in several sites. A program that incorporates the patient in self-monitoring and pressure relief is described in a later section of this chapter.

Bladder Management

Although significant progress has been made in the management of neurogenic bladder and prevention of renal failure, bladder disorders continue to be an important cause of mortality and morbidity. They also contribute to secondary causes of death with septicemia. This area continually needs to be targeted for ongoing diligent medical care. The goals are (1) to achieve continence, (2) to prevent illness due to infection and stone formation, and (3) to achieve and maintain low pressure within the bladder system to prevent ureteral reflux and hydronephrosis. The process of bladder rehabilitation involves retraining the bladder and re-educating the patient.

The peripheral pathways (afferent and efferent) of the urologic system involve three systems. Figure 5-2 depicts the innervation of the urinary system. The autonomic nerves are both the pelvic (parasympathetic) and hypogastric (sympathetic) nerves along with the pudendal (somatic) nerve. The detrusor muscle is primarily under parasympathetic control by the cholinergic receptors that arise from S2–S4, and receptors are diffusely distributed in the bladder, trigone, and urethra. These receptors are activated during bladder contraction. The sympathetic outflow derived from the thoracolumbar T11–L2 segments has an inhibitory effect on the bladder. It promotes relaxation of the bladder for urine storage via β-adrenergic receptors. The proximal urethra and internal sphincter have predominantly α-adrenergic receptors, and with sympathetic stimulation the bladder neck smooth muscle contracts and urine is retained. The external sphincter and pelvic floor muscles are under somatic control via the pelvic nerves that are responsible for contraction during bladder filling and relaxation during bladder emptying.[43]

Central control of the bladder is at multiple levels. The bladder reflex center is in the pons. Another reflex with afferent neurons arises from the bladder and synapses on the pudendal nerve nucleus at S2–S4. This reflex allows inhibition of pelvic floor muscles during voiding. Voluntary control over pelvic floor muscles is transmitted by afferents that ascend to the sensory cortex of the brain and descending fibers from the motor cortex to the synapse on the pudendal nerve nucleus.[44]

As the bladder fills in normal voiding, involuntary inhibition of the micturition reflex occurs via the suprapontine center pathways. Once the bladder distends to approximately 50% of the normal capacity of 300–600 ml, the urge to void is transmitted to the cerebral sensory centers. As a result, voluntary activation of the micturition reflex occurs when voiding is necessary and appropriate to occur. This results in relaxation of the external sphincter and detrusor contraction and relaxation of the internal sphincter. Sympathetic pathways are inhibited during voiding. Voluntary contraction of the external sphincter allows discontinuation of voiding on command and triggers reflex inhibition of detrusor contraction.

Management of the neurogenic bladder depends on the neurologic level and the completeness of the lesion. The residual problem may be either a failure to store or a failure to empty the bladder with

Figure 5-2. Innervation of the urinary tract. The parasympathetic, sympathetic, and somatic nerve supply to the bladder, urethra, and pelvic floor are displayed. N = nerve. (Reprinted with permission from DD Cardenas, ME Mayo, JC King. Urinary Tract and Bowel Management in the Rehabilitation Setting. In R Braddom [ed], Physical Medicine and Rehabilitation. Philadelphia: Saunders, 1996;556.)

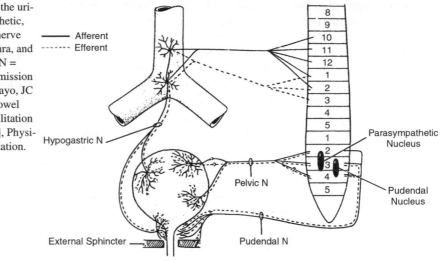

overflow incontinence. In spinal cord lesions above the sacral cord, a reflexic bladder develops. Sensory nerve input and motor output are preserved; however, function is not under conscious control. A reflexive emptying pattern eventually develops in these patients, and an incontinent state exists. They run the risk for development of detrusor hyperreflexia, which can lead to high bladder pressure and eventual renal damage. In patients with spinal cord lesions at the level of the sacral plexus or below, a lower motor neuron bladder develops with bladder areflexia or a flaccid bladder-emptying pattern.

During the acute phase of SCI, in the presence of spinal shock, flaccid paralysis of the bladder occurs. Urine retention develops, and overflow voiding occurs when the intravesicular pressure is greater than the sphincter. The risk is present for residual atonic bladder if prolonged distention persists. An indwelling Foley catheter is used to provide adequate bladder drainage. During this time the patient is at increased risk for UTI, bacterial colonization, epididymitis, prostatitis, periurethritis, and urethrocutaneous fistula formation if the catheter is used for a prolonged period.

The majority of patients use the preferred intermittent catheter program or reflex voiding, with the goal of maintaining a balanced bladder, which refers to a low pressure, low postvoiding residual volume, and relative continence.[45] In subsequent years after injury, use of the intermittent catheter program declines in men, with a concomitant increase in the use of external condom catheter drainage. In women, use of intermittent catheterization decreases with the increased use of indwelling urethral catheterization.

Recurrent UTI or bacteriuria is the most frequent secondary medical complication or illness. Inadequate emptying is the major source for the proliferation of bacteria to occur in the bladder. Illness in the form of bacteremia and clinical UTI occurs when bacterial concentration rises to a significant level. Management may require adequate urinary volume for dilution along with adequate emptying. Appropriate antibiotic treatment for 7–10 days is initiated for symptomatic UTI, that is, urinary incontinence, increased spasticity, fever, general malaise, pain over the bladder, or autonomic dysreflexia. Treatment of asymptomatic bacteriuria remains controversial. Such infections are not treated routinely unless the incidence of bacteriuria is the first occurrence and is accompanied by pyuria, urease-producing organisms are present, or the patient is immunocompromised or has vesicoureteral reflux.[45]

Upper tract urologic complications can impair long-term health and survival. These complications include hydronephrosis, renal insufficiency and failure, renal calculi, and vesicourethral reflux. Increased frequency of renal calculi, a serious complication, is seen with indwelling catheters. Regular evaluations of the urinary tract (yearly or every few years) are advised to reduce mortality and morbidity and maintain normal renal function.

A major opportunity for maintenance of health is afforded by patient participation in the monitoring of agreed-on goals such that in the presence of early signs of clinical infection, appropriate treatment is initiated promptly to reduce the degree to which illness interferes with life. A program plan designed to bring about such patient participation is described in the second section of this chapter.

Bowel Management

Neurogenic bowel dysfunction with impaired ability to control elimination of stool is a major issue in individuals with SCI. It has the potential to affect social, emotional, and physical well-being and can lead to life-threatening complications. Levi et al.,[46] in the Stockholm SCI study, found that bowel dysfunction was reported as a moderate to severe life-limiting problem in 41% of individuals. Neurogenic bowel dysfunction has been related to depression, and up to 23% of people with chronic SCI have required hospitalization as a result of these problems. Multiple complications are reported and commonly include constipation, diarrhea, hemorrhoids, ileus, gastric ulcer, gastroesophageal reflux, pain, autonomic dysreflexia, incontinence, diminished appetite, and delayed evacuation time. Diligent, effective management of bowel function needs to be implemented to decrease illness, disability, or handicap.

Menter et al.,[47] in evaluating outcomes of bowel management in individuals with chronic SCI, found that 42% of subjects reported constipation, 35% reported gastrointestinal pain, and 27% reported bowel accidents. Constipation was greatest in paraplegics using digital stimulation, with an increased incidence of hemorrhoids seen in those who used suppositories and enemas. Fecal incontinence and diarrhea were diagnosed three times more often in tetraplegics. These findings support the need for ongoing long-term management in people with chronic SCI.

The colon starts at the ileocecal sphincter. An internal anal sphincter (IAS), consisting of smooth muscle, is located in the distal colon. The external anal sphincter (EAS) consists of a circular band of striated muscle that contracts the pelvic floor. The puborectalis muscle travels around the proximal rectum and provides a 90-degree anorectal angle.

Fecal continence is maintained by coordination of the IAS, EAS, and puborectalis muscle.[44]

Intrinsic innervation of the colon is supplied by the parasympathetic, sympathetic, and somatic nerves. An enteric nervous system, located in the wall of the colon, coordinates all segmental movement to advance stool throughout the colon and mixes the stool. This highly organized system consists of Auerbach's plexus (intramuscular myenteric) and the submucosal Meissner's plexus. The vagus nerve supplies the parasympathetic innervation from the esophagus to the splenic flexure of the colon. Parasympathetic nerve fibers from S2 to S4 travel in the pelvic nerve to supply the descending colon and rectum and promote colonic motility. Sympathetic innervation arises from the superior and inferior mesenteric nerves from T5 to T12 and from the hypogastric nerves (T12–L3). The EAS is innervated by the somatic pudendal nerve (S2–S4), which also provides the nerve supply to the pelvic floor.[44,48]

Continence in a normal resting state is maintained by closure of the IAS and the puborectalis sling in the anal canal. IAS tone remains increased to promote storage by sympathetic nerve stimulation from L1 to L2. Dilatation by stool and digital stimulation can both inhibit the IAS. Stool incontinence with cough or a Valsalva's maneuver is inhibited by reflex contraction of the EAS and the puborectalis muscle. With intact bowel function, defecation is initiated with involuntary movement of stool into the rectum. The urge to defecate is perceived after rectal and puborectalis stretch. Voluntary contraction of the EAS can retain stool temporarily. Defecation follows relaxation of the EAS and the puborectalis muscle, triggered by peristalsis and intra-abdominal pressure via a Valsalva's maneuver.[48,49]

Spinal shock refers to the temporary loss of all reflex activity below the level of injury. It can last for hours to weeks. Initially, reflex-mediated defecation is decreased. Rectal tone is diminished. The anal and bulbocavernosus reflexes are absent. Resolution of shock occurs with return of the bulbocavernosus reflex. The type of neurogenic bowel dysfunction that results from SCI depends on location and completeness of the injury.[49] If the SCI is above the sacral spinal cord segment, an upper motor neuron reflexive bowel pattern develops. Voluntary control with relaxation of the EAS is lost, along with the inability to modulate descending inhibitory impulses in the spinal cord. This results in pelvic floor musculature and EAS spasticity, which contributes to stool retention. Resting pressure of EAS and IAS is sustained, which ensures continence most of the time. Reflex coordination of stool propulsion in the colon is preserved because the intrinsic innervation of the colon remains intact.[44]

A complete spinal cord lesion located at or below the sacral segment leads to the development of a lower motor neuron or areflexic bowel pattern. The sacral defecation center and related nerve supply to the anus and rectum are destroyed. Reflexive peristalsis, which is typically mediated by the spinal cord, is lost. Slow stool propulsion from the colon into the rectum may lead to impaction. Fecal incontinence is increased due to the laxity of the anal sphincter as a result of the denervated EAS.[49] Resting anal tone is reduced due to loss of parasympathetic control and reflex innervation of the IAS.

Management of the neurogenic bowel involves an individualized program. The overall goals of such a program are to promote stool continence, achieve simple independent defecation in a timely manner, and prevent gastrointestinal complications. In the case of an upper motor neuron–type bowel, the patient is trained in reflex bowel elimination with digital stimulation of the anal reflex. This relaxes the sphincter and causes evacuation of the stool contents. In addition, a suppository can be used, which provides chemical stimulation. In the case of a lower motor neuron–type function, digital stimulation is performed followed by gentle manual disimpaction to avoid trauma and prevent over-dilatation of the sphincter. A regular bowel program is recommended, which is performed every night or every other night, preferably to limit interference with other activities.

Typically, the program is performed shortly after meals to facilitate gastrointestinal motility with the aid of the gastrocolic reflex. This reflex is triggered by eating, especially fatty or protein-rich meals, and produces peristalsis in the colon and small intestine. The mechanism is not clearly defined and may include neural or hormonal influences. Studies have been inconsistent in showing a predictable gastrocolic response to meals after SCI.[48] The person with SCI or family members, or both, can make important contributions toward achieving control, particularly the patient with lesions that involve the

sacral outflow, where incontinence is more likely. Developing independence in this area is crucial when planning for the individual with SCI to return to a more normal lifestyle in his or her community.

Regular and complete evacuation at the appointed time and place requires management to prevent stool from remaining too long in the gut. Water reabsorption occurs during the stay in the colon, resulting in impaction followed by loose stools around the area of blockage. The person with SCI must understand the mechanisms by which bowel contents may have a relatively short transit time. Exercise is helpful, as it is for those with an intact spinal cord. Adequate dietary fiber coupled with fluid intake leads to bulk in the stool. This enables the musculature in the bowel wall to be more effective. The amount of fiber in the diet and its sources cannot be predetermined, but 20–30 g of fiber per day is the general recommendation, although the need may vary. Effective management requires input from the patient in monitoring his or her results and adjusting the amount and type of diet. Many can identify particular foods that cause them to have an almost immediate bowel evacuation. Although most find it desirable to forgo such foods, some find it useful to use such foods deliberately when they wish to have a bowel evacuation. Table 5-6 lists the fiber content of some common foods to enable patients to design their own diet.

Illness or medical complications as a result of neurogenic bowel dysfunction contribute to life-limiting problems for an individual with SCI. Severe chronic constipation can develop with accompanying nausea, vomiting, and abdominal pain and obstruction. Chronic laxatives eventually lose their effectiveness over time. Constipation can result from a poor diet, side effects of medications such as oxybutynin chloride (Ditropan) for treatment of bladder incontinence, and a prolonged interval before performing the bowel program. This inadequate bowel program may be secondary to lack of caregiver support to perform the task or psychological maladjustment of the individual in managing his or her bowel function in this manner. For example, a person may limit food intake and perform a bowel program once a week to avoid the issue. Other limiting factors may include a lack of funds to pay for an attendant or strained family relationships that would preclude performance of this intimate task. A poorly regulated bowel pro-

Table 5-6. Dietary Fiber Content of Foods in Commonly Served Portions

Food Group	<1 g	1.0–1.9 g	2.0–2.9 g	3.0–3.9 g	4.0–4.9 g	5.0–5.9 g	>6 g
Breads (1 slice)	Bagel White French	Whole wheat	Bran muffin (1)	NA	NA	NA	NA
Cereals (1 oz)	Rice Krispies Special K Cornflakes	Oatmeal Nutri-Grain Cheerios	Wheaties Shredded Wheat	Most Honey Bran	Bran Chex 40% Bran Flakes Raisin Bran	Corn Bran	All-Bran Bran Buds 100% Bran
Pasta (1 cup)	NA	Macaroni Spaghetti	NA	Whole-wheat spaghetti	NA	NA	NA
Rice (1/2 cup)	White	Brown	NA	NA	NA	NA	NA
Legumes (1/2 cup), cooked	NA	NA	NA	Lentils	Lima beans Dried peas	NA	Kidney beans Baked beans Navy beans
Vegetables (1/2 cup unless stated)	Cucumber Lettuce (1 cup) Green pepper	Asparagus Green beans Cabbage Cauliflower Potato without skin (1) Celery	Broccoli Brussels sprouts Carrots Corn Potato with skin (1) Spinach	NA	NA	NA	NA
Fruits (1 medium fruit unless stated)	Grapes (20) Watermelon (1 cup)	Apricots (3) Grapefruit (1/2) Peach with skin Pineapple (1/2 cup)	Apple without skin Banana Orange	Apple with skin Pear with skin Raspberries (1/2 cup)	NA	NA	NA

NA = not applicable.
Source: Reprinted with permission from JL Slavin. Dietary fiber: classification, chemical analyses, and food sources. J Am Diet Assoc 1987;87:1164.

gram with stool incontinence and diarrhea secondary to chronic laxative use can cause skin irritation and breakdown. Anticipation of potential incontinence can contribute to an impaired QOL such that a patient may remain confined to his or her home because of these issues. Effective training in bowel management must be built on patient participation in monitoring results and making adaptations in diet and other factors that are specific to the person.

Sexual Function

The effects of SCI on sexual expression are more far-reaching than those that affect the ability to carry out sexual acts that involve the genitalia. Human sexual activity serves a complex need for personal expression and gratification, with numerous psychological, social, and aesthetic implications.

The differential effects of the level of neurologic impairment vary in a way similar to that of micturition and defecation in terms of suprasacral (upper motor neuron) and sacral (lower motor neuron) involvement. The character of the functional impact of the changes reflects not only the physiologic issues but also the person in whom those changes have occurred. The person's sex, age, and previous pattern of sexual intimacy and the availability of a mate all contribute to making the character of the disabilities almost unique to each individual. A significant disability for one person may involve problems related to vaginal penetration; for another, the ability to sire a child; and for another, the ability to bear a child. Alternative means are available that are specific to each goal.

Analogies can be made to the innervation of the other perineal functions. Both cholinergic and sympathetic fibers as well as striated muscles are involved. Erection of the penis (or clitoris) comes about with both tactile and cerebral stimuli and with sustained vasodilatation of the corpus cavernosus. Vasodilator adrenergic fibers serve psychogenic arousal. Stimuli from the bladder, rectum, or skin lead to vasodilatation via parasympathetic cholinergic fibers, which causes reflexogenic arousal. Although these two channels for erection generally work synergistically, they may not. For example, psychogenically induced stimuli may serve to inhibit reflex arousal.

Emission depends on the pooling of the bolus of sperm and fluid preparatory to ejaculation. It relies on adrenergic fibers, which also simultaneously cause closure of the internal sphincter of the bladder, preventing the admixture of urine and sperm. Ejaculation occurs from stimuli carried by adrenergic fibers coupled with innervation via the pudendal nerve of the striated musculature (ischiocavernosus and bulbocavernosus). The contraction of the striated muscles propels the seminal bolus forward. Although orgasm is sometimes considered to be synonymous with ejaculation, it can be a separate event. *Orgasm* refers to the subjective feelings associated with emission and ejaculation and may potentially occur without the physical act of ejaculation.

The likelihood of disabilities in the various functions associated with sexual performance varies, in general depending on the pattern of impairments. The presence or absence of the anal wink and the bulbocavernosus reflexes and the finding of perineal pinprick sensation are determinants. A reflexic (upper motor neuron) and areflexic (lower motor neuron) pattern can be coupled with complete or incomplete injury. The majority of men with reflexic-complete status have erections on a reflex basis with tactile stimuli, and a large percentage of these can have successful coitus. Most are not able to ejaculate or have an orgasm during coitus, and psychogenic erections are almost unknown. The incidence of both erections and penetration increases for those who are reflexic incomplete.[50]

Most areflexic-complete men do not have erections of any type. The relatively small percentage who do have them, have them on a psychogenic basis. If the injury is below T12, some of the adrenergic fibers with supraspinal connections can reach the requisite organs. Success in coitus for patients who have these erections is lower than for those with reflexogenic erections. Approximately one-third of those who have successful coitus also ejaculate, albeit not forcefully. For those who are areflexic incomplete, the incidence of erections is high, with the majority also successful in coitus and approximately one-half able to ejaculate and also have orgasm.[50] Tachycardia and hypertension may occur on ejaculation particularly in those with lesions above T5 and with a tendency toward autonomic dysreflexia.

Infertility in men with SCI is primarily due to ejaculatory failure (seen in 95% of cases) and poor semen quality, particularly reduced motility.[51-53] Technological advances provide methods to retrieve sperm and bypass ejaculation problems. The most commonly successful techniques include penile vibratory stimulation in men with spinal cord lesions above T10 (80% effective) and electroejaculation by rectal probe stimulation (nearly 100% effective).[52,53] Direct sperm aspiration can also be used. Assisted reproductive techniques are subsequently performed, such as intrauterine or intravaginal insemination, and in vitro fertilization with or without intracytoplasmic sperm injection.

In women, the ability to conceive, carry, and give birth is not affected solely by the SCI. Menstruation may not be affected or may resume within 6 months to 1 year. Counseling with regard to contraception is important before the first home visit. The ability to engage in sexual activity is preserved; however, additional lubrication and alternative positioning may be needed. Arousal and sensory response depend on the level and completeness of the injury. The ability to experience an orgasmlike feeling depends on the degree of sensation that remains in the secondary erogenous zones. A physiologic increase in heart rate or blood pressure is noted, as in able-bodied women.[54]

Pregnant women with SCI typically do not experience increased risk of birth defects. Miscarriage rates are no different than they are for nondisabled women. Birth weights are within normal limits. Potential medical complications include UTI, pulmonary dysfunction, anemia, lower extremity edema, pressure ulcers, impaired mobility, constipation, and autonomic dysreflexia. Patients have an increased risk for premature labor and unattended delivery, such that weekly monitoring after 28 weeks may be recommended.[55] The type of delivery is generally determined by standard obstetric indications; however, the rate of cesarean delivery is increased over the current rate of 25% for nondisabled people in the United States.

The expression of one's sexuality after recovery from the acute effects of SCI requires, in many instances, a reorganization of one's sense of self. Sexual reintegration requires development of ways to deal with the implications of the impairments not only in the sexual act but in terms of one's overall physical appearance. In addition, sex is not only a physical act, but also a social one. The term *sexuality* can encompass how one expresses one's social role as a man or woman.

The treatment of disabilities related to sexual function illustrates to a particular degree what the characteristics of any rehabilitation program should be. It must serve to develop within the person (and partner) an ability to monitor one's own signals, to communicate one's own needs, and to continue to learn to solve problems as they arise. It is particularly important to identify the difference between goals or ends and the means or actions by which one can go about achieving them. In addition to defining one's goals as clearly as possible, it is necessary in this area of disability, as well as all others, to develop a sense of options, of alternative means by which one can accomplish one's goals whether they be sexual intimacy, siring a child, or whatever the goal may be. Being informed about what others with similar impairments have done can be helpful, but ultimately it is the sense that a range of alternatives exist that is most important. Each couple must determine what is appropriate for them.

Pain

Pain is a frequent complication of SCI. It is a complex phenomenon that causes emotional and physical stress and can stagnate the rehabilitation process. The reported incidence is quite variable, ranging from 11% to 94% of patients, often with disabling consequences, and the exact prevalence is not known. Pain is considered to be an impairment. Efforts should be devoted to reduction of the resultant functional consequences or disabilities.

Management of pain in SCI requires some basic understanding of the neuroanatomy and neurophysiology of pain perception. A full discussion is beyond the scope of this chapter. However, three main types of afferent (sensory) axons extend from the periphery (skin, muscles) and terminate in the dorsal gray matter of the spinal cord. Type A delta fibers conduct slowly and generate sharp pain, and type C fibers are nonmyelinated, conduct slowly, and carry diffuse pain. Type A beta fibers conduct quickly and carry low-intensity proprioception sensation. According to the gate control theory for pain, stimulation of large fast fibers via touch or vibration blocks small pain fibers at the first synapse level of the dorsal horn. The dorsal horn is comprised of a complex multilayered sensory processing center in which information is either inhibited or facilitated. Secondary afferents arise from the dorsal horn and project to the thalamus. Most pain fibers cross over in the spinal cord, and others that carry touch and proprioception are in the dorsal column. Tertiary afferents project from the thalamus to terminate on the somatosensory area of the cerebral cortex. Pain perception is also influenced by chemical substances in the nervous system, such as substance P, serotonin, norepinephrine, histamine, and prostaglandin-mediated and endogenous pain opiates that cause pain suppression.[56,57]

Many classifications of pain have been proposed in persons with SCI. Brittel and Mariano[57] describe the main categories of pain as follows: (1) mechanical pain with localization at the injury site; (2) radicular pain with a radiating dermatomal pattern, caused by injury to the peripheral nerve; and (3) dysesthetic pain that is perceived below the level of the lesion and is characterized by diffuse burning, stinging, and stabbing.

Determining an accurate diagnosis with localization of the pain generator allows for a more favorable treatment outcome. It is important to perform a thorough diagnostic evaluation, with a full explanation to the patient regarding the nature of pain and the available safe therapeutic interventions, reassurance, and regular physician follow-up, all of which assist in decreasing the intensity of pain and improving the patient's pain tolerance and QOL.[56,57]

The level of injury has been shown to affect the prevalence of pain, with the greatest pain complaints occurring in patients with the cauda equina syndrome followed by thoracic and then tetraplegic patients. Psychological and social factors appear to clinically affect perception of pain intensity as well as activity level. The higher the individual's activity level, the fewer complaints of pain. Depression and adjustment to disability issues are related to severe pain.[56,58] In a study by Cairns et al.,[58] a relationship between pain and depression was established. Changes in pain appeared to affect depression to a greater degree than depression affected increased pain perception. Limited social support and lack of financial resources also contributed to depression and increased complaints of pain.

Musculoskeletal Pain. Musculoskeletal or mechanical pain may be caused by acute or chronic injury to the bones, tendons, muscles, or ligaments, and typically occurs early, within days after injury. The pain is characterized as a dull ache or penetration-type pain. The location of pain may be at or above the level of injury. It may be increased by activity or prolonged activity and decreased with rest.[58] In a study by Sie et al.,[59] upper extremity pain in a population with chronic SCI occurred in 55% of tetraplegics; the shoulder was the joint that was most commonly involved. The most frequent clinical diagnoses for shoulder pain (45%) included tendonitis, bursitis, capsulitis, and osteoarthritis. Referred pain from cervical origin represented 33%. Upper extremity pain was seen in 64% of paraplegics, with the most common complaints due to carpal tunnel syndrome followed by shoulder pain. Other causes of pain at the level of the cord lesion include myofascial pain, arthritic changes, spinal instability, deformity, infections, and tumor. Appropriate therapy is based on the underlying diagnosis and may include a short course of non-narcotic medicine, trigger point injections, joint or bursa injections, soft tissue mobilization, strengthening exercises, spinal orthoses, and other modalities.[59]

Radicular Pain. Radicular pain originates from damage to the nerve roots either unilaterally or bilaterally. It has a paroxysmal, lacerating quality and is usually distributed along one or more nerve dermatomes. Patients also describe variable feelings of burning, aching, and feelings of tightness. Injury to the nerve root is variable and may be a combination of contusion, laceration, compression, and traction. Arachnoiditis due to scar formation may develop. Radicular pain appears to be more prevalent in cases of penetrating or comminuted spinal injuries compared with nontraumatic closed injury.[56,57]

Characterization of segmental pain is similar to that of radicular pain. It is due to damage of gray matter of the dorsal horn in the spinal cord with hyperactivity of the nociceptor cells.[60] Pain is usually bilateral, and distribution varies with completeness and level of injury. Incomplete injuries experience more intense severity and wider distribution. Cervical lesions present with more tingling, burning, numbness, and pain in the upper extremities. Thoracic spine lesions tend to have a squeezing tightness and pain around the thorax. Lumbar lesions have segmental pain to different parts of the lower extremities and groin. A combination of a hypersensitivity and hyperalgesic area of skin may exist at the border between normal and absent sensation.[56]

Damage to the conus medullaris, cauda equina, or both can give rise to "cauda equina" pain, which is a type of radicular or segmental pain. It is usually symmetric, with greater occurrence in incomplete lesions, and it affects the sacral dermatomes, that is, the buttocks, anus, and genitals. Burning or tingling symptoms are most common.

Central Pain. Deafferentation central pain (DCP) originates from a spinal cord or brain source. It is the most common type of pain and the most refractory to treatment. This phenomenon is seen in both complete and incomplete injured patients. It is characterized by diffuse nondermatomal pain and other sensations, such as dysesthesias (unpleasant abnormal sensation), allodynia (pain from non-noxious stimuli), and hyperpathia (exaggerated pain from noxious or non-noxious stimuli) below the neurologic level.[56,57] Other descriptive sensations include abnormal cold feeling, burning, tingling, shooting, pressure, aching, and squeezing.

The character and intensity of DCP may vary significantly. DCP is usually continuous; however, it fluctuates in frequency and intensity. Changes in weather appear to exacerbate symptoms, and DCP tends to be chronic. The actual mechanism is not clearly understood; however, the pain is thought to be due to absent sensory input and hyperexcitation of the spinal cord neurons in segments of the spinal cord at or just above the cord lesion. These neurons subsequently transmit impulses to the thalamus in the brain, which are perceived as pain.[56] Some investigators have proposed that misinterpretation of the preserved dorsal column sensation sends impulses to the thalamus, giving rise to a pain response. Deafferentation—that is, absent or impaired sensory input from the perceived pain region—is believed to change chemical substances that are important for pain perception. Substance P is depleted, which alters transmission of nerve impulses in the spinal cord and changes the concentration of catecholamines, opioid peptides, and γ-aminobutyric acid–like substances. The overall effect is increased facilitation with decreased inhibition, which allows perception of painful stimuli in supraspinal centers.

Visceral Pain. Visceral pain can occur and is usually ill defined. It is perceived to be located within the abdomen or pelvis. It may have a neuropathic or nociceptive origin, and differentiation is difficult. Potential treatable underlying etiologies must be ruled out, such as kidney or ureteral stones, cholecystitis, bowel obstruction, UTI, and bowel ischemia. With cervical and high-level thoracic lesions, signs and symptoms of abdominal pathology may be atypical in nature, such as an increase in spasticity, autonomic dysreflexia, decreased appetite, and change in bowel function. The lower the cord lesion, the more accurate are abdominal pain complaints.

Pain Management. The management of pain in individuals with SCI is often difficult. In achieving an accurate diagnosis, one must rule out and remove any factors that may be influencing the pain. The majority of patients with neurogenic pain have no specific etiology other than the initial injury. Although the degree and type of impairment may vary, even more variable is the degree to which pain may be disabling, even in the presence of similar impairment. One can define pain as causing moderate disability if it is annoying enough to use medication for relief or to modify one's behavior to relieve discomfort, such as going to bed. Severe disability due to pain is present when it is even more difficult to bear; the person is unable to divert attention from it and cannot pursue daily activities when the pain is present.

In any individual, the disabling aspects of pain and, thus, the goals of its treatment vary. For example, one person with disabling cramping pain after injury to the cauda equina was most concerned about the frequency of the episodes. Although the pain was extremely severe, it lasted for a very short time and only occurred during the day. His initial goal was to have at least 5 minutes between episodes. Only after having achieved a 20-minute interval between episodes did he begin to address the intensity of the pain as one of his concerns. Another person with an incomplete cervical lesion had pain present intermittently throughout the day but found it particularly disabling at night when it interfered with his ability to fall asleep. His goal initially was to fall asleep within 60 minutes without the need for sleep medication or alcohol. Still another person with a lesion at T12 had stabbing pain in the legs and burning pain in the buttocks. The latter was particularly troublesome. He found that he could function satisfactorily when his pain was at the level of 5/10. His goal was to have that lowered level of intensity for the several hours he needed to transact personal business.

Once one determines the goals, one can assess the proper means for achieving them. The unique character of pain is its susceptibility to modulation. Appropriate pharmacologic treatment is determined to some degree, but not entirely, by the character of the pain, considered as the impairment. In all instances, the particular medication and its dosage vary with the person in whom the pain occurs and with its specific functional consequences or the type and degree of the disabilities.

One of the first lines of intervention is to encourage activity that may decrease the perception of pain. The individual should participate in appropriate therapeutic interventions to maximize independence in ADL and mobility. Increased pain is noted with depression, poor adjustment to disability, and decreased social support. Supportive counseling and effective communication with the patient in the process of planning and ongoing review of the treatment plan is integral to effective treatment. The patient must participate defining the functional problem and goals that are meaningful and measurable. Treatment of underlying medical illness, such as constipation, spasticity, or urinary retention, may assist with decreasing pain. Pain perception may also be influenced by removal of chemical agents such as nicotine, ethanol, caffeine, and cannabis.[56] A comprehensive approach is needed.

Pharmacologic management of pain is undertaken when it interferes with overall function and mood and affects sleep, which ultimately influences QOL. Tricyclic antidepressants, such as nortriptyline and amitriptyline, are used frequently for dysesthetic and central pain. Both are nonselective inhibitors of serotonin and catecholamine uptake. The initial dosage is typically 25 mg every night; however, a 10-mg dose is recommended for the elderly. The dose is titrated upward to 50–100 mg as tolerated until the desired therapeutic goal is reached or significant side effects occur. Major side effects include sedation, dry mouth, constipation, palpitations, cardiac arrhythmias, and orthostatic hypotension. The effective dose for pain relief may vary from person to person. The effectiveness of newer antidepressants that involve the serotonin system, such as fluoxetine (Prozac), paroxetine (Paxil), and sertaline (Zoloft), for neurogenic pain in SCI is less known.[56,61]

Anticonvulsant treatment is frequently used for radicular, dysesthetic, or central pain and includes medications such as gabapentin (Neurontin), carbamazepine (Tegretol), phenytoin sodium (Dilantin), and divalproex sodium (Depakote). Gabapentin has been prescribed for neurogenic pain with some success; however, the efficacy has not been confirmed by scientific data, and the mechanism of action remains unclear. Clinically, dosages start at 300 mg per day with titration to achieve therapeutic effect or until significant side effects occur. Carbamazepine is effective in treating radicular pain with lacinating DCP-type pain. Initial dosages are 100 mg twice a day with titration to a schedule guided by pain control and side effects. Major side effects include bone marrow suppression, which necessitates periodic monitoring of white cell count. The mechanism of action involves suppression of neuronal transmission by altering sodium conduction. Phenytoin has been used, although less effectively than carbamazepine. Divalproex sodium has had limited success with treatment of pain, and its major side effect is liver failure.[57]

Still another level of analysis is necessary to define the elements of any effective program for persons with chronic pain. The element of suffering is the additional component. One cannot separate the person who is experiencing the suffering related to the pain from either the definition of the disability or the goals, as in the several cases cited. Even more important can be participation by the patient in helping to define the actions by which the problem is solved. Chapter 11 illustrates the application of these principles to the management of other sources of chronic pain. Medication can become far more effective as part of an approach that seeks to develop in the person with chronic pain the ability to manage the self—to monitor the body and to implement strategies on a more immediate basis.

Spasticity

Spasticity is a common occurrence in persons with SCI lesions above the conus medullaris. The management of spasticity can be clarified by distinguishing between the impairments based on the neurologic examination and the disabilities as defined with the aid of the person with SCI. It is defined as a motor disorder, characterized by a velocity-dependent increase in tonic stretch reflexes with exaggerated tendon jerks, resulting from hyperexcitability of the stretch reflex.[62] However, the major disabilities that result from the loss of supraspinal controls can be attributed to the disinhibition of flexor reflexes in the lower limbs rather than the disinhibition of the stretch reflex.

Flexor reflex afferents are no longer subject to tonic inhibition from the brain stem by the dorsal reticulospinal pathways. The Babinski-type response is associated with isolation of this tract from supraspinal control. The resulting disabilities described by persons with SCI are problems such as trouble in maintaining sitting balance in the wheelchair, interference with transfer, or difficulty in maintaining control of a powered chair. The signs of spasticity found on neurologic examination that reflect disinhibition of the stretch reflex do not necessarily relate to those problems.

What is particularly relevant is the change in the response to noxious cutaneous stimuli. The normal flexion response of withdrawal to cutaneous stimuli in the lower extremity has its threshold reduced and its receptive field enlarged. After SCI, brisk flexor reflexes are produced by more natural non-noxious stimuli that do not produce flexor movements in normal subjects. *Spasms* is the term used by patients to describe the overwhelming quality of the response. They arise from spinal afferent input because they are abolished by dorsal rhizotomy. Their frequency is much higher when the limb is a site for a pressure sore or other source of noxious stimuli even in the absence of any awareness of pain.

In evaluating an SCI patient with spasticity, one must bear in mind that all spasticity need not be treated. Some beneficial effects of spasticity include an increase in muscle bulk, assistance in regulating bowel function by maintaining tone in the external sphincter, decreased osteopenia, and aid in performing standing pivot transfers or ambulation by way of extensor spasms in the lower extremities. Gross hand grip, which is needed for picking up objects or grooming, may be facilitated by finger flexor spasms.

On the other hand, the presence of spasticity can create some functional disadvantages that are quite disabling to the individual. Involuntary movement and painful spasms can interfere with the ability to perform daily living skills, such as dressing, grooming, and transfers. Prolonged spasms can lead to abnormal posturing, which contributes to joint contracture, pressure ulcer formation, and impaired perianal hygiene. Increased urethral sphincter tone can facilitate the development of hydronephrosis and renal damage. Severe paroxysmal spasms can cause a person to fall from a chair or bed. A change in spasticity can act as a diagnostic tool. It may represent an underlying new noxious stimuli, such as UTIs, urethral stones, pressure ulceration, bowel impaction, or acute abdomen. Other potential areas of involvement include DVT, heterotropic ossification, tight clothing, or secondary lesions, such as tumors and spinal stenosis.

Some common indications for treatment are (1) spasticity that prevents or interferes with the ability to perform daily living skills, such as driving, transfers, and dressing; (2) painful spasms that interfere with movement or activities; and (3) spasticity that interferes with sleep. The major goals of treatment are to relieve pain or discomfort and to improve function. The patient must also be an integral part of the planning and treatment team. Educating the patient as to the etiology of spasticity, the advantages and disadvantages of spasticity, and preventive management to reduce the underlying medical complications and understand the treatment options available is crucial. Clear functional goals for treatment of spasticity should

be identified. Clinical improvement in spasticity does not always correlate with improved function. Significant weakness often underlies spasticity, and the overall level of function will not change drastically.

As an example, a 40-year-old woman had a history of multiple thoracic spine surgeries for chronic pain and kyphoscoliosis, with resultant incomplete paraplegia after failed back surgery. She presented with moderate to severe spasticity despite intensive therapeutic intervention and a combination of baclofen and clonidine therapy. A multiple drug regimen with antiepileptics, tricyclic antidepressants, and narcotics as limited additional oral medication was prescribed for management of spasticity. Motor control in the lower extremities was dominated by increased extensor tone and significant underlying weakness in the 1–2/5 range, especially in the proximal muscles. She was independent at the wheelchair level for mobility and daily living skills. Discussion with the patient revealed her goal of functional ambulation. Even with modest control of spasticity, her ambulation would be limited to short distances at best, given her extent of weakness. This dialogue with the patient and treatment team was crucial in further clarifying the approach to treatment of spasticity.

The mainstay of treatment for SCI patients with spasticity is sustained stretching techniques, which are taught to the patient and his or her caregiver. Positioning in inhibitory postures has been shown to reduce spasticity and maintain proper body alignment. For example, positioning in the wheelchair with the hips and knees fully flexed to 90 degrees can decrease extensor tone patterns, maintain comfortable postural alignment, and facilitate more normal patterns of movement. Other physical modalities, such as heat, cold, vibration, electrical stimulation, therapeutic exercise, and splinting, are incorporated by the therapist. Ultimately, any of these modalities and exercises can best be accomplished with the patient collaborating in their use.

Pharmacologic treatment with oral agents is added if therapeutic treatment is limited or ineffective in relieving generalized spasticity. Efficacy of treatment is assessed by clinical and functional evaluation as well as by economic considerations. Functional improvement is the most important element. Common agents act either centrally or peripherally to influence the stretch reflex. Medications used include baclofen, benzodiazepines, tizanidine, clonidine, and dantrolene sodium. These agents can be used alone or in combination. The choice of agent should be based on patient clinical presentation, cost, and the side effect profile of the medication. The following case illustrates improving effectiveness while lowering the cost in terms of medication and its side effects and also illustrates the frequent association of pain and spasms.

A 33-year-old man with a long-standing lesion at T5 had recent worsening of long-term pain in the back starting at the level of his spinal fusion. Pain was almost always present but was intermittently more severe. If this pain lasted as long as 60 seconds, it would then be followed by spasm of the abdominal muscles and lower extremities. The spasms interfered with sitting in his wheelchair and would awaken him at night. He was unable to get out of the house because of these difficulties, despite the ingestion of 60 mg diazepam each day in divided doses. His initial goal was to feel well enough to go outdoors without taking any more diazepam than he already was taking.

One month later, the patient reported that he had met his goal on 3 days. On those days, the pain did not last as long as usual and therefore did not result in spasms. He noted that what may have helped was a feeling that his back became looser after he heard a popping sound while carrying out his ordinary stretching routine. He had been following a prescribed daily 10 repetitions with use of a 140-lb weight. His goal now was to increase the number of days in which he was able to go out while simultaneously reducing the total dose of diazepam to 45 mg per day. He also agreed to continue to use the stretching exercises because they seemed to be helpful and to try to achieve the popping sound several times each day.

At the end of the next month, the patient reported 8 days, several in a row, in which he had done well enough to go outdoors. Pain was lasting as little as 15 seconds, and the spasms did not occur. He had added ice rubs to his treatment to numb the area in his back from which the pain seemed to arise when he was awakened at night. He continued to use the stretching exercise several times each day, seeking to achieve the popping sound he had associated with good results.

Over the next several months, the patient had an increasing number of good days, as many as 20

each month. He continued to use the ice cubes but on a more regular basis. On those occasions when he had been sitting up all day, he would use ice at night before going to sleep to reduce the number of times he would need to use it after being awakened. He also modified his stretching exercises to perform them with a lesser weight and at a time when he began to feel pain during the day. He was also able to reduce the dosage of diazepam to 20 mg per day.

Although these procedures were not new, they had become far more effective as measured by the number of days he was able to go out and by the reduced dose of medication. He was able to develop a more fine-tuned use of both the ice and the stretching in response to his becoming better able to monitor his results.

Localized spasticity can be treated with local injections to targeted muscles or small muscle groups. These injections can be combined with physical modalities and splinting and serial casting techniques. Beneficial effects include limiting the risks of systemic side effects, improving specific functional skills, and reducing muscle contracture and local pain as well as facilitating hygienic care.

Botulinum toxin is a neuromuscular blocking agent that is injected into the end plate zone of a muscle.[63] It blocks and inhibits the release of acetylcholine from presynaptic motor axons, causing a reversible denervation atrophy. The degree of denervation is determined by the dose and volume of medicine injected. Local muscle weakness results, and effects may be seen after 48–72 hours. The clinical effect may last up to 2–6 months as a result of axon sprouting and reinnervation. Advantages include ease of injection, short duration of action, and no significant pain or dysesthesia. Botulinum toxin allows treatment of isolated spastic muscle groups while preserving areas in which increased muscle tone is beneficial for function. The primary side effect is weakness, and cost may limit frequency of use.

Local injection of alcohol or phenol into the nerve has been used to cause axonal destruction and demyelination. It generally produces an effect of variable duration that is incompletely reversible. A common side effect with mixed sensorimotor nerve blocks is the development of dysesthetic pain. This usually resolves within a few weeks. Motor point blocks avoid this complication and may include transient side effects, such as muscle pain, swelling, and muscle nodules.

Neurosurgical intervention can be considered for patients who have a poor response or intolerance to oral antispasmodic medications. Most notably, an implantable intrathecal baclofen pump is available for treatment in SCI patients with severe spasticity. Baclofen is delivered directly to its site of action via intrathecal administration. Systemic side effects are minimized. The major benefit is the ability to titrate medication dosage to fit the needs of the patient. Oral baclofen is gradually reduced after implantation to decrease the risk of hallucinations and seizures. Potential complications include pump, battery, or catheter failure and infection, with the need for surgical intervention for pump, catheter, or battery removal or replacement.

Heterotopic Ossification

Neurogenic heterotopic ossification (HO) is a condition in which mature lamellar bone is laid down in soft tissues adjacent to neurologically affected joints. The actual etiology is unknown; however, it is proposed that mesenchymal cells are transformed into osteoblasts. It forms below the level of spine lesion in complete and incomplete SCIs. The most common site is at the hip, followed by the knee, shoulder, and elbow. Signs and symptoms in the acute phase include loss of range of motion, pain, unilateral leg swelling, erythema, fever, and local inflammation. The interval between the SCI and onset of HO ranges from 4 to 12 weeks, with peak occurrence at 2 months. Differential diagnosis includes thrombophlebitis, abscess, hematoma, unrecognized fracture, osteomyelitis, neoplasm, and cellulitis. Of these, DVT is the most serious condition to be ruled out because it can mimic or coexist with HO. In the chronic phase of the disease, pain and stiffness may be the only sign or symptom. Ankylosis of the joint was reported in 5% of cases.

Diagnosis is suggestive with elevated serum alkaline phosphatase, which occurs after 3 weeks along with limited range of motion and pain in the joint. Phase I of a three-phase bone scan permits early diagnosis of HO within 2–4 weeks. Ultrasonography may provide earlier diagnosis than an x-ray and can be used to differentiate HO from a DVT or abscess. Plain x-ray films become positive in 4–6 weeks after clinical presentation. Conservative treatment involves early active and passive range-of-motion exercises. Etidronate disodium has been effective in reducing the extensiveness of HO as long as treatment is given. It delays the mineralization of osteoid but has no significant effect on already formed HO. Nonsteroidal anti-inflammatory drugs such as indomethacin can be helpful. Surgical resection and radiotherapy can be considered only once bone matures and the HO limits a patient's functional mobility.[64]

The nature of the problem in the management of persons with SCI lies in the severity of the impairments and their extent. The level of injury and the transverse extent are the major determinants of severity. Injury to the sensory and motor systems affects the ability to carry out basic human functions such as mobility and ADL but also frequently extends to the excretion of bodily wastes, maintenance of skin integrity, and sexuality. The nature of the problem faced by these persons is also the result of their gender and relative youth and the extent to which the injury is the result of trauma and violence. The opportunities for leading a long and healthy life require management of medical problems that can lead to illness and early death. A fruitful and satisfying QOL requires major changes in priorities and the development of new organizational skills. The greatest opportunity for such to occur is based on health care that provides continuity of broad-based comprehensive care in a fashion that recognizes and reinforces the ability of the person to become his or her own self-manager. The next section in this chapter illustrates some methods used to bring this about.

Character of the Solution

Overall Plan

The organization of this chapter is analogous to the planning process exemplified throughout this book. In working with any patient, after identification of the problem comes the plan for the design of a treatment program. The identification of the problems caused by SCI, as described in the previous section, can now provide the basis for the appropriate design of services. Four principles underlie the design. First, management of people with a chronic neurologic illness such as SCI requires continuity of care. As aging occurs, new problems arise. Second, the process of planning care is a collaborative one in which the patient learns to be proactive in his or her health care. It involves identification of problems, establishment of goals, and formation of activities to reach the goal along with a time line for ongoing evaluation, review, and revision as needed. This approach is described in detail in Chapter 2. Third, individuals with SCI also require a comprehensive range of services that deal not only with the physical and medical needs but also with the psychosocial aspects as well. Maintenance of the relationship with the caregiver is frequently essential for ongoing community living. Fourth, one must seek to optimize the results achieved with concern for costs. What is ultimately cost-effective is an approach that seeks to involve the patient in his or her own care, particularly as it relates to the maintenance of health. This section illustrates the application of each of these principles.

Continuity of Care

Recovery from SCI is a lifelong process. It includes three major phases of recovery of varying lengths. In each stage the problems differ, and, thus, the goals and the methods differ as well. One variable is the frequency and intensity of the contributions by the professional versus the patient and family both in the planning and the treatment process. During these various stages, the opportunity is present for development of the patient's ability to grow in his or her own management.

The *initial acute care phase* primarily involves medical and neurologic stabilization and lasts from a few days to a few weeks. The primary goal is to limit the degree of injury and impairment. In relation to the evolution of the role of the patient versus the professional, it is the latter who is primarily responsible for the definition of the problem and design of the treatment plan. The patients with SCI and their families have the opportunity to be kept informed about their status and to consent to any treatment plan. The sources of information are the neurologic assessment and other methods in which the patient is a relatively passive participant.

The *rehabilitation phase* may last for weeks to months. A major goal at this time is to reduce the degree of disability and retrain the individual in preparation for community reintegration. The goal of information collection becomes the identification of problems in terms of the person rather than the impairments as measured by the neurologic assessment of the professional. Identifying the character of the disabilities requires a contribution by the patient and family.

Any particular impairment such as paraplegia can have substantially different consequences for different people. One man mentioned his concern about being able to keep up with other members of his family when they went out together. Another man mentioned his concern about being able to go fishing in a boat. Still another man, with a similar level of injury and degree of weakness, was far more concerned about his appearance. He was worried about having to use a cane or appear otherwise impaired. His disability arose from his sense of being different from the way he was before his injury. Although the neurologic findings were similar, the significance of those findings to each individual was unique.

The success of any restorative program depends on the extent that it helps each person to deal with his or her specific concerns. Unlike the neurologic assessment in the hands of the professional who is seeking objective data, the assessment that leads to the design of a rehabilitation plan seeks subjective data. By identifying the problem in terms that are meaningful to the individual, each person can then participate in setting goals that he or she is more likely committed to achieving. The goals for training during this rehabilitation phase include the ability to conduct one's life by the use of assistive devices and alternative ways of doing things using what remains unimpaired. A primary objective in persons with SCI must be training in the methods of prevention of medical illness that can interfere with the ability to maintain a quality life.

Major recovery from impairments usually occurs within 6 months. During this time, a new plan is established to facilitate the next phase after discharge from rehabilitation care. As a result of major adjustment issues related to the injury, premorbid antisocial behavior, and significant residual disability, some patients resist the routine structure and interaction with health professionals to reach appropriate goals during the rehabilitation phase. Consequently, the rehabilitation physician and team often need to expand their traditional training to incorporate treatment approaches that are more relevant to the patient's sociocultural reality. A better understanding of the psychosocial issues and team flexibility are crucial in establishing a true partnership for long-term care.

The following case illustrates the complexity that must be dealt with during the rehabilitation phase. A 19-year-old man sustained a C3 ASIA A tetraplegia with ventilator dependency as a result of a gunshot wound. Multiple medical complications developed during his acute care and rehabilitation hospitalization, including pneumonia, severe spasticity, heterotopic ossification, joint contractures, pressure ulcers, and depression. He frequently refused attempts by the rehabilitation team to perform passive range of motion, facilitate seating times, and take medication at scheduled times. Family training attempts were strained by multiple child care needs for his single mother and lack of transportation. The secondary caregiver (his aunt) was unable to continue because of the violent death of her son. This was a devastating blow to the patient. To maintain participation in the rehabilitation process, the physical therapist and the occupational therapist accompanied him to the funeral and provided the supportive care: ventilator management, suctioning, mobility, and self-care support.

Individual psychological counseling was implemented. First, a supportive approach was used with the goal of helping the patient overcome or at least manage the grief associated with the loss of most of his physical functions. Because he had significant medical setbacks and limited premorbid support resources, this process took an extended length of time and had to be reinstituted periodically.

Second, an ego-strengthening approach was used with the goal of helping the patient to identify and accept positive social role functions that he could still fulfill. Key among these was his role as a father to his young son, whose mother was also a teenager with limited knowledge of parenting and child development issues.

Third, an insight-oriented approach was used with the goal of helping the patient understand some of the premorbid issues that contributed to his injury, including choices he made that increased the chances for the type of violence to which he was exposed. This was also done to help the patient make more choices in the future, such as choosing to be an active participant in his son's life and social development and avoiding the repetition of the fatherless existence he knew as a child.

Finally, a behavioral approach was used with the goal of increasing the patient's consistent compliance with rehabilitation goals. This was difficult to implement to a significant degree because of the few enjoyable activities (e.g., television time, outdoor time) that could be made contingent on his compliance.

A behavioral contract was instituted late in the patient's stay (approximately 3–4 weeks before discharge) when it became evident that the patient's medical status was fairly stable, and the critical obstacle to discharge home was family training and the patient's inconsistent compliance with nursing care (e.g., turning, bowel and bladder program, and rehabilitation tasks such as getting out of bed to the wheelchair, range-of-motion exercises) that would be necessary to maintain physical and medical stability at home. Through discussions with the patient, it became clear that he harbored some resentment toward family members (e.g., his mother) for not coming in on a regular basis for psychosocial and physical support. The contract hinged on the possibility that the patient would be forced to go to a nursing home if family training was not completed. This was discussed fully with the patient and his mother.

The components of the contract involved the following:

1. The primary patient behaviors included awakening by a reasonable time to be washed, fed, and ready for therapeutic range of motion by midmorning followed by being placed in his wheelchair for progressively longer sitting periods.
2. Family behaviors included having the patient's adult cousin arrive at agreed-on times to learn nursing care procedures, range of motion, turning, and transfer techniques. Training of this secondary caregiver was a requirement by the home care agency as a condition of acceptance of the case.
3. Team behaviors included ensuring that consistent staff would be available to provide the patient with the nursing and therapy tasks mentioned previously and to supply the training described above to his cousin. In addition, assurance of

home care services was to be arranged, and acquisition of necessary durable medical equipment for discharge home would be arranged.

Although imperfect, the contract/agreement, bolstered by the team's previous allowance and support of the patient's attendance at a relative's funeral, gave the patient the sense that his efforts and compliance would result in his desired goal of returning home, where he could enjoy some semblance of normalcy and have some hope of reestablishing previously enjoyable and potentially positive social role functions. For the most part, he complied with training and therapeutic tasks, and his cousin was consistent in attending training sessions. Close to the team's projection, he was discharged home within a reasonable period after institution of the contract/agreement.

The *continuing care phase* lasts for the lifetime of the patient. With increased longevity, issues of superimposed medical illness extend beyond those that are directly related to the SCI. Crucial to this phase is the patient's ability to be sufficiently knowledgeable to avoid regression of functional level and the ability to carry out a self-directed program with limited supervisory intervention from the therapist or rehabilitation physician. The goal is to maintain an optimal level of function, reduce further impairment or recurrent illness, and maintain a supportive system that is conducive to successful community living. The major problems during this continuing care phase are the prevention of intercurrent illness and dealing with the depression and withdrawal from community living that occur.

The following case illustrates the changes in the character of the problems faced. A 50-year-old woman presented with a left C5 Brown-Séquard's syndrome that resulted from a stab wound to the posterior cervical spine. She underwent a left C4 laminotomy and dural repair. She remained in acute care for 5 days and subsequently transferred to the inpatient rehabilitation hospital. There she received intensive physical therapy and occupational therapy treatments as well as vocational rehabilitation evaluation, because her prior job was as a cook. She progressed in neurologic recovery and regained functional motor control of the left lower extremity with the use of an ankle foot orthosis for ambulation. Her left upper extremity, however, continued to display significant deficits.

Functional use of her left lower extremity was limited to gross control of her elbow flexion muscles. She remained an inpatient for approximately $3^{1}/_{2}$ weeks, and at discharge she was independent for feeding and grooming with one-handed techniques but required supervision for bathing and dressing. She was independent for bed mobility, transfers, and ambulation, using a single-point cane.

The early continued care phase consisted of outpatient medical follow-up at least once a month while the patient received ongoing physical therapy for mobility and gait training and occupational therapy for homemaking skills, splinting, and range of motion to the left upper extremity. Subsequent development of focal spasticity in the left upper extremity necessitated botulinum toxin injection on two occasions followed by serial casting to improve range of motion at the elbow. Because the patient was no longer participating in an active outpatient program by then, a home program that she can carry out on her own was added to maintain her functional status.

The frequency of ongoing medical follow-up depended on whether active medical or rehabilitation issues continued to exist. During her first year, she was seen once a month; then the transition was to every other month and then every 6 months as needed. Her long-term issues centered around orthotic management, maintaining functional range of motion and independence with ADL. She will continue to need further local treatment for spasticity management in the left upper extremity and must address return-to-work issues with vocational rehabilitation intervention. This case illustrates the importance of continuity of care with appropriate reassessment along the continuum while the patient recovers from this incomplete SCI.

Another example of the importance of continuity of care and of how limited patient participation can affect health outcomes is illustrated in the next example.

A young adolescent boy sustained a spinal cord infarct that resulted in T4 paraplegia. He underwent comprehensive inpatient rehabilitation for approximately 3 weeks. The hospital course was significant for treatment of recurrent UTI. Although he achieved independence in basic mobility and ADL at the wheelchair level, he did not achieve full independence with bowel, bladder, and skin management. He tended to rely significantly on his caregiver (mother) for assistance in these areas. He did not develop ownership over his bodily functions and remained resistant in assuming responsibility in these areas. This was further complicated by major unrelated family issues that affected his emotional state and sense of security.

After discharge home, the patient experienced a major interruption in consistent caregiver support, and he became emotionally withdrawn, which resulted in multiple complications. He required treatment for recurrent UTI and viral flulike symptoms. Severe spasticity in the bilateral lower extremities developed in the presence of underlying heterotopic ossification followed by hip flexion contractures. The limited range of motion in the hip limited his ability to lie prone and contributed to superficial ulcers over the knee. A stage III sacral pressure ulcer formed as a result of inadequate pressure relief and prolonged sitting on surfaces other than his wheelchair cushion in a slouched position. Subsequent bed rest resulted in bilateral stage II–III trochanteric ulcers.

This case illustrates that successful community reintegration remains a formidable challenge for people with SCI. A smooth transition to the community requires these patients to learn organizational and communication skills to navigate the health care system to manage their changing medical needs. They must become knowledgeable managers of their bodily functions and recognize early signs and symptoms of medical problems and develop strategies to manage them. It is important to learn how to avoid predictable problems and to know when to obtain professional consultation. Appropriate psychological support to assist in adjusting to the disability cannot be overemphasized. The ability to problem solve at multiple levels, to manage caregivers, and to apply compensatory strategies to varied, less predictable community settings is key to successful independent living.

Comprehensive Care

An interdisciplinary team approach is required to implement a comprehensive range of services to manage a person with SCI. The active members of the rehabilitation team vary, depending on the phase of recovery that a person is undergoing, which, in turn, is influenced by the severity and extent of the problems. The medical and health issues are greatest in the acute rehabilitation phase. The interdisciplinary team usually consists of a physician and nurse and physical and occupational therapists who deal with mobility and daily living skills. Speech and language therapists are typically involved for dysphagia or cognitive issues, or both, as well as for speech and language issues related to prolonged tracheostomy management. Psychological services are crucial in the acute rehabilitation phase to deal with adjustment issues related to disability as well as with cognitive problems if concomitant TBI is present. Psychologists also assist with patient-caregiver–related issues to promote continuity of care. Social workers and rehabilitation care coordinators are instrumental in implementing plans for the subsequent return to community living.

The comprehensive care process begins early in the acute care phase and continues with the greatest intensity in the rehabilitation phase. The family, friends, and caregiver are involved in the rehabilitation planning stages from the beginning. During this process of patient participation, the ability of the patient to self-manage his or her functional rehabilitation and health promotion is fostered. This is further illustrated by the following example.

A 30-year-old man sustained C4 tetraplegia ASIA B after a sports-related injury. He had a C5 fracture with retropulsion of bony segments into the spinal canal and subsequently underwent C5 corpectomy, fusion of C4–6, and a diskectomy at C4–5 and C5–6. On admission to the inpatient rehabilitation hospital, comprehensive evaluation and treatment were initiated by the team, which included a physiatrist, a physical therapist, an occupational therapist, and a psychologist. The patient was maintained in a semirigid collar for immobilization until cleared by neurosurgery. Due to his high-level injury with inherent respiratory dysfunction including poor cough and excessive pulmonary secretions, aggressive pulmonary toileting continued. He underwent pharmacologic treatment for spasticity as well as range of motion and positioning to reduce tone. The development of neuropathic pain in the extremities required pharmacologic treatment and desensitization techniques by the therapists. Despite placement of an inferior vena cava filter before admission and DVT prophylaxis with subcutaneous heparin, bilateral DVTs developed, and the patient was subsequently anticoagulated with coumadin.

Neurologically, the patient improved, with a change in neurologic classification to ASIA C, that is, motor-incomplete status. He underwent intensive training in health promotion by the rehabilitation nurse, including training in bowel, bladder, and skin management. He initially required intermittent catheterizations, which later improved to spontaneous voiding with the use of an external catheter because of limited hand function. The caregiver training with his wife was initiated within the first week of rehabilitation admission. The patient was able to direct his wife in how to perform skills such as transfers, bed positioning, and pressure relief, as well as management of his bowel, bladder, and skin program. The patient and his wife were successful in independent completion of both inhospital and out-of-hospital therapeutic passes in preparation for discharge home. The patient participated in intensive physical therapy and occupational therapy sessions with an emphasis on mobility and daily living skills. He was also involved in individual psychological counseling at least two to three times a week, and his wife attended sessions on occasion. He also participated in weekly SCI support group discussions, which allowed him to share with other spinal cord–injured patients the various concerns, adjustment issues, frustrations, and accomplishments experienced during this acute rehabilitation phase. The patient's strong religious faith and positive attitude contributed significantly to his subjective well-being despite the residual disability. This case also illustrates the major opportunity available to maintain community living despite a high-level lesion by means of family training and a comprehensive coordinated approach.

Caregiver Training Plan

Nature of the Problem

Favorable outcomes for people with SCI after discharge from rehabilitation revolve around the ability to return to the community in the least restrictive environment and to remain there. This is dependent on the degree of the disability and the caregiver's availability to provide ongoing care to compensate for the disabilities. Progress during hospitalization is linked to the ongoing social support of family and friends. The greater the support during the rehabilitation process, the better the out-

comes. Those with premorbid social isolation or dysfunctional support systems often experience poor outcomes. The patient often regresses in his or her functional status and withdraws from the rehabilitation process.

The caregiver and social support become major risk factors in prognosis and clinical management. Support systems must be identified early and integrated into the rehabilitation plan. Caregiver training focuses on all components of SCI education, including knowledge about SCI, secondary medical complications, and specific skills for mobility and ADL that can be transferred to the home setting. The process should include training in how to identify problems and find solutions on an ongoing basis. Concurrent counseling may be needed for the patient and caregiver to assist in adjusting to disability and newly established roles. These are essential elements of training for the patient and caregiver.

In dealing with the younger population with SCI, especially in urban or lower socioeconomic levels, identification of one caregiver is often difficult. The spouse or family members often have one or more jobs out of financial necessity, and child care responsibility makes it difficult to come in for training. Language and cultural barriers may further exacerbate or complicate the issue.

For example, a C4 Hispanic man who is married with three young children, one a newborn, experienced significant difficulty with the family training process. The patient lives with his brother, sister-in-law, and their children. All the adults work except for the patient's wife, who is non–English speaking and is responsible for care of all the children in the household. The newborn child had to accompany her during the training sessions, which was quite disruptive. Special arrangements also were made with the brother because he was unable to attend regularly timed sessions due to his job responsibilities.

The three major caregiver training goals include (1) basic SCI information in reference to the disease process, impairments, prognosis for recovery, and need for self-monitoring to prevent secondary medical complications; (2) skilled training in areas of mobility, ADL, and bowel, bladder, and skin management for safe function at home; and (3) problem-solving techniques to promote independence, patient advocacy, and ability to access resources in the community as needed.

Method

The caregiver component is crucial to the entire rehabilitation process and is implemented early on admission. It is one of the essential criteria to determine the appropriate level of care after injury, along with the patient's functional disability. Initially, the caregiver is given information regarding the acute rehabilitation process and SCI injury in general. During the first team conference with the patient or at the patient-family conference, the physician and rehabilitation team shares updated information on medical and rehabilitation status. The rehabilitation case manager also deals with discharge plans and the potential need for assistive devices and medical equipment. Scheduled times for caregiver training are arranged with each member of the professional rehabilitation team.

Ongoing communication is maintained between the caregiver(s) and the rehabilitation case manager to address concerns and answer questions. The caregiver(s) and the patient are encouraged to identify community resources and initiate contact. Discharge arrangements are established for medical rehabilitation follow-up, primary care evaluation for general medical care, and outpatient or home-based care for therapy or nursing treatment, or both, if indicated.

Evaluation

The caregiver training module implementation is evaluated throughout the hospital stay. The caregiver participation is documented at the team conference and the family conference and at the scheduled training sessions with the nurse and physical and occupational therapy team members. The patient's ability to direct care and the caregiver's ability to perform skills are reassessed during team conferences. This is further evaluated after a therapeutic day pass, preferably out of the hospital, in which the patient and caregiver independently practice these skills. Inhospital therapeutic passes are available, with the use of the family room as an alternative. The therapeutic pass experience is shared with the team, and the areas identified that require further training are incorporated into the rehabilitation plan. In some circumstances, a home evaluation with caregiver training is required because of unusual family circumstances, architectural barriers, and potential limited caregiver availability. During the first follow-up visit and subsequent re-evaluations, the caregiver training status is reassessed.

Cost-Effective Care

The direct costs of SCI are related to the extent of services provided and the phase of recovery. In addition, the changing health care environment necessitates appropriate allocation of resources to achieve optimal outcome. Hospital LOS for tetraplegia was greater than 6 months in the 1970s. Length of acute rehabilitation stay has been reduced significantly, from 115 to 46 days in 1997.[2] Previous studies have linked a shorter LOS with fewer complications when treatment occurred in specialized SCI units. However, economic restraints dictated by some insurance companies are challenging this concept. Alternative methods are being used to reduce rehabilitation LOS and subsequent cost per day, such as earlier discharge to outpatient or day treatment programs or initial admission to a nursing home or subacute rehabilitation. This is being observed most commonly with paraplegic patients. These choices are determined by the severity of the disability, caregiver availability, and accessibility of the home environment. Clearly defined criteria have yet to be established.

The shorter LOS can adversely affect patient education and adjustment to disability. Patients often express feelings of being overwhelmed by the amount of information being offered. Often the patient is experiencing a limited state of readiness to hear what is being conveyed. Instead of concentrating on basic issues of understanding SCI, the patient is often preoccupied with questions such as the following: Will I walk again? How will I be accepted by my family and peers? How will I make a living?

The overall goal of rehabilitation is to discharge the patient to the community with minimal disability and decreased burden of care. The continuing care phase is essential to provide ongoing medical and rehabilitation management throughout the life span of an individual to prevent reinstitutionalization. A patient-managed health promotion plan with a caregiver support component is essential to minimize recurrent medical illness, maintain a good QOL, and minimize the degree of handicap. The major opportunity for reducing costs and maintaining QOL lies in the appropriate design of training in the prevention of medical illness.

Health Promotion Plan

Nature of the Problem

People who are recovering from SCI have a high prevalence of medical symptoms and illness. Levi et al.[65] report bowel and bladder dysfunction in 41% of SCI subjects as moderate to severe life problems. The frequency of reported medical illness requires a lifelong comprehensive management approach. Avoidance of this aggressive management can lead to further impairment, disability, and handicap.

Methods

Establishment of a health promotion plan is integral to the rehabilitation process. With the inception of such a plan, the person with SCI becomes empowered and slowly develops a sense of control over the body. Goals are clearly identified, reinforced, and measured on a regular basis. Table 5-7 describes a typical plan that can be implemented during the inpatient rehabilitation phase. Similar plans can be modified for an outpatient setting as well.

In this plan, three major areas of concern are identified, including skin, bowel, and bladder management. For example, development of a pressure ulcer is a major complication in people with SCI. Pressure sores have contributed to 44% of rehospitalizations in people with SCI, with substantial costs.[66]

After discussion between the patient and the health care professional, the patient expresses agreement to pursue a management plan. The patient will know the goal and how to monitor the

Table 5-7. Spinal Cord Injury Health Promotion Module Planning Form

	Date/Time Initial TC	Date/Time TC No. 1 with Patient	Date/Time Interim TC	Date/Time Discharge Conference	Date/Time Follow-Up Postdischarge
Objectives	1. Integrate HP into IDP 2. Initiate specific first priority	1. Review and revise first priority area (skin) 2. Initiate second priority (bladder) 3. Integrate patient into IDP	1. Review and revise first and second priority areas (skin and bladder) 2. Initiate third priority area (bowel) 3. Increase patient participation	1. Review and revise all areas 2. Review and revise caregiver training by patient if tetraplegic	1. Review and revise all areas
Activities	1. Identify problem areas with patient and caregiver 2. Identify priority areas (skin, bladder, bowel) and establish mutually agreed on goals	1. Review goals and status with patient and caregiver 2. Identify what is working 3. Develop and revise goals 4. Initiate caregiver training 5. SCI education classes begin	1. Review goals and status with patient and caregiver 2. Identify what is working 3. Develop and revise goals 4. Continue caregiver training 5. SCI education classes continue until completion	1. Evaluate caregiver training 2. Retrain and reinforce skills	1. Review status of goals with patient and caregiver if tetraplegic 2. Revise goals
Evaluation	Team conference sheet Nursing database	Team conference sheet	Team conference sheet	Team conference sheet	HP questionnaire

TC = team conference; HP = health promotion; IDP = interdisciplinary plan; SCI = spinal cord injury.

goal with the assistance of the health professional. The patient will use a mirror to monitor skin integrity and keep a log to document the status of the skin and the frequency of pressure reliefs. In addition to monitoring the extent to which the goal is being accomplished by the patient, an agreement is obtained by the patient as to what techniques and methods are to be used that are effective in maintaining the goal.

Educational materials are provided in written form, and a verbal discussion is held as part of the SCI educational series, which involves a group-individual discussion. The patient learns the goal of the skin program in addition to why and how to perform pressure reliefs. He or she learns how to perform and direct proper bed and wheelchair positioning, the areas at risk for pressure sores, and the etiology of skin breakdown. The patient is also able to verbalize what to do if a pressure sore seems to be forming. A written pretest and posttest on basic skin, bowel, and bladder management are given to establish a baseline and provide feedback as to understanding of the material given. Before each team conference, a patient coordinator (rehabilitation team professional) discusses the status of the identified area and re-establishes the goal for the upcoming week. At the team conference, the patient reiterates this information, and the degree of patient participation is documented.

The patient's participation in his or her health promotion program is reinforced by all members of the rehabilitation team. This is done informally while on physician rounds or as part of the therapeutic sessions. For example, for bladder management, the patient is asked what the bladder program consists of and is expected to verbalize his or her specific bladder goal. The patient is asked the volume of urine that is obtained during catheterization and whether it is within his or her goal of management. The patient is also asked what does or does not work in attempting to keep within his or her goal of the bladder program.

Evaluation

The participation in health promotion is documented during the team conference. The criteria for the particular levels of participation are defined in Chapter 2. The patient is to discuss the current status and contributing factors in reaching a goal, and a new goal is established. Inherent in this process is the measurement of the patient's verbal participation based on the previously described scale. The patient keeps the health promotion planning form for reference at the end of the conference. A bedside log sheet is maintained and is brought with the patient at the follow-up visit.

The health promotion plan is evaluated based on three criteria. The first is the implementation of the health promotion plan with documentation on the team conference report. The second criterion includes the assessment of the degree of patient participation at the team conference and at the follow-up evaluation. The patient's long-term implementation of the health plan and the effect and reduction of medical morbidities compose the third potential level of evaluation at the time of follow-up visits.

Collaborative Care

Long-term management of people with SCI requires a collaborative relationship between the patient and medical professionals. Participatory planning on the part of the patient is an approach that can be used to facilitate follow-through of instructions or recommendations regarding care. Lack of follow-through by the patient can lead to impaired health and rising health care costs due to the development of serious medical complications, which can be prevented.

The patient is more likely to adhere to a treatment plan and follow through with treatment if an agreement has been reached between the patient and the health care provider. The better the patient is able to understand the relevance of the treatment approach, the more likely it is that he or she will engage in the process. If the treatment regimen is presented in a functional way, the patient tends to have a clearer understanding of the goals.

As an example, a 16-year-old boy sustained a C6 ASIA C (motor incomplete) tetraplegia after a diving accident. During his acute rehabilitation phase, he developed bilateral lower extremity spasticity, UTI, hyperreflexic bladder function with incontinence, neurogenic bowel, and healing of his sacral pressure ulcer.

Adjustment issues arose related to the significant residual deficits from the patient's injury, especially related to loss of bladder control. However, as early as the second team conference, the patient had the opportunity to verbalize his status and progress made for the week; he was beginning to understand how his bladder functioned and components of a bladder program. He was able to discuss issues related to his progress, such as the obvious need to learn how to direct others in performing intermittent catheterizations because he lacked sufficient arm and hand function. With assistance from the rehabilitation team, he was able to establish new goals to be accomplished for the upcoming week, that is, keeping track of his fluid intake and output and learning how to make adjustments in his program, dependent on the results. The team and the patient agreed on newly set goals. In this milieu, the patient is an active participant in the development of his or her rehabilitation program and goals. This planning process allows for re-establishment of a sense of control over one's body and life situation.

Along with the goal of minimizing the disability that arose out of the motor and sensory impairments, the rehabilitation phase must prepare the patient to enter into the long-lasting continuing care phase. A disabled person is not necessarily an ill person merely by the nature of the continued disability. The maintenance of health, however, requires a high degree of independent action, ideally with short and only intermittent interaction with health professionals. The goal is to maintain QOL. One measure is the ability to get out of the house. One can measure the degree of health by the days lost as well as the need for rehospitalization and other measures of use of health care services.

This self-management of overall health includes the identification, in collaboration with the professional, of what are appropriate criteria as to the existence of a problem that requires professional advice and intervention. For example, because skin ulceration is a major source of illness, it has been helpful for the patient and professional to agree on a criterion as to when the patient is to relieve pressure by resting in bed to the extent possible. If the ulcer continues to progress despite bed rest, the appropriate response is to proceed to seek hospitalization rather than permit the ulcer to worsen. The overall results in terms of days lost were far better than when the patient would remain at home and seek professional care only when the ulcer had reached a more severe stage. In a similar fashion, one should establish criteria for a significant change in urinary status that would require antibiotic treatment. Criteria could include changes in urine odor, pH, or frequency or difficulty in emptying.

The characteristics of spinal management may bring about not only a change in the frequency and severity of particular illnesses but also a change in the mode of presentation of any illness. It is important for the individual to become a monitor who can evaluate his or her own response to illness to aid the professional in making decisions. For example, the normal body temperature of a person with SCI may vary from the usual temperature for those without SCI. The significance of an elevation from the normal for that particular person is an important criterion that the patient can best contribute to the assessment of the existence of illness. Similarly, it is not at all uncommon for the patient to be aware of subtle changes that may be missed by the professional who is relatively unfamiliar with SCI and certainly less familiar than the patient with his or her own characteristics. One such situation is the ability to recognize the signals of bone fracture. An increase in the degree of spasticity may be the signal, or swelling in a joint may be an indication.

Another example of the value of the person with SCI contributing to his or her own management is the ability to intervene early in the course of a developing illness. For example, many persons become able to abort a UTI by increasing their fluid intake and, thus, their urinary output on the basis of any of the early signs of urinary infection that they have come to know. One man would increase his urinary output whenever he noted sweating and headache just before micturition. Another had learned to change his indwelling catheter, using as a criterion an increase in the pH of the urine that signified an increase in the concentration of pathogenic bacteria.

Measuring Effectiveness

This section replicates the general process of planning, in which this third review-evaluation step is integral to the implementation of any individual treatment plan. The management of persons with SCI requires the measurement of outcomes. The WHO model of disablement is an important and widespread standard that aids us in understanding potential outcomes after an SCI.[67] This model differentiates among three major outcome domains, including (1) impairment at the organ level (extent of sensory loss and motor paralysis), (2) degree of disability at the person level (inability to perform ADL), and (3) degree of handicap at the societal level. This section discusses a variety of the more common clinical outcome measures that are used in the presence of SCI. Each of the measures is described and evaluated in terms of its relevance for the management of persons with SCI.

Measurement of Impairment

Frankel Classification or Grade

The Frankel classification or grade was one of the earlier widely accepted systems of classifying neurologic impairment. It was introduced in 1969. Injuries were classified into four categories of quadriplegia (complete and incomplete) and paraplegia (complete and incomplete). The severity of the SCI was further subdivided into five groups, A–E. Grade A refers to motor and sensory complete, grade B to motor complete and sensory incomplete, grade C to preserved useless motor strength, grade D to preserved useful motor strength, and grade E to full recovery. The majority of the studies on neurologic outcome that compare changes from admission to discharge use the Frankel grade.

American Spinal Injury Association Impairment Scale

In response to the need for a uniform measure of SCI severity, the ASIA impairment scale replaced the Frankel grade in 1982. These international standards for neurologic classification were revised by the ASIA Committee in 1992 and endorsed by the International Medical Society of Paraplegia. The definition of neurologic levels was more precise, developing key muscles and key sensory points for use as end points in motor and sensory scores. (Details of the scale have been described in the previous section, Nature of the Impairments.)

The motor index score is a key component of the ASIA impairment scale. It has been used in studies to measure neurologic change. When clinical trials were performed with methylprednisolone,[16] 487 spinal-injured patients were studied, with 52 complete quadriplegic patients used as the control group. A 4.2 to 26.5 change was seen in the motor score at 6 months after injury. The important area of self-care function was not necessarily correlated with motor recovery.

In 1994, Waters et al.[68] showed that lower extremity ASIA motor scores strongly correlated with walking ability. Key muscles are measured in the lower extremities, and a maximum of 50 points can be scored and represent myotome levels from L2 to S1. A score of less than or equal to 20 was seen with limited ambulators, who had lower than average velocity, higher heart rate, greater peak axis load exerted on assistive devices, and greater energy expenditure than patients with lower extremity ASIA motor scores of greater than or equal to 30 who were community ambulators.[68]

Measurement of Disabilities

The primary goal of rehabilitation is to decrease disability by maximizing functional independence in performing daily living skills. The ability of a person with SCI to return to the community is significantly affected by the level of functional performance, caregiver support and availability, and the presence of an accessible environment. Determining an adequate measure of disability is important for patient care, clinical research, assistance in determining compensation, describing changes in functional status, assistance in predicting outcome, estimating amount of care required, and placement planning.[68] The following are common measures of performance that are available to assess function in people with SCI.

Functional Independence Measure

The FIM is one of the most widely used measures in rehabilitation. It was developed to provide a uniform basis for the evaluation of function in patients with a variety of disabilities. Multiple studies have shown that it has overall good reliability, validity, sensitivity, and practicality when applied to SCI patients. The functional assessments of spinal cord–injured persons have been shown to correlate well with the modified BI.[69] The index has also been used as a disability measure for SCI Model Systems databases and has been incorporated in the revision of the ASIA standards in 1996.[25]

The FIM consists of 18 items to assess self-care (eating, grooming, bathing, dressing, toilet, sphincter management, bladder management, and bowel management), mobility (transfer to bed, chair, or wheelchair; to toilet; and to tub or shower), locomotion (walking, wheelchair propulsion, and stair climbing), communication (comprehension and expression), social cognition (social interaction), and problem solving (memory) on a seven-level scale.[70] Each item is scored from 1 to 7, with the lowest rating of 1 representing total dependence and 7 representing complete independence. The measure also incorporates the extent of physical assistance, supervision, and use of adaptive equipment. For example, the score of 3 indicates moderate assistance with the patient providing 50% of the effort, a score of 5 indicates the need for supervision, and a score of 6 indicates independence with the use of aids. The patient who achieves a score of 4, which is a task that requires only 25% of physical assistance, has a greatly enhanced likelihood of returning to the community with a lesser burden of care for the caregiver.

A study by Middleton et al.[71] supports the finding that functional performance, assessed using the FIM, in people with SCI is reduced in the presence of greater neurologic impairment. However, inherent limitations are noted. The FIM cognitive subscale inadequately detects the neurocognitive sequelae of TBI as well as other cognitive aspects, such as psychological adjustment, adaptive coping style, and self-efficacy. This is especially important in patients with high tetraplegia. Second, the important ability of a patient to direct his or her care, that is, to perform or assist in tasks, is not measured. This is of key significance with high-level tetraplegic patients because they are unable to show significant gains in FIM physical function items. Third, a ceiling effect is seen in wheelchair locomotion items, that is, no difference is noted between individuals with varied neurologic levels. Most patients scored 6 regardless of whether they were paraplegic in a manual wheelchair or tetraplegic in a power wheelchair. Actual skills needed for independence in the community are not truly reflected, because the FIM score does not incorporate effects of architectural barriers, uneven surfaces such as curbs or inclines, or surface variations such as carpet thickness. A floor effect is noted on the stair item as well because most patients scored a 1 at discharge from inpatient rehabilitation.[71]

Modified Barthel Index

The modified BI (MBI) is a widely accepted 100-point scale that assesses functional ability. This scale has been shown to be sensible and reliable. Fifteen tasks are scored. Nine are self-care activities, including dressing, grooming, bathing, bowel and bladder incontinence, drinking, and feeding. The mobility subscores are composed of six mobility skills, including chair, toilet, and tub transfers; walking 50 yards; wheelchair propulsion; and stair climbing. Each task is given a numerical scale based on the level of assistance, and the patient's performance is rated as dependent, assisted, or independent.

The MBI has only three levels by which the patient can be rated for a task; therefore, it may lack sensitivity to small changes in functional status.[69] The MBI also does not include communicative and cognitive skills, and, subsequently, a person may score well on this scale but still remain unable to live alone or function socially.[72]

Spinal Cord Independence Measure

Unlike the MBI and the FIM, the spinal cord independence measure (SCIM) is a disability scale specifically for persons with SCI. Areas of function on this scale include self-care (0–20 subscore), respiration and sphincter management (0–40), and mobility (0–40). Cognitive abilities are excluded. Each functional area is evaluated and scored according to proportional weight relative to overall activity. The ultimate score falls between 0 and 100.

In a study by Catz et al.,[73] the reliability and sensitivity of the SCIM to functional changes in people with SCI were compared to those of the FIM in 30 patients. Results showed high inter-rater reliability among the multidisciplinary team members. The SCIM was found to be more sensitive than the FIM with its ability to detect all the functional changes that the FIM scoring obtained as well as an additional 26% of functional changes missed by the FIM. Some of the SCIM tasks had less impressive inter-rater reliability, and sensitivity among scores in functional changes of the SCIM and the FIM were not statistically significant. The scoring criteria for these items will most likely need to be adjusted.[73]

Quadriplegia Index of Function

In contrast to other disability measures, such as the FIM and the MBI, the Quadriplegia Index of Function (QIF) was designed specifically to measure the self-care function of persons with cervical SCI. It has been observed that tetraplegic patients in particular make small but significant functional gains during rehabilitation that may not be adequately reflected by the FIM or MBI scores. The QIF was developed in 1980 as a functional assessment tool to address this issue.

The QIF comprises 10 variables (transfers, grooming, bathing, feeding, dressing, wheelchair mobility, daily activities, bladder program, bowel program, and understanding of personal care).[74] Several items are included in each category and are scored from 0 to 4 in order of increasing independence.[75] The total category scores are weighted to obtain a final score from 0 to 100.

In addition, the QIF contains a questionnaire that samples the level of understanding about such significant health issues as respiratory function, skin care, and UTI. For example, in the last area, questions deal with signals of infection, what to do if an infection is suspected, and how to prevent infection. The use of these questions is innovative in recognizing that one of the goals of the rehabilitation phase is the ability to deal with health problems during the continuing care phase.

In a comparison study performed on 30 quadriplegic patients, the QIF was found to be more sensitive, that is, 46% improvement versus 20% improvement, compared with the BI.[74] Marino et al.[75] compared the QIF with the FIM in performing self-care skills in people with cervical SCI. The QIF feeding category had a significantly better correlate than the FIM in the upper extremity motor scores that were derived from the manual muscle test to measure neurologic function. However, both the QIF and the FIM showed significant and similar correlations to the upper extremity motor score in the bathing and grooming areas. The study suggests that further modifications of the FIM with incorporation of more sensitive portions of the QIF may be beneficial.

Measurement of Handicap and Quality of Life

In the WHO model, handicap exists when individuals with an impairment or disability are unable to fulfill one or more roles that are considered normal for their age, gender, and culture.[67] The successful outcome of persons with SCI includes the ability to fulfill the societal role and community reintegration. It is one of the three major outcome domains: impairment, disability, and handicap. However, such a classification does not realistically reflect all the important outcome domains in people with SCI.

QOL measures have increased in importance to evaluate rehabilitation program outcomes. It can be measured through the objectives that deal with impairment, disability, handicap, medical complications, survival, and health status.

Whiteneck[76] proposes two additional outcome domains to the WHO model, subjective well-being and maximizing health status. *Subjective well-being* and its synonym, *subjective QOL*, refer to the degree to which an individual has positive thoughts and feelings about his or her life experience along a continuum. An individual's subjective appraisal of the quality of his or her life may be quite different from the assessments made by others.[77] In addition, subjective well-being is not solely related to the degree of impairment and disability but appears to be more strongly related to successful community reintegration. The ability of an individual to assess his or her own satisfaction with life is believed to be an important aspect in the eventual outcome, as opposed to assessments made by researchers, clinicians, and other outsiders.[76]

Maximizing health status refers to the ability to limit the incidence of secondary complications that may occur over a lifetime. It may also encompass the survival of the person with SCI and the number of days rehospitalized as a reflection of significant illness. Achieving a favorable health status involves effective medical and psychological rehabilitation as well as the ability to provide a specialized continuum of care over a lifetime. It includes determining the individual risk for secondary illness and the potential influence of environmental factors as well.

Life Satisfaction Index A

Life satisfaction index A (LSIA) is a widely used, multi-item, 20-question scale that assesses well-being. Multiple studies that use the LSIA-A (an 18-item version of the LSIA) have shown that life satisfaction in people with SCI correlated positively with self-assessed health, perceived social support, and perceived control of one's life, expressed as a level of satisfaction with the quality and quantity of social contacts. LSIA-A scores were found to be unrelated to the degree of paralytic impairment or degree of disability with daily living activities.[77] In rating satisfaction with specific aspects of life, Furher et al.[77,78] found the highest average satisfaction ratings in families, relationships, spiritual life, and daily living tasks. Employment, sex life, and money matters were associated with the lowest satisfaction.

Multiple studies have reported conflicting findings regarding QOL because of methodologic problems such as small sample size and lack of uniform measures. For example, a study by Evans et al.[79] showed no clear evidence that rehabilitation affected QOL. Poor QOL was noted with more severe injuries. In contrast, Dijkers[80] performed a meta-analysis of 22 QOL studies in SCI. Overall, a lower subjective well-being was reported by individuals with SCI than other disabled populations. A stronger correlation was noted between QOL and handicap, whereas no statistically significant relationship was found between QOL and impairment. It was again emphasized that further research in areas of subjective QOL measures is indicated to truly reflect the person with SCI.

Boswell et al.,[81] in a qualitative study of 12 people with SCI, examined the meaning of QOL as defined by these individuals. The majority strongly agreed that QOL meant degree of satisfaction with life, that is, how close one comes to meeting life's goals. QOL was thought to be subjective and to mean different things to different people. In addition, it had a developmental component in that it changed as life priorities changed. Further research is needed to understand the impact of subjective well-being on medical rehabilitation outcome such as independence in performing ADL or preventing secondary medical complications. The three most important domains of QOL were attitude toward life, work opportunity, and level of resources.[81]

Craig Handicap Assessing and Reporting Techniques

The Craig Handicap Assessing and Reporting Techniques (CHART) was specifically designed to measure handicap. It measures all six dimensions of handicap previously identified by WHO. It uses a 100-point scale that has been normed with the general population. The CHART dimensions include cognitive independence, physical independence, ability, occupation, social integration, and economic self-sufficiency. The CHART has been found to be reliable and has been validated in spinal cord–injured individuals.[81] The cognitive independence component assesses the degree of supervision needed to perform tasks due to lower cognitive function and communication skills. The physical independence dimension is determined by the number of hours of attended care services required. The mobility component deals with the number of hours out of bed daily, days a week out of home, nights away from home, access to home independently, and use of transportation. The occupation dimension measures the number of hours spent in work, school, active homemaking for others, volunteering, recreation, and self-improvement. The social integration scale assesses romantic involvements as well as number of other people interacted with in the home and the number of regular contacts outside the home. The economic self-sufficiency scale measures total family income of all sources not used for medical care. Items in each dimension are given a weighted value, and each dimension has a maximum score of 100 points. The maximum total CHART score is 500 points, which indicates no handicap at all.[82]

References

1. Go BK, Devivo MJ, Richards JS. The Epidemiology of Spinal Cord Injury. In SL Stover, JA Delisa, G Whiteneck (eds), Spinal Cord Injury: Outcomes from the Model Systems. Gaithersburg, MD: Aspen, 1995;21–55.
2. SCI Facts and Figures at a Glance, April 1999. Birmingham, AL: National Spinal Cord Injury Statistical Center, 1999.
3. Devivo MJ, Rutt R, Black K, et al. Trends in spinal cord injury demographics and treatment outcomes between 1973 and 1986. Arch Phys Med Rehabil 1992;73:424.
4. Price C, Makintubee S, Herndon W, Istre GR. Epidemiology of traumatic spinal cord injury and acute hospitalization and rehabilitation charges for spinal cord injuries in Oklahoma, 1988–1990. Am J Epidemiol 1994;139:37.

5. Gordon S, Lewis D. Psychological challenges of drugs, violence, and spinal cord injury among African-American inner city males. SCI Psychosocial Process 1993;6:53.

6. Devivo M, Stover S. Long-Term Survival and Causes of Death. In SL Stover, JA Delisa, GG Whiteneck (eds), Spinal Cord Injury: Clinical Outcomes from the Model Systems. Gaithersburg, MD: Aspen, 1995;289–316.

7. Devivo M, Black K, Stover S. Causes of death during the first 12 years after SCI. Arch Phys Med Rehabil 1993; 74:248.

8. Krause JJ, Sternberg M. Mortality after SCI: an 11-year prospective study. Arch Phys Med Rehabil 1997;78:815.

9. Gerhart K, Bergstrom E, Charlifue S, et al. Long-term SCI: functional changes over time. Arch Phys Med Rehabil 1993;74:1030.

10. Whiteneck GG, Charlifue S, Frankel HL, et al. Mortality, morbidity and psychosocial outcomes of persons with SCI more than 20 years ago. Paraplegia 1992;30:617.

11. Menter RR, Hudson L. Effects of Age at Injury and the Aging Process. In SL Stover, JA Delisa, GG Whiteneck (eds), Spinal Cord Injury: Clinical Outcomes from the Model Systems. Gaithersburg, MD: Aspen, 1995;272–288.

12. Devivo M, Karus PL, Stover SL, Fine PR. Influence of age at the time of spinal cord injury on rehabilitation outcomes. Arch Neurol 1990;47:687.

13. Devivo M, Whiteneck G, Edgar C. The Economic Impact of Spinal Cord Injury. In SL Stover, JA Delisa, GG Whiteneck (eds), Spinal Cord Injury: Clinical Outcomes from the Model Systems. Gaithersburg, MD: Aspen, 1995; 235–271.

14. Tator CH, Fehlings MG. Review of the secondary injury theory of acute spinal cord trauma with emphasis on vascular mechanisms. J Neurosurg 1991;75:15.

15. Tator CH. Biology of neurological recovery and functional restoration after spinal cord injury. Neurosurgery 1998;42:696.

16. Bracken M, Shepard MJ, Collins WF, et al. A randomized, controlled trial of methylprednisolone or naloxone in the treatment of acute spinal cord injury. Results of the Second National Acute Spinal Cord Injury Study. N Engl J Med 1990;322:1405.

17. Bracken MB, Shepard MJ, Holford TR, et al. Administration of methylprednisolone for 24 or 48 hours or tirilizad mesylate for 48 hours in the treatment of acute spinal cord injury. Results of the Third National Acute Spinal Cord Injury Study. JAMA 1997;277:1597.

18. Ozer MN. The Management of Persons with Spinal Cord Injury. New York: Deinos, 1988;1–20.

19. Bohlman H, Ducker T, et al. Spine and Spinal Cord Injuries. In RH Rothman (ed), The Spine (3rd ed). Philadelphia: Saunders, 1992;973–1011.

20. Waters R, Adkins R, Yakura J, Sie I. Profiles of spinal cord injury and recovery after gunshot injury. Clin Ortho Related Res 1991;267:14.

21. Yoshida G, Garland D, Waters R. Gunshot wounds to the spine. Orthop Clin North Am 1995;26:109.

22. Waters R, Apple D, Meyer P, et al. Emergency and Acute Management of Spine Trauma. In SL Stover, JA Delisa, GG Whiteneck (eds), Spinal Cord Injury: Clinical Outcomes from the Model Systems. Gaithersburg, MD: Aspen, 1995; 56–78.

23. Waters R, Adkins R. The effects of removal of bullet fragments retained in the spinal canal. Spine 1991;16:934.

24. Waters R, Adkins R. Firearm versus motor vehicle related spinal cord injury: preinjury factors, injury characteristics, and initial outcome comparisons among ethnically diverse groups. Arch Phys Med Rehabil 1997;78:150.

25. Maynard FM. International Standards for Neurological and Functional Classification of Spinal Cord Injury (revised). Chicago: American Spinal Injury Association, 1996;1–26.

26. Waters R, Adkins R, Yakura J. Definition of complete spinal cord injury. Paraplegia 1991;29:573.

27. Marino R, Crozier K. Neurologic examination and functional assessment after spinal cord injury. Phys Med Rehabil Clin North Am 1992;3:829.

28. Kirshblum S, O'Connor K. Predicting neurologic recovery in traumatic cervical spinal cord injury. Arch Phys Med Rehabil 1998;79:1456.

29. Brown PJ, Marino RJ, Herbison GJ, Ditunno JF Jr. The 72-hour examination as a predictor of recovery in motor complete quadriplegia. Arch Phys Med Rehabil 1991; 72:546.

30. Ditunno J, Stover S, Freed M, et al. Motor recovery of the upper extremities in traumatic quadriplegia: a multicenter study. Arch Phys Med Rehabil 1992;73:431.

31. Penrod L, Hedge S, Ditunno J. Age effect on prognosis for functional recovery in acute, traumatic central cord syndrome. Arch Phys Med Rehabil 1990;71:963.

32. Crozier KS, Graziani V, Ditunno JF Jr, Herbison GJ. Spinal cord injury: prognosis for ambulation based on sensory examination in patients who are initially motor complete. Arch Phys Med Rehabil 1991;72:119.

33. Apple D. Spinal Cord Rehabilitation. In RH Rothman (ed), The Spine (3rd ed). Philadelphia: Saunders, 1992; 1225–1246.

34. Hartkopp A, Bronnum-Hansen H, Seidenschnur AM, Biering-Sorensen F. Suicide in a spinal cord injury population: its relation to functional status. Arch Phys Med Rehabil 1998;79:1356.

35. Depression Following Spinal Cord Injury: A Clinical Practice Guideline for Primary Care Physicians. In Paralyzed Veterans of America, Clinical Practice Guidelines, Spinal Cord Medicine. Washington, DC: Paralyzed Veterans of America, 1997;8–30.

36. Weitzenkamp DA, Gerhart KA, Charlifue SW, et al. Spouses of spinal cord injury survivors: the added impact of caregiving. Arch Phys Med Rehabil 1997;78:822.

37. Ragnarsson K, Hall K, Wilmot C, Carter CR. Management of Pulmonary, Cardiovascular, and Metabolic Conditions after Spinal Cord Injury. In SL Stover, JA Delisa, GG Whiteneck (eds), Spinal Cord Injury: Clinical Outcomes from the Model Systems. Gaithersburg, MD: Aspen, 1995;79–99.

38. Paralyzed Veterans of America. Prevention of Thromboembolism in Spinal Cord Injury. In Paralyzed Veterans of America, Clinical Practice Guidelines, Spinal Cord Medicine. Washington, DC: Paralyzed Veterans of America, 1997;1–14.

39. DeVivo M, Stover S. Long-Term Survival and Causes of Death. In SL Stover, JA Delisa, GG Whiteneck (eds), Spinal Cord Injury: Clinical Outcomes from the Model Systems. Gaithersburg, MD: Aspen, 1995;289–316.

40. Paralyzed Veterans of America. Acute Management of Autonomic Dysreflexia: Adults with Spinal Cord Injury Presenting to Health-Care Facilities. In Paralyzed Veterans of America, Clinical Practice Guidelines, Spinal Cord Medicine. Washington, DC: Paralyzed Veterans of America, 1997;4–12.

41. Yarkony G. Pressure ulcers: a review. Arch Phys Med Rehabil 1994;75:908.

42. Yarkony G, Heineman A. Pressure Ulcers. In SL Stover, JA Delisa, GG Whiteneck (eds), Spinal Cord Injury: Clin-

ical Outcomes from the Model Systems. Gaithersburg, MD: Aspen, 1995;100–119.

43. Cardenas D, Hooton T. Urinary tract infection in persons with spinal cord injury. Arch Phys Med Rehabil 1995; 76:272.

44. Cardenas D, Mayo M, King J. Urinary Tract and Bowel Management in the Rehabilitation Setting. In R Braddom (ed), Physical Medicine and Rehabilitation. Philadelphia: Saunders, 1996.

45. Selzman A, Hampel N. Urologic complication of spinal cord injury. Urol Clin North Am 1993;20:453.

46. Levi R, Hultling C, Nash MS, Seiger A. The Stockholm Spinal Cord Injury Study. 1. Medical problems in a regional SCI population. Paraplegia 1995;33:308.

47. Menter R, Weitzenkamp D, Cooper D, et al. Bowel management outcomes in individuals with long-term spinal cord injuries. Spinal Cord 1997;35:608.

48. Paralyzed Veterans of America. Neurogenic Bowel Management in Adults with Spinal Cord Injury. Consortium for Spinal Cord Medicine, Paralyzed Veterans of America. Washington, DC: Paralyzed Veterans of America, 1998;8–30.

49. Stiens SA, Bergman SB, Goetz LL. Neurogenic bowel dysfunction after spinal cord injury: clinical evaluation and rehabilitative management. Arch Phys Med Rehabil 1997;78:86.

50. Comarr AE. Sexual concepts in traumatic cord and cauda equina lesions. J Urol 1971;106:375.

51. Lisenmyer T, Perkash I. Infertility in men with spinal cord injury. Arch Phys Med Rehabil 1991;72:747.

52. Sønksen J, Sommer P, Biering-Sørenson F, et al. Pregnancy after assisted ejaculation procedures in men with spinal cord injury. Arch Phys Med Rehabil 1997;78:1059.

53. Seager SWJ, Halstead L. Fertility options and success after spinal cord injury. Urol Clin North Am 1993;20:543.

54. Sipski M, Craig JA, Rosen R. Physiological parameters associated with psychogenic sexual arousal in women with complete spinal cord injuries. Arch Phys Med Rehabil 1995;76:811.

55. Baker E, Cardenas D. Pregnancy in spinal cord injured women. Arch Phys Med Rehabil 1996;77:501.

56. Ragnarsson KT. Management of pain in persons with spinal cord injury. Spinal Cord Med 1997;20:186.

57. Brittel CW, Mariano AJ. Chronic pain in spinal cord injury. Phys Med Rehabil 1991;5:71

58. Cairns DM, Adkins RH, Scott MD. Pain and depression in acute traumatic spinal cord injury. origins of chronic problematic pain. Arch Phys Med Rehabil 1996;77:329.

59. Sie IH, Waters RL, Adkins RH, Gellman H. Upper extremity pain in the post-rehabilitation spinal cord injured patient. Arch Phys Med Rehabil 1992;73:44.

60. Nashold BS Jr, Bullit E. Dorsal root entry zone lesions to control central pain in paraplegics. J Neurosurg 1981; 55: 414.

61. Sandford PR, Lindblom LB, Haddox JD. Amitriptyline and carbamazepine in the treatment of dysesthetic pain in spinal cord injury. Arch Phys Med Rehabil 1992;73:300.

62. Stolov WC. The concept of normal muscle tone, hypotonia and hypertonia. Arch Phys Med Rehabil 1966;47:156.

63. Brin M. Botulinum toxin: chemistry, pharmacology, toxicity and immunology. Muscle Nerve 1997;6(suppl):S146.

64. Garland D. A clincial perspective on common forms of acquired heterotropic ossification. Clin Orthop 1991;263: 13–29.

65. Levi R, Hultling C, Nash MS, Seiger A. The Stockholm Spinal Cord Injury Study. 1. Medical problems in a regional SCI population. Paraplegia 1995;33:308.

66. Frost F, Lee S, Simmons A. The true cost of spinal cord injury and comorbidity analysis in 131 acute hospital readmissions (abstract). J Am Paraplegia Soc 1993; 16:92.

67. World Health Organization International Classification of Impairments, Disabilities and Handicaps: A Manual of Classification Relating to the Consequences of Disease. Geneva: World Health Organization, 1980.

68. Waters RL, Adkins R, Yakura J, Vigil D. Prediction of ambulatory performance based on motor scores derived from standards of the American Spinal Injury Association. Arch Phys Med Rehabil 1994;72:756.

69. Roth E, Davidoff G, Haughton J, Arden M. Functional assessment in spinal cord injury: a comparison of the modified Barthel index and the "adapted" functional independence measure. Clin Rehab 1990;4:227.

70. Heinemann AW, Linacre JM, Wright BD, et al. Relationships between impairment and physical disability as measured by the functional independence measure. Arch Phys Med Rehabil 1993;74:566.

71. Middleton J, Truman G, Geraghty T. Neurological level effect on the discharge functional status of spinal cord injured persons after rehabilitation. Arch Phys Med Rehabil 1998;79:142.

72. Grey N, Kennedy P. The functional independence measure: a comparative study of clinician and self-rating. Paraplegia 1993;31:457.

73. Catz A, Itzkovich M, Ring H, Tamir A. SCIM—spinal cord independence measure: a new disability scale for patients with spinal cord lesions. Spinal Cord 1997;35:850.

74. Gresham GE, Labi MLC, Dittman SS, et al. The quadriplegia index of function (QIF): sensitivity and reliability demonstrated in a study of thirty quadriplegic patients. Paraplegia 1986;24:38.

75. Marino RJ, Huang M, Knight P, et al. Assessing selfcare status in quadriplegia: comparison of the quadriplegia index of function (QIF) and the functional independence measure (FIM). International Medical Society of Paraplegia. Paraplegia 1993;31:225.

76. Whiteneck G. Evaluating outcome after spinal cord injury: what determines success? J Spinal Cord Med 1997;20:179.

77. Fuhrer MJ. Subjective well-being: implications for medical rehabilitation outcomes and models of disablement. Am J Phys Med Rehabil 1994;73:358.

78. Fuhrer MJ, Rintala DH, Hart KA. Relationship of life satisfaction to impairment, disability, and handicap among persons with spinal cord injury living in the community. Arch Phys Med Rehabil 1992;73:552.

79. Evans RL, Hendricks RD, Connis R, et al. Quality of life after spinal cord injury: a literature critique and meta analysis (1983–1992). J Am Paraplegia Soc 1993;17:60.

80. Dijkers M. Quality of life after spinal cord injury: a meta analysis of the effects of disablement components. Spinal Cord 1997;35:829.

81. Boswell B, Dawson M, Heininger E. Quality of life as defined by adults with spinal cord injuries. J Rehabil 1998:64;27.

82. Whiteneck G, Charlifue S, Gerhart K, et al. Quantifying handicap: a new measure of long-term rehabilitation outcomes. Arch Phys Med Rehabil 1992;73:519.

Chapter 6

Management of Persons with Brain Injury

Andrew D. McCarthy

Nature of the Problem

Extent of the Problem

Incidence and Prevalence

TBI has been, is, and will remain a common event and tragedy. It causes a significant amount of morbidity and mortality throughout the world and, in particular, in the United States. This tragedy directly affects patients and their families and indirectly affects all Americans in regard to the medical and supportive care required.

The traditionally accepted incidence rate of TBI is 200 cases per 100,000 persons per year. (This represents primarily the number of hospitalized cases.) If this figure is accurate, then TBI occurs in approximately 540,000 individuals each year in the United States (with a current U.S. population of 270 million). This rate varies in regard to urban or rural communities, socioeconomic status, gender, age, and specific causes. Mild brain injury cases represent approximately 80% of this number.[1] At least 400,000, and probably more, cases of mild brain injury occur each year. The 80,000 cases that remain are the more serious brain injuries and are classified as either moderate or severe. This is the population in which lifelong impairments and disabilities secondary to brain injury develop.

On a more hopeful note, some indications suggest that the incidence of brain injury is on a downward trend. For example, the incidence of brain injury in the state of Utah between the years 1990 and 1992 was 108 cases per 100,000.[2] This number may be related to changing admission criteria, however. The National Center for Injury Prevention and Control and the National Center for Environmental Health are working to develop brain injury surveillance programs. It is hoped that this effort will show that the incidence of hospitalized brain injury cases is truly declining. A good synopsis on this subject can be found at the Web site of the National Center for Injury Prevention and Control.[3]

The number of deaths each year from brain injury is estimated at 22 cases per 100,000. In the United States, approximately 50,000 to 60,000 persons die each year from brain injury.[4] A general decrease in the number of deaths was seen between 1972 and 1992.[5] The death rate decreased from 24.6 in 1979 to 19.3 in 1992. A 25% decline in motor vehicle–related deaths occurred in this period. Firearms-related deaths, however, increased 13% in the same period.[6]

Few studies have been done that show the prevalence of brain injury in the population. In regard to mild brain injury, probably a very large but undocumented number of patients continue to experience the effects of a mild brain injury.[7] Most patients with mild brain injury recover uneventfully,[8] although a significant number of people continue to have lingering cognitive-behavioral and physical symptoms. In regard to the more serious cases, the federal Interagency Head Injury Task Force has given an estimate of prevalence. Each year, approximately 70,000–90,000 people develop a lifelong disability secondary to brain injury.[9] This converts to an annual rate of approximately 27 cases per 100,000 persons per year. In comparison, the Australian rate of serious brain injury is approximately 25 cases per 100,000 persons per year.[10] In a report to the U.S. Congress in 1995, it was estimated that the overall number of persons with a disability from brain injury was approximately 5 million individuals.[11] This report confirms the prevalence of persons with brain injury–related disability to be approximately 2% of the U.S. population.[3] In general, the risk of brain injury is highest between the ages of 15 and 30 years. Also, the rates remain higher than average for the elderly.[12] Moreover, the brain injury rate is approximately twice as high in men as in women.[13] Even with age taken into consideration, it has been found that the incidence of TBI remains higher in the lower socioeconomic groups.[14]

Age and gender characteristics reflect the causes of head injury. Motor vehicle accidents account for a significant number of injuries in all studies, ranging from a little less than one-fourth to approximately one-half of all cases in most surveys.[15] Another common cause of traumatic brain injury is injury as a result of falls. Falls account for approximately 20–30% of all cases and can be of two distinct types. Most falls occur at standing distances and are usually less than 6 ft. The elderly are particularly susceptible to this common type of fall. Younger adults, on the other hand, can fall from greater distances, which often occurs at work-related incidents. This type of injury can be similar to motor vehicle accidents in that a significant incidence of diffuse axonal injury results from the acceleration-deceleration forces.

Other causes of TBI include assaults, firearms, and other miscellaneous sources. Violent causes of brain injury often result in more serious injuries as well as increased incidence of death. In a 1992 report on deaths from brain injury, firearms caused 44% of all deaths, with motor vehicles at 34%, falls at 9%, and other causes at 14%.[6] Those who incur brain injury due to assaults and firearms have a much higher likelihood of living alone and being male, unmarried, less educated, and unemployed.[16]

Burden

The burden of care reflects the age and longevity after head injury as well as the gender and the severity. Psychosocial disability is seen in persons with brain injury as well as in their families long after the initial injury. Families commonly complain of a decrease in pleasurable activities as well as increasing behavioral dysfunction.[17] They have increased emotional stress as well as increased aggressiveness. These families also have added financial strain. Approximately 47% of the caregivers had to change their jobs or even give up their jobs 1 year after injury.[17]

The costs of TBI are hard to calculate. Although the reasons for this difficulty are many, one very important reason is that one cannot put a cost on a tragedy that can only be reduced or adapted to but never eliminated. No amount of money, time, or effort can ever restore patients and families to their previous level of function. Also, no matter how well one deals with brain injury, there will always be a sense that society may not get the best "outcome" for its money. That is a danger in today's world: Sometimes we estimate costs only through money when, in fact, other human costs exist.

Nevertheless, one has to look at the economic costs to the health care system and to the community. The treatment of brain injury includes costs that are directly related to care resources. However, one needs to emphasize the economic burden placed on the patient and the family from lost wages of the injured, as well as lost wages of the caregivers. Max et al.[18] estimated that, in 1985 dollars, brain injury and its consequences cost up to 37.8 billion dollars a year.

It is clear that brain injury is a major burden to families and the health care system and may become even more of a burden given increased survival rates among those who have experienced the more severe injuries. With the diminution in the incidence of injuries from auto accidents, an increase nevertheless exists in injuries due to violence in the lower socioeconomic group.[19] With the expected increase in the aged population, falls should continue to be a major source of head injury.

Nature of the Disease

Common predisposing characteristics of the at-risk population can include an aging or an immature brain. If alcohol is a factor, it may have a deleterious effect on recovery.[20] A correlation can also be found between psychiatric disease and TBI.[21] Those who have had a brain injury are susceptible to recurrent injury as well. Suffice it to say that the majority of brain injuries occur in individuals who already possess some characteristics that make recovery, as well as limitation of impairment and disability, difficult. No two injuries are exactly the same because of the unique characteristics of the injured person. Patients with similar presentations can have vastly different clinical outcomes. Thus, it is important to learn the classification strategies but not to make gross assumptions about individual cases.

Processes of Injury

Several types of primary damage to the brain and the brain stem can occur. The most common type of diffuse injury is damage from acceleration-deceleration forces. This is most often seen in cases involving motor vehicle accidents. This type of force causes different degrees of axonal injury and, at its worst, is termed *diffuse axonal injury* (DAI). CT and MRI scans do not always identify all of these lesions. Also, it can be hard to identify these axonal injuries unless special care is taken with routine autopsies.[22] Larger samples of tissue are indicated for more accuracy in diagnosis. One can probably assume the presence of axonal injury by the mode of clinical presentation and should understand that it may be under-represented.

Even the "trivial" brain injury seen in concussion can sometimes result in permanent axonal injury.[23] Generally, the more extensive the injury, the greater the amount of axonal shear injury. In the more severe cases, diffuse damage is seen in the corpus callosum, corona radiata, and brain stem.[24] Patients who present with immediate coma are thought to have severe DAI.

The second type of injury is direct contact in which a force is applied to a specific area using a club, baseball bat, fist, or other object. This is the most common type of injury seen with assaults. Usually, most of the damage occurs in the area of brain underneath the site of contact. In this area, one can find contusions and bruising as well as tissue injury to the gray matter. Even in more diffuse types of injuries, focal injury is often seen at the inferior frontal and anterior temporal poles. These areas of brain sit on rough, hard, bony surfaces of skull and get bruised quite easily.[24]

This initial injury also occurs at a time when the brain is at risk for further bleeding from stretched vessels secondary to torsional forces and can result in small contusions and/or large bleeds such as epidural and subdural hematomas as well as intraparenchymal hemorrhages. The primary processes of direct contact, along with acceleration-deceleration forces, set into motion a cascade of bleeding, bruising, and swelling that can cause clinical deterioration. This is important to keep in mind, especially in patients with a low level of response. Sound clinical practice is to recheck brain CT scans in these patients on a periodic basis. It is not uncommon to find a subdural hematoma or some other treatable condition.[25]

Anoxia is also a contributing factor. Patients can experience this more global insult when a period of decreased oxygen flow to the brain has occurred. This can happen when a respiratory arrest, cardiac arrest, or both are present that causes anoxia or hypoxia. Although this is a diffuse process, some areas of the brain, including the hippocampus, cerebellum, and basal ganglia, are very susceptible to lack of oxygen.[26] Other areas that are susceptible include the third and fourth layers of the cerebral cortex and many of the basal ganglia, as well as the Purkinje cells of the cerebellum.[27] Clinically, this can be seen when a patient does not progress as expected and all other treatable causes are ruled out. Still, it is hard to distinguish between the lack of recovery from anoxia and DAI.

Falls, the second most common cause of brain injury, can give a different clinical picture than that seen in motor vehicle accidents. Falls of less than 6 ft are more commonly seen in the young and the elderly.[28] The risk is present for an acute focal contusion, a depressed or nondepressed skull fracture, and/or an extradural bleed. These injuries usually present with acute, focal neurologic findings in the nonelderly population. The presentation in the elderly population may be more subtle. No obvious physical or neurologic changes may be present but, instead, a change in personality skills, thinking skills, or both, may be brought on by a slow-developing subdural hematoma.

Most sports-related head injuries are in the mild brain injury or concussion category. These patients present with the mildest form of reversible symptoms, but permanent changes can sometimes develop. The exact cause for this is undetermined but is probably related to altered anatomy and physiology and its effects on cognitive function.[29] Usually these cases clear uneventfully. Because of the risk of second impact syndrome, however, it is important to diagnose these cases in a timely fashion to prevent further harm.[30] Second impact syndrome is when the brain remains at risk for a further and perhaps a more devastating second brain injury. This can result if further head contact occurs in the symptomatic phase. The symptomatic phase may vary from patient to patient, and provocative physical tests are recommended to identify these individuals before they are allowed to resume previous activity.

Firearms-related injuries are on the upswing in regard to fatalities, as stated earlier. The pathophysiology of this type of injury is often quite incompatible with life, and clinical deterioration quickly occurs. The bullet creates missile tracks, severe swelling, and hemorrhagic contusion within the vicinity. Damage can also occur in areas far from the missile track.[31] The type of pathology seen in these sorts of injuries includes bone fragments and edema.

Clinically, if these patients can survive the massive amount of injury and edema, they have a chance for recovery. One case that comes to mind is that of an 18-year-old high school student who received a gunshot wound. The bullet entered and exited along the right hemisphere. Severe focal edema quickly developed that spread to cause an extremely elevated intracranial pressure. He had a Glasgow Coma Scale (GCS) score of 3 for several days. This is the lowest score possible and signifies no motor or verbal responses as well as no eye opening. His family was told he would not survive. Yet he recovered fairly quickly once the intracranial pressure began to return to normal. Within 2 weeks he woke up in a confused, agitated state and had a hemiparesis. He entered rehabilitation but instead of staying for the estimated 6 weeks, he went home in 3. He had no noticeable weakness within a 4-month period, and he was able to attend college after sitting out the year. He now has only minimal cognitive impairments and no obvious disability. Physically, he lost only his ability to play competitive tennis at the collegiate level. Neither seizures nor focal cognitive or motor deficits, often seen in this group of patients, developed. Although such a case is rarely seen, it demonstrates that some people recover despite severe injury.

In summary, the type of common pathology seen is generally associated with the type of injury. Motor vehicle accidents as well as falls from a distance greater than 6 ft are typically seen in young men and have associated DAI. Falls from less than 6 ft occur in those with impaired mobility. This includes the very young and the elderly, who usually seem to develop the focal type of contact injuries. The brain injury secondary to a sporting event occurs primarily in the young. It is important to recognize individuals at risk for presumed second impact syndrome. Finally, assaults and gunshot wounds are seen in young men and are associated with certain characteristics. It is important to recognize the type and degree of injury and correlate them with the type of individual who is susceptible to that type of injury. Finally, the mode of injury and degree of pathology do not always predict the clinical presentation and, even more important, the clinical outcome.

Nature of the Impairments

Common Medical Conditions

Seizures and Epilepsy. One condition that causes worry for the patient, his or her family, and the treating physician is epilepsy after TBI. Chapter 10 discusses this topic in depth. This condition has some special characteristics in brain injury. The incidence ratio of seizures in comparison with that of the general population risk of 3.1 is as follows[32]: The population with severe brain injury is thought to have a risk of 17; moderate injuries, approximately 3; and mild brain injury, less than 2, according to Annegers et al.[32] These figures are for the population as a whole, but what about prediction in the individual patient? Although many studies have shown that early seizures, depressed skull fractures, and acute intracranial hematomas can increase the risk of seizures, prediction is not always correct in individual cases.[33]

The pitfalls of seizure management are illustrated in a 68-year-old man who was admitted with a serious but uncomplicated brain injury secondary to a car accident. He was in a coma for 6 hours and remained confused for several weeks. He had been placed on anticonvulsant medication in the acute care setting, and it was thought that some of his confusion could be a result of this medication. An electroencephalogram (EEG) showed diffuse slowing but no epileptiform activity. Physicians also had concerns about the elevation in his liver enzymes, and therefore his phenytoin (Dilantin) was stopped. He had a seizure 7 days after the medication was discontinued. The family was quite upset that this seizure occurred. Although no error was made in stopping the Dilantin, this case emphasizes the need to explain the seizure risk in detail before discontinuation. The family needs to know that when a patient stops taking an anticonvulsant, he or she remains at risk for having a seizure because of the brain injury.

Another case illustrates the importance of appropriate management of seizures as a complication of brain injury. A 20-year-old man with injury and removal of blood clot in the left frontal region was initially placed on anticonvulsant medication. Approximately 6 months after his injury, his medication was stopped. He had a grand mal seizure and went into status epilepticus, requiring general anesthesia to control the status. He had a resultant retrogression in motor control with reappearance of his right hemiparesis. Since then he has been on multiple medications, and, despite varying signs of drowsiness and ataxia, there has been an ongoing problem with adequate control. The goals initially were to prevent the appearance of the generalized seizures. This was not possible with medications because of side effects that limited his function. Fifteen years after injury, the goals have become not to control the seizures fully but to use the knowledge of the consistent prodromal symptoms to seek safety.

It is generally taught that prophylaxis with a traditional anticonvulsant such as Dilantin is not effective in reducing the risk of epilepsy.[34] Some patients, however, do not want to take any risk of having even a first seizure and may wish to remain on the anticonvulsant for various reasons. Those who want to continue taking an anticonvulsant, at least for the short term, need to know the risk of allergic reactions or dose-related side effects.

The mainstays of treatment are Dilantin, carbamazepine (Tegretol), and divalproex sodium (Depakote). Some newer medications are available, but none has been used extensively with TBI. One of these, gabapentin (Neurontin), has been used more commonly, and one of its strengths is that it does not affect the liver as do the previously mentioned three.[35] In the author's experience, however, it has sometimes caused symptoms of lethargy and ataxia in persons with brain injury. Dilantin can cause a tremendous amount of behav-

ioral impairment in brain injury patients. It can also affect balance, even at therapeutic levels. Sometimes Depakote may be the drug that makes the patient "feel groggy." The physician has to be willing to try different anticonvulsants or to take the patients off the drugs entirely.

In the patient who has an accelerated behavioral problem or manic state, Tegretol and Depakote are probably more helpful than Dilantin, although a true study in the TBI population has yet to be done.[36] It is always important to make sure that the family is kept informed of the risk of seizures and the risks of treatment versus no treatment and to consider the psychosocial, community, and work impact of the decision. The family, along with the patient, can contribute to the decision-making goals in terms of seizure control versus side effects and in monitoring status. It is hoped that some of the newer agents may prove to be effective both at controlling the seizures and reducing unwanted side effects. The general management of persons with seizures is described in greater detail in Chapter 10.

Hydrocephalus. Ventricular dilatation is seen fairly commonly in the post-traumatic phase of injury. In most cases, this is due to a severe brain injury with cerebral atrophy, but it also can be a sign of the development of hydrocephalus. Obstructive or tension hydrocephalus is fairly easy to diagnose. The patient has a change in the level of consciousness and awareness, and the ventricles get quite large. Harder to diagnose is a partial tension hydrocephalus or communicating/normal pressure hydrocephalus, especially in the concurrent presence of cerebral atrophy. One clinical indication that we have found helpful is the presence of variability of performance. These patients are able to walk without assistance, speak in a coherent manner, or have no behavioral problems on one day. Then, the next day, they are much worse, needing more assistance and supervision.[37]

One example of this is a 57-year-old man who had a TBI in an automobile collision and remained comatose for 6 weeks. He was admitted to a subacute rehabilitation unit and showed no reported change for several months. Finally, the patient was transferred to acute rehabilitation for a second opinion. His condition of unawareness and drowsiness appeared to be quite variable. He would go from needing minimal assistance for self-care to being almost "akinetic" the following day. His CT scan of the brain had been read as showing only "atrophy." He improved with serial lumbar punctures and had a dramatic improvement with shunt placement. He was able to attend his thirtieth high school reunion 2 weeks later, unattended!

The clinician is still the best person to make the clinical diagnosis of hydrocephalus. One has to be willing to consider it and to perform the serial lumbar punctures even if only a remote chance exists that the diagnosis is possible. A patient review done at the National Rehabilitation Hospital (NRH) several years ago revealed that patients who had the above clinical finding and responded well to serial lumbar punctures (remove 30 ml fluid 2–3 times in a week) showed improvement with a ventricular peritoneal shunt in the majority of cases.[37] Failure to improve with serial lumbar punctures can make one more certain that no diagnosis of communicating hydrocephalus is present. Still, some question remains that patients who have a meningeal type of partial tension hydrocephalus may not respond to serial lumbar punctures yet still need a shunt. Currently, the effectiveness of other diagnostic tools such as MRI flow studies and cerebrospinal fluid (CSF) dynamics are being studied but without any overwhelming acceptance.[38,39]

It is also important to mention that the usual triad of confusion, incontinence, and gait ataxia in normal pressure hydrocephalus is not very helpful in making the diagnosis of hydrocephalus in the TBI population. Most of these patients admitted to a rehabilitation facility already have trouble with confusion, incontinence, and an inability to walk. Overall, the determination of patients that would benefit from a shunt remains elusive. It is the author's belief that one must use all means to help assess the situation. The most important signs are usually clinical, and one has to be looking for them. If this condition is missed, the patient may have a lifelong condition of abnormal CSF flow with its resultant cognitive deficits. The tragedy is that the patient has had a brain injury, and the deficits are attributed solely to the brain injury and not to the underlying hydrocephalic condition. Although this condition is reported to be rare (only 18% of patients), it is very important that it is not missed.[40]

Post-Traumatic Head and Neck Pain. Headaches secondary to trauma are not too common in the

patient with moderate to severe injury but are quite often seen in the mild brain injury patient, at least in my experience. When they do appear, they can be broken into the usual classification of headaches. They can be migraine or tension related, or both. The diagnosis of migraine can actually be associated with the brain injury.[41] Many times, headaches are due to a musculoskeletal derangement. Often, the patient has related cervical pain, and x-rays are indicated to rule out a cervical injury.[42] The most important thing to consider when head or neck pain develops is that no serious neurologic complication is present, and a neck fracture is one of the most important things not to miss. Also, it should not be assumed that no fracture exists just because the previous x-rays were normal.[42] When the pain syndrome is associated with changes in cognition and behavior, it is important to do a brain CT scan.

One case that demonstrates this point is that of an elderly man who had fallen at home. He was admitted to the acute brain injury rehabilitation unit in a mildly confused state approximately 3 weeks after drainage of a large, chronic subdural hematoma. He was progressing well until one day the speech therapist informed the physician that "he was complaining of a headache and [was] just not himself" while she was doing her cognitive treatment session. The only thing noticeable when he was examined was the complaint of headache and a mild decrease in attentional skills. No focal findings were found. A CT scan of the brain was done and showed a reaccumulation of the subdural hematoma with a large left-to-right shift. He was immediately transferred to the neurosurgical unit for further surgery. Although rare, the development of a late subdural or a symptomatic hydrocephalus should be ruled out when such changes are noticed. (Also, this case demonstrates the need to listen to members of the rehabilitation team. They spend quite a lot of time with the patient and can pick up subtle changes in cognition.)

Once all serious causes of headaches are ruled out, one can treat the head and neck pain symptomatically. The usual medications work quite well. We tend to use nonsteroidal anti-inflammatory drugs such as naproxen (Naprosyn), ibuprofen (Motrin), and other over-the-counter pain-relief medications, and/or antidepressants. Amitriptyline (Elavil) and other classic antidepressants are very effective in treating patients with brain injury who have these types of pain syndromes. Elavil can help calm patients down as well as help them to sleep. One should be careful, however, in ensuring that the medication does not cause unwanted anticholinergic effects such as hypotension, tachycardia, and bowel or bladder dysfunction. This can be a problem in the elderly and should be kept in mind. Again, the proper treatment depends on the patients and their symptoms as well as their history and the individual doctor's preferences for treatment of headache. The management of persons with disabling headache is discussed in greater detail in Chapter 12.

Dizziness. Dizziness is a fairly common symptom after TBI, occurring in up to 78% of these patients.[43] It may be present whether the brain injury is serious or mild. This condition requires a full history and physical examination. Causes of dizziness can be broken into four major categories: cardiovascular causes, peripheral nerve/inner ear disorders, central disorders, and psychogenic factors. The first is general dizziness or lightheadedness. This can be due to a cardiovascular cause and may be related to medications. One should check for orthostatic hypotension and consider a cardiac arrhythmia, especially if the patient is elderly. Once the general conditions of lightheadedness are ruled out, the causes of disequilibrium or vertigo should be considered. These causes can be divided into two major areas: inner ear disorders and central disorders. In regard to the inner ear disorders, one can have post-traumatic endolymphatic hydrops, benign paroxysmal positional vertigo as well as a concussion to the labyrinth, and/or semicircular canal paresis. A perilymphatic fistula can also be the cause. Usually, the post-traumatic endolymphatic hydrops and the labyrinthine concussion and semicircular paresis improve slowly on their own, but this is not always the case with the fistula. These conditions can be complicated and may require referral to an ear-nose-throat (ENT) clinic.

One condition that needs to be given special consideration in the workup of dizziness due to a traumatic cause is a perilymphatic fistula. With this condition, common symptoms include hearing loss, tinnitus, and frequent vertigo and disequilibrium, which may be intermittent. The diagnosis is a fairly difficult one to make, and it is best to refer to a very competent otolaryngologist; some disagree-

ment often occurs with the diagnosis of this condition. It is important not to overlook this possibility, however. Current recommendations in regard to this condition were published in 1996 and include watching for fluctuating dizziness, re-examining if symptoms persist for longer than 6 months, and being vigilant in pursuing this diagnosis if the patient has any evidence of hearing loss.[44] At the NRH, many patients with this disorder have been treated successfully.

The symptoms of dizziness can make the entire clinical picture cloudy. Patients in whom severe dizziness develops can continue to show cognitive and behavioral impairments out of proportion to their injury, making it difficult to determine what the primary disorder is. For example, a young woman fell down some steps while at work and was thought to have incurred only a minimal brain injury. Before the fall, she was very successful at her job despite tendencies to work at an excessive pace. She took a few days off from work because of the injury and felt "sort of groggy." Then she noticed that she would experience severe attacks of dizziness and that she "couldn't think very well." She saw a neurologist and was sent for further tests. Her neuropsychological testing demonstrated not only definite cognitive changes suggestive of a brain injury but also other cognitive deficits that were not expected. A perilymphatic fistula was also diagnosed. After the surgery, she was able to go back to work and to resume normal activities. Her symptoms of poor concentration and forgetfulness dramatically improved after her fistula repair. She had two simultaneous processes occurring at the same time, a brain injury and a fistula, but the fistula appeared to make her cognitive deficits worse.

Patients who experience a TBI remain very sensitive to conditions that affect them in a general way. Changing cognition or behavior or the reappearance of weakness or ataxia may be the first sign of overwork or development of a condition as simple as a cold. Patients who are recovering from a hemiparesis may notice that they get increased weakness or increased tone when they develop a concurrent viral infection or experience any other general medical condition. It is not uncommon to see patients return to the clinic with symptoms of dizziness, headaches, neck spasms, or increased weakness when they return to work

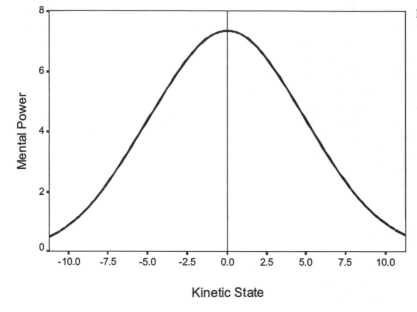

Figure 6-1. Kinetic syndromes.

too soon. They must listen to the body and its signs and symptoms. If such deleterious changes occur, it usually is because patients are trying to do too much too soon.

Cognitive and Behavioral Deficits

The area of cognitive deficits in brain injury is a complex one. It underlies much of the disruption of life that occurs long after the other more obvious effects clear. The spectrum of cognition is quite variable, and the ways to measure cognitive "impairments" are still fairly crude. We can only make an approximate measure of its function. It can be broken into several categories that are somewhat arbitrary, and it must be understood that these categories cannot simply stand by themselves. They are just descriptions of multiple interactions that leave each person with unique mental abilities as well as unique impairments. It is useful sometimes to break these functions into categories that help guide treatment. Ultimately, to deal with these deficits and to compensate for their effects on the person and the family, it is necessary to define them in terms of their functional consequences.

Kinetic Disorders. Brain injury shows how cognition and behavior are directly interrelated. One depends on the other, almost as if they are the

speed (cognition) and acceleration (behavior) of a race car. No activity is present at rest. Yet, once the car is turned on and starts to move, the speed gives this race car its cognitivity, and the acceleration applies the emotional forces. Similarly, human cognition and behavior remain intertwined much like the kinetics of the car, and therefore the term *kinetic disorders* is used in this section to help explain some of the common cognitive and behavioral disorders seen especially in the early recovery of serious brain injury (Figure 6-1).

After a TBI, with or without a period of coma, many patients display abnormal cognitive and motor activity. One pattern is that the patient can be withdrawn and apathetic with little initiative. These patients have been described in traditional neurologic literature as being akinetic or abulic. Also, they can appear to be depressed and exhibit psychomotor retardation. The other extreme is the patient who is restless, agitated, and trying to move without proper awareness of risk of injury. He or she is impulsive and lacks pragmatic thought. These patients show elements of a very active mental state. The closest diagnosis would be a patient in a manic phase.

Sometimes patients have a mixture of the two, going from a state of abulia to one of extreme restlessness or agitation, or both, in a very short period. Also, almost all of these patients show signs and symptoms that lead to a preliminary estimation that some element of emotional discomfort or depression of mood is present. These can be described as *kinetic disorders* to try to differentiate them from the equivalent mood disorders seen in non–brain-injured persons.

The kinetic syndromes are talked about first because they have to be brought under control before one can deal with other mental functions. The race car needs to be controlled before it can get back into the race. In the kinetic syndromes, great interplay occurs between the pure cognitive tasks of the individual and the emotional state. It is believed that the ideal cognitive state is brought about when the extremes of the emotional and behavioral features are brought into equilibrium.

The proper treatment can include changing the environment or adjusting the medications, or both. For hyperkinetic patients, the symptoms can be thought of as being quite similar to those of the classic delirium seen in traditional neurology textbooks. The treatment is also quite similar in that one tries to place the patients in a calm, comforting environment and adjust the medications. The environment should be changed to facilitate a reduction in stimuli. This includes reducing the noise level, reducing the number of visitors, changing staffing needs, and so forth. Another opportunity for changing the environment can be the availability of persons who are familiar to the patient.

One case that illustrates the opportunities provided by family and home environment is that of a 20-year-old man who was injured in the left parietotemporal area during an assault. His agitation and aggressive behavior during the early weeks after injury led to excessive use of phenothiazines while he was in the hospital. His parents were excluded from his care. Also, the staff believed that he would be permanently impaired, and this information was relayed directly to the patient and his family. The family therefore decided to remove the patient from the institution, and they took him home. After he returned home, approximately 8 weeks after injury, he was successfully withdrawn from the drugs used, with marked improvement in his cognition as well as reduction in the agitation for which the phenothiazines had been used. Also, more normal motor function returned. Another reason for improvement is that he was put in a caring environment and was treated by people who encouraged

him to get better. This case illustrates that adjusting the environment before using medications can help return a patient to an improved mental state.

Medications that can cause unwanted behavioral-cognitive activity include anticonvulsants, beta blockers, and/or a multiplicity of medications.[45–47] Removing the offending medications should be the first step. Once this has been done, one can consider adding other medications. For the hypokinetic patient who is abulic, withdrawn, or slow to respond, stimulants can be very helpful. Methylphenidate (Ritalin), dextroamphetamine (Dexedrine), pemoline (Cylert), and other alerting-type medicines can cause a dramatic change in a patient's alertness and, subsequently, great improvements in both physical and mental activities. This can result in a significant functional improvement. Cylert, however, has been shown to cause liver toxicity.[48] Other medications, such as amantadine, levodopa, and bromocriptine, have also shown some success in improving arousal and performance.[49] Traditional antidepressants, including trazodone (Desyrel), Elavil, and nortriptyline (Pamelor), are helpful in these patients.[49–51] Other medications that are used to control manic symptoms include the anticonvulsants Tegretol and Depakote.[52,53] Both of these are quite effective in manic-depressive disease. Lithium can also be an effective medication for patients in an aggressive state.[54] The antianxiety medications such as buspirone (BuSpar) and short-time use of benzodiazepines are also helpful, especially if panic symptoms are present.[55–57] Treatment of symptoms that may be consistent with an underlying thought disorder includes use of major tranquilizers, but these medications should be used with caution because they may impair recovery.[58,59]

It is important to remember that even with our knowledge concerning the properties of neuroactive medications, we never truly know how a given medication (let alone a combination of medicines) is going to affect a particular patient. Medications can sometimes be harmful in the recovery stage. For example, a young man had a severe hyperkinetic syndrome with severe bouts of agitation as well as obvious signs of depression. It seemed that the more medications that were added, the worse he got. Finally, he was taken off almost all medications, and he then began to show better cognitive and behavioral control. The goal must be to use the least amount of medication consistent with the other behavioral objectives. It is again important to explain to families what one is trying to accomplish and to elicit their contributions to defining the goals and monitoring the degree to which the goals are being met. A choice of medications may be able to be used, and a trial-and-error approach with judicious selection of medications is needed. When goals can be identified that are clear enough to the individuals involved, ongoing evaluation of the effects can minimize the excessive use of medication.

Mental Power. Patients with brain injury who achieve balanced "kinetics" still must deal with the loss of mental power. These individuals may be able to carry out some high-level executive skills but find that they have trouble with divided attention as well as an inability to sustain maximal levels of performance over an extended length of time. Mental power is the amount of "work" that the brain can sustain. It gives the brain its cognitive endurance almost like it is the combustion of the engine, and it directly affects both the acceleration and the speed. Early in the recovery state, this lack of mental power exhibits itself via kinetic disorders. The hypokinetic patient may have trouble staying awake, whereas the hyperkinetic patient is awake all night. In regard to simple thinking skills, the hypokinetic patient may seem to have a void of thoughts or to be very perseverative and abulic, whereas the hyperkinetic patient may have racing, and possibly manic, thoughts. Both of these types of patients may feel depression but for different neurophysiologic reasons. Later in the recovery period, mental power deficits are seen in more subtle ways. The patients have a decreased ability to work as before, also described as poor cognitive endurance, and symptoms may arise that seem to be unrelated to a brain injury such as pain and other bodily complaints. They can have a return of quality work, but the amount of work must be greatly reduced.

A case that comes to mind is a lawyer with a seemingly uncomplicated concussion that occurred while on an extended vacation. After several days, her headache went away, and she was able to sleep without problems. On going back to work after a 2-month hiatus, however, she began to find that her previous mental stamina did not return. Finally, after approximately 2 years of having no sign of improvement, she went to get a medical opinion. On testing, it was found that she had only minimal loss of language and comprehension skills and fairly well-preserved motor and visual spatial skills. Her ability to sustain these for periods longer than 3–4 hours a day was significantly diminished, however. It appears that she will have a lifelong disability. Her mental power skills have been permanently diminished. Her rehabilitation nevertheless has been moderately successful. The rehabilitation team worked with her employer to modify her work environment. She now has her own office in a quiet part of the building, and she is allowed extra work breaks. These seem to be working so far, at 6 years after injury.

Attention and Memory Disorders. A common impairment and complaint of patients with TBI is a memory disorder. This can happen to patients ranging from those who have a severe TBI with a long period of coma to those with a mild brain injury. These conditions are brought on by injuries to the frontal, temporal, and brain stem areas. The most disabling memory impairment involves short-term memory dysfunction. Post-traumatic amnesia is common in the acute phase but usually clears in a patient who is making a good recovery.[60] Memory, however, can be also be affected by a patient's ability to attend to a task. Thus, an attentional disorder can also affect short-term memory. These impairments are highly significant when learning new strategies and adapting them to other deficits.

How does this disability cause trouble and how can adaptive techniques help compensate for this disability? This can be demonstrated by the case of a college-aged student with a severe brain injury. He was in the acute rehabilitation hospital for approximately 4 months. He made an adequate physical recovery, and even cognitively he appeared to have most of his previous functions intact. On return to school, however, he demonstrated two types of deficits. The first thing he complained about was an inability to remember. He attended class yet seemed to forget everything he learned. In individual therapy sessions with the speech therapist, he did not appear to have an overwhelming problem with auditory memory, but a breakdown with this type of memory appeared to happen in class. This was then postulated to be a problem of attention. The patient was placed on Dexedrine and experienced a dramatic improvement in functional auditory memory. Still, his overall test scores were greatly diminished; he just did not receive the grades he did before. The speech therapist then had him tape all the classes and turn the information from auditory into visual data. After doing this, he had an immediate improvement in his grades. This case demonstrates how both improvements in memory and attention can help improve function in demanding environments. This case also demonstrates how pharmacologic and behavioral interventions potentiate one another.

One other aspect of attention and memory as well as mental power is that sometimes patients are not very good at giving reliable information. What they say may not actually be the case. An example of this is a 52-year-old woman who was placed on two different stimulants at different times for a hypokinetic state with obvious elements of depression. She just did not seem to function efficiently. It was agreed that she would try two different stimulants, to measure her subjective feelings and her performance in testing, and interview her family members who were always keeping her under supervision. With stimulant A, she felt that she was "thinking better," but her family reported a decrease in functional cognitive skills in comparison to when she was taking stimulant B. The patient was sure, however, that she was better on stimulant A. The automated neuropsychological assessment metrics (ANAM) test (see Measuring Effectiveness, later in the chapter) demonstrated that stimulant A improved her reaction times but also increased her error rate, whereas stimulant B produced no improvement in her performance speed but did result in a substantial reduction in her error rate. In essence, stimulant A, which the patient liked enormously, made her fast but error prone, whereas stimulant B, which her family considered the better medication, "tightened" up her behavior. She performed better on stimulant B, and it appeared that her family was more accurate in describing her function than she was. Thus, again, one must be cautious when deciding what is best for the patient without adequate information from the caregivers.

Problem-Solving and Judgment Deficits. Problem-solving and judgment deficits are higher-level problems that are quite common. Patients often demonstrate breakdown either when a task gets too complicated or the environment is too stimulating. Problem-solving ability is difficult to separate from problems of divided attention or of mental power deficits. Also, because the inherent individual cognitive abilities are usually not known, it is again vital to obtain family information before establishing what kind of problems the rehabilitation team is facing. Thus, it is once again wise to have family members give some background on the patient's preinjury capabilities.

It is helpful to assume that patients will not do well in more stimulating environments until this is proven otherwise. Even with mild brain injury, it is wise to be cautious about returning these patients back to work too quickly. In the postacute period, an inpatient brain injury unit is quite helpful both in treating these patients and in keeping them safe. They can be treated and cared for by a rehabilitation team of nurses, therapists, and physicians who are experienced in dealing with patients who have similar problem-solving deficits. Patients may be unable to recognize their own deficits. They can benefit best when able to accept suggestions as to adaptive strategies from a person whom they have come to trust. Willingness to accept strategies from a coach can mark the beginning of what is frequently a necessary ongoing support system.

Higher-level problem-solving situations are quite variable, depending on the environment and level of the task. Once the patients have shown themselves to be safe in a hospitalized setting, it is important to demonstrate safety in the home as well as in the community. Sometimes being at home is the only option, and they cannot tolerate the community, especially going into malls, stores, and so forth. Not only do problem-solving skills break down, but significant problems with judgment and safety arise. Judgment is a very high-order skill; it is usually required when human drives conflict. This is exactly when the most significant problems develop in patients with brain injury. Because of this, another individual sometimes needs to be the constant supervisor of the patient, as a cognitive prosthesis. This person is particularly valuable at times when judgment is needed.

Patients' problem-solving and judgment deficits can be a lifelong burden to their families. One case that demonstrates these problems is that of an individual who was living independently at least 10 years postinjury. He was able to maintain his work schedule and was well received by his fellow workers. He managed his finances satisfactorily under usual conditions. When his place of work moved, however, he was required to change his established pattern of getting to work. In response, under more stress, he bought a car but did not know if he could safely drive it. He had not driven in 10 years but had kept his driver's license. Also, in this time of stress he did not realize that he did not have enough money to pay for the car in addition to his normal expenses. It was a humiliating situation for him and difficult for his family to then reverse his commitment for loan payments and return the car. Thus, even when these patients are "better," they remain at risk.

Another type of patient who deserves mention is one who uses or abuses alcohol. It is not uncommon to find that alcoholic patients experience extremes of memory impairment and have increased agitation and aggression.[61] These patients present with memory and behavioral disorders that are quite similar to those of individuals with Korsakoff's syndrome. Treatment is difficult, and some of the patients with the worst outcomes come from this group. It can put the brain at risk for poor recovery even in individuals who would not be classified as alcoholics.

Neuromotor Impairments

Neuromotor impairments are related to the neurologic and musculoskeletal systems that cause disorders of sensorimotor and mechanical systems. Although possibly less debilitating and more straightforward in regard to disability than the behavioral and cognitive impairments, they still are problematic, especially when severe.

Cranial Nerve Impairments. Sensory and motor impairments involving cranial nerves can occur as the result of a combination of cerebral injury, brain stem injury, and cranial nerve injury. This includes injury to the special senses of sight, smell, and hearing. Common motor dysfunction includes slurred speech, swallowing problems, and double vision.

Visual impairments are quite common and can be secondary to either a motor or a visual deficit. Motor deficits usually result from an injury to the three cranial nerves involved in eye movement— the oculomotor, trochlear, or abducens nerves. Also, double vision can result from an injury to the

brain stem–cerebellar region, resulting in a skew deviation. Treatment of this is primarily time and the use of an eye patch.

In regard to visual dysfunction, injury can be either prechiasmal or postchiasmal. It is more common to see an injury to one of the optic nerves than to get a simple field cut. Many times, however, one can come across quite rare impairments. One case that comes to mind is a patient who had a severe occipital injury that left him with cortical blindness. (Of interest is the fact that he was not aware of the condition, which is described as Anton's syndrome.) He would run into objects and comment, "How did that get in the way?" Also of interest is the fact that he still could protect himself from an object thrown in his direction. His reflex mechanisms were still intact via the optic nerves, but he had no cortical perception of vision.

The first cranial nerve is quite commonly injured. This is due to its location at the base of the frontal floor. It is easily jarred from its place, and commonly the condition is permanent.[62] With loss of both vision and the sense of smell, the patient does not always become aware of the deficits until far into the recovery stage. It is very common for these patients not to complain about the inability to taste food until they go home.

Swallowing disorders are quite common after brain injury. Approximately one-fourth of patients have disorders of swallowing and require enteral feedings.[63] Usually with time, however, the condition improves, although some individuals do require long-term gastrostomy tubes. Once the patients have had significant improvement in alertness and basic cognitive functions, one can see if they are able to tolerate oral feedings. The modified barium swallow examination is usually performed by the radiologist and is helpful in clarifying these disorders.

Extremity Impairments. Extremity impairments usually occur from a combination of injuries. Impairments can result from upper or lower motor neuron injury, cerebellar damage, frontal injury, and/or basal ganglia injury. These areas of injury present themselves clinically with varying degrees of weakness, ataxia, and abnormal tone and posture. This is then mixed in with the various combinations of fractures and joint limitations possibly from heterotopic ossification, and/or other musculoskeletal disorders. One can see that a complex variety of extremity dysfunctions may occur and that they can result in impaired mobility and self-care.

Various problems with tone, weakness, or loss of joint movement can develop. The direct injury to the brain can cause trauma to the frontal area, giving patients either leg weakness or frontal ataxia. It is typical to see a patient with a brain injury exhibit trouble with balance and develop some type of gait disorder. Several syndromes of weakness, such as quadriparesis, hemiparesis, or monoparesis, can also develop. The patterns of weakness do not usually follow the typical stroke patterns. They are more varied, and it may be more difficult to determine where the injury is located. Also, the CT scan of a brain injury patient with weakness can be confusing. It may show a contusion or an area of encephalomalacia that does not always correlate with the clinical examination. Because the neurologic deficit may be from a neuronal or axonal injury that cannot be seen on CT scan, it is wiser to rely on the neurologic examination to determine the location of injury, whether in a cortical, subcortical, brain stem, and/or spinal cord location.

A lower motor neuron injury may also be present in a TBI. Concurrent trauma may occur to either the shoulder or the leg area, causing either a brachial plexus, lumbosacral, or even a root injury. Again, one must rely on the examination to determine what has been injured. Both an upper motor neuron injury and a lower motor neuron injury can occur in the same patient, and the examination is quite important in making the right diagnosis. Laboratory testing with electromyography (EMG) or evoked potentials, or both, can help to confirm the diagnosis.

In regard to abnormal tone, both spasticity and dystonia are quite common and sometimes occur in the same patient. Patients who develop an upper motor neuron injury also can damage the other motor systems, including the deep parts of the brain, the basal ganglia, and brain stem nuclei. This can lead to a combination of tonal disorders, including both spasticity and dystonia. Interventions may include medications such as dantrolene, baclofen, diazepam (Valium), and tizanidine hydrochloride (Zanaflex). These are well described in most rehabilitation textbooks. Because many of these medications can cause unwanted cognitive side effects, this needs to be watched, as described in each medication's *Physicians' Desk Reference* (*PDR*) description.

Extremity tone problems and loss of extremity motion can also be treated with physical modalities, including serial casting and bracing. Also, botulinum toxin injections can be helpful if the disorder is limited to a certain area. Still, tone problems can be quite discouraging. Patients who have severe tone dysfunction usually have severe weakness along with it, and the treatment for these individuals can be quite limited. Surgery should only be considered if some function is present in the limb that can be improved or if hygiene is an issue. It is very important that a good orthopedic surgeon is available who can help plan out with the rehabilitation physician the different surgical techniques that can help improve function if the medical and rehabilitative treatments are limited.

A common orthopedic problem is heterotopic ossification. This occurs when abnormal calcification is present in joints. Also, fractures of skeletal bones can often be missed in the acute care setting. This is understandable because patients often cannot express their discomfort concerning an area, or they may not be able to move the limb due to the weakness. X-rays are indicated whenever the patient has decreased range of motion or pain on movement. A good rule of thumb is that if it hurts or it cannot be moved in the normal range of motion, a follow-up x-ray may be indicated.

Autonomic Impairments. Autonomic impairments include bowel and bladder dysfunction as well as abnormal temperature regulation. Bladder problems include both incontinence and retention, and it is usually wise to get early urologic evaluation to rule out anatomic or physiologic causes. Bowel dysfunction can be complicated by tube feedings or by infections such as Clostridium difficile. Once treatable causes are ruled out, it is important that the rehabilitation team put these patients on a bowel program and a bladder schedule. It is important not to call a patient "incontinent" when the problem is actually the team's failure to set up the environment in such a way that the patient can access the bathroom or the portable commode.

The following case demonstrates how a memory disorder can complicate bladder function. A 14-year-old boy returned home approximately 6 weeks after an auto accident. He would go to the toilet to urinate every few minutes. He did not have a bladder problem, but, rather, he did not seem to remember that he had just gone to the toilet. He had a similar problem with eating. As soon as he left the table, he would turn around to ask when it was time to eat.

Nature of the Disabilities

The impairments described in the previous section can vary with the sites of injury in the brain and also with the severity of the injury. Most devastating are those impairments in cognition and judgment that interfere with the ability of the person with head injury to carry on an independent life. The disabilities are the functional consequences in the life of the person that result from the impairments, the end result of the pathologic processes. Not only are the disabilities the consequences of the impairments, but they also take into account the individual differences in people and environments. This is especially true when one deals with cognitive and behavioral issues. For example, it is one thing to break a bone but to have a memory disorder is an entirely different impairment. Unless a person is a world-class athlete, the fracture usually causes similar impairments and disabilities in healthy individuals. A cognitive injury secondary to frontal and temporal lobe injury is very unique to each patient and results in varying degrees of disability.

It is also important to know who the patient was before the injury. Only then can the real mental deficits be gauged. For example, what were the premorbid characteristics of the patient regarding emotional control, intelligence, problem solving, and so forth? What did the brain injury affect? Does the patient now swear? Does he or she have a problem with word choices? Does the patient get angry when speaking, or does he or she rarely speak and is simply silent and withdrawn? How is this accepted in the patient's home, community, or work? The answers to these questions are very personal, which makes it difficult for professionals to accurately measure patients independent of those who are familiar with the patient. Family members and, ultimately, the patients themselves to the fullest extent possible are vital to understanding the injury. It is important to attempt to personalize each brain injury case.

Important aspects of each patient include premorbid physical and cognitive strengths and weaknesses, school history, family support, place of residence, insurance coverage, and state and federal support programs that are available. Knowledge of these aspects can give a better idea of ways to lessen the impact of the impairments that would otherwise result in disability. Also, it is imperative that the rehabilitation team include a neuropsychologist as well as a person trained in vocational aspects. Both of these individuals are quite helpful in reducing the roadblocks that may confront the patient.

Goals should be minimal at first. When the patient initially comes to the rehabilitation hospital, the first questions the family usually asks after the injury are the following: Will she live? Will he be the same? Will she be able to go back to the previous level of function? The answer about survival is usually known at the time of admission to rehabilitation. The answers to the latter two questions, however, are difficult to predict. In the meantime, all the above-mentioned personal factors need to be explored.

It is also essential that the rehabilitation team be practical. It is important not to try to teach patients a skill that they can never master. For example, if they never did well in school, had trouble with reading, or both, it is inappropriate to measure their impairments with written tests. Instead, these patients should be treated in a more practical manner, with the ultimate goal of returning them to their previous level of functioning. If this cannot be achieved, then they should be taught practical ways of adaptation.

It is also important not to tell the family that the patient's outcome will be poor. Too many times, this is said to families and never forgotten. Even if a patient has no appreciable cognitive activity or any purposeful movement, one nevertheless does a disservice to the family by stating that the predicted outcome is poor. It is better to say that the longer a patient does not demonstrate activities of movement or thinking, the higher the likelihood of severe impairments in these areas, but any improvement in these areas can be a "good outcome" for that individual family.

An example of this is a young man who experienced a serious brain injury and who, for many months, could not move purposefully and had limited but significant mental responses. Many years later, the family remained angry that all the medical specialists gave their son a poor prognosis. He walks with a limp and has some memory problems, but his family remains ecstatic over his recovery and is still resentful toward the medical profession. It should be remembered that, although the impairment may be present, its effect in relation to the person and his or her individual disabilities cannot be estimated simply by a relatively brief neurologic evaluation. Also, it is sometimes better to err on the side of realistic hope than to give an early doom-and-gloom report.

One area of disability that is difficult to pinpoint involves cases of mild brain injury. Sometimes it is easier to deal with the moderate to severe cases because the physical and cognitive changes are easily observable. With mild brain injury, however, the impairments are often only felt by the individuals and are not noticed by others. It is crucial to have a neuropsychologist involved in these cases. The neuropsychologist can both diagnose the condition with testing and interview and aid the patient in adapting to and coping with the disability. With the neuropsychologist's help, the rehabilitation team can educate the family and employers on better ways to enable the patient to do well on returning to home and work.

Nevertheless, facts of brain injury are that it causes profound changes in the patient. Such changes include a higher incidence of divorce, a higher rate of depression, and a higher rate of unemployment.[64-66] The reasons for this involve all the previously discussed impairments, but the cognitive impairments are what seem to be the most frustrating. The patient can have a loss of intelligence as well as a change in personality,[67,68] with increased emotional distress and emotional lability.[69] Long-term relationships are invariably altered and sometimes ended.[64] Social isolation is increased, which can affect the caregiver as well.[68,69]

Fundamental to the major disabilities, limiting opportunities for employment and interpersonal relationships, are the problems in cognition and judgment that arise from brain injury. These problems are a function not only of the extent and severity of the impairments but also of the person in whom these impairments exist. Moreover, the ability to compensate for these disabilities derives from the skills that remain in that person and in his or her environmental supports—the availability of family members and other supports, their continuity, and their variety. Perhaps most important is the willingness of the person with brain injury to trust the input of those caregivers who function as coaches. Particularly relevant to the management of persons with more severe brain injury is the degree to which the family is enabled to provide that support by being provided the information and the training to participate in their care.

Character of the Solution

Overall Plan

Brain injury and its myriad of problems cannot be eliminated but can be managed more effectively. The majority of these traumatic cases are usually self-limited. This includes most of the mild brain injury cases as well as a small percentage of moderate and severe cases. A significant number of individuals with more serious brain injuries will not achieve a full recovery.

The management of the person with brain injury is an example of the management of a person with chronic neurologic illness. Illness continues to exist when there has been and will continue to be a need for ongoing care and supervision within the health care system. This can be the result of medical illness due to seizures and other medical problems. The relationship based on this management of medical problems can provide the basis for dealing with the wider range of emotional and other difficulties. Such difficulties include the area of ongoing interpersonal relationships and carrying on a productive life.

Care of the person with brain injury can be considered to be an ongoing planning process. Problems are identified, goals set, activities designed including the use of medication, and time established for review and revision of the initial plan. At the time of review, any progress is identified as well as the process by which those results have occurred. One then makes a new plan. The value of this recurrent planning and treatment process is measured by two factors. The first is the degree to which the client(s), in many instances the person with brain injury and the family member(s), are able to accomplish and maintain life in the least restrictive setting. The other is the degree to which they are enabled to participate in this planning process and thus learn to carry out their own management as a major component of community living. The role of the professional is that of a consultant in planning, especially in the chronic stage of recovery. The structure of this recurrent planning system is described in detail in Chapter 2.

This format of ongoing assessment and problem solving has particular value in the management of persons with brain injury. It can provide a model for those individuals whose major impairment is that of the executive-type function. Undergoing such a model with the professional staff provides a learning experience. It illustrates the ability to plan and evaluate oneself, which can in turn be a strategy for compensating for one's disabilities. Various components of the structure of the planning process can be seen as useful and can be used more independently.

One example is that of a 14-year-old boarding school student injured in an automobile accident. Initially, he had been in a coma. He made a fast recovery physically, within a few weeks, but was left with residual memory problems. When he first left the acute care hospital, he could not recall when he had eaten just after having done so. He found it useful to use a clock and calendar to compensate for his difficulty with time. His special education program had clearly defined objectives, which were reviewed at the end of each day. He was able to return to regular school classes within 6 months of injury and eventually graduated from boarding school. Now at the age of 40, he continues to follow a procedure similar to the one he learned after his accident. He has found it particularly helpful to have a clear idea of what he has to accomplish each day and when. He now is able to maintain himself in a hospital job dealing with seriously ill patients. He has done so by establishing a routine in his life so that he adheres to a relatively rigid time-line schedule to accomplish tasks. He has been putting into practice for himself what he experienced as working for him in school.

Another example is a 35-year-old man injured 15 years ago who still has significant cognitive and communication problems. He had been a champion swimmer at college. He was able to compensate for multiple cognitive deficits and was eventually able to return to school, earning an associate degree in graphic arts. He now lives independently and works part time in a photo shop. What worked for him was to set goals and search for alternative ways to accomplish them. Once he had met one goal, he would set another. He describes his experience in setting goals as a swimmer as giving him the basis for his strategy to be used in relation to problems with his head injury.

Another example is a 19-year-old man injured several years ago. He had been in a comatose state for 4 months. He continued to have severe motor impairments with balance problems as well as impaired use of fine hand movements. He could not write very well. Also, he struggled with depression for many years. The depression actually became worse as his insight improved. He was very troubled with the depths of his impairments that at times were only realized by his own inner self. He had prided himself on his athletic ability, and skiing was particularly important to him. He was able to successfully deal with his depression, and he began to consider strategies by which he might compensate for his other problems only after a plan was made with him to ski once again. He was enrolled in a special sport program for disabled persons. He went on the ski slope with a person on each side of him. As he began to go down the slope, he was able to tell them to let go. He succeeded in once again going down the slope independently, although he still required help in getting on and off the ski lift. His participation in defining the priority goal to ski again seemed irrational to the professionals in his rehabilitation program. Yet this irrational goal was achieved. This accomplishment, or perhaps the fact that his priorities were taken seriously, was crucial in enabling him to deal with the other overwhelming losses he had undergone.

Four fundamental principles of care must be followed. First, such care must be provided over the course of the person's life. Problems change, and different levels of ongoing support may be needed over the individual's lifetime. The second principle is that such care must be comprehensive and coordinated. The brain-injured person requires expert care yet in a selected fashion. The team may vary but, at least in the acute rehabilitation setting, should include physicians, nurses, and therapists who have a working knowledge of brain injury and its consequences. Especially important is that those with serious brain injuries be treated appropriately by expert staff and allowed the opportunity to succeed. This does not mean that the health care professionals should have an open checkbook in the treatment of these conditions. It does mean that knowledgeable people usually do a better job.

The third principle is that such care must be responsive to cost constraints and to methods that can maximize cost effectiveness. One opportunity to do so is to recognize the importance of family involvement in enabling the person with head injury to live in community settings relatively independent of the need for health professionals. The fourth principle is the process by which the patient and family are involved. Their involvement must be focused on in a collaborative manner so that they are enabled to be managers of their own lives once again.

Continuity of Care

Acute Care

The brain injury survivor is in recovery for the rest of his or her life. The life of the person and family member, or both, is divided into three phases of unequal duration wherein the frequency and intensity of treatment and the planning process that supports the treatment vary. The following is helpful in seeing the choices of care at different times.

The acute care hospital works vigorously to maintain the proper homeostasis to enable recovery. Due to the number of possible complications, the length of the acute care hospitalization can vary, lasting from days to months. Primary goals at this stage are identification of medical and functional deficits in addition to saving the life of the person injured. Both of these should occur at the same time. Too often the functional assessment is put off as unimportant and left to the rehabilitative phase. Yet the admission to the next phase depends on this assessment. Also, one underlying principle is that the faster one attempts to return patients to the routine tasks, the better they are going to do. The faster that patients learn to sit up in a chair or begin mobility tasks, or both, the better are the chances that they will not encounter any serious medical setbacks, such as a deep vein thrombosis or a pneumonia. Also, it is hard to evaluate cognitive impairments at the bedside. Often, it is only when a therapist can stress a patient in real-life environments that such deficits appear, and can be treated.

Before admission to the rehabilitation phase, it is important to have a well-trained professional evaluate potential patients in the acute care setting. This evaluation should include a complete medical review, psychosocial assessment, and functional evaluation. It is helpful if the physician can actually see the patient, especially in borderline cases. It is essential to clarify with the family of the patient their goals and potential resources. Many times, families say they plan to take the patient home but have no idea what that actually means. The admissions office, with the help of the physician, can serve everyone by educating the family on what the burden of care might actually be. Also, sometimes the reviewer can see that the support that would truly be needed is not available and realizes that acute rehabilitation may not be the answer.

Medical-neurologic condition, functional status, premorbid situation, and postdischarge support are all important in assessment. Patients who appear to have very poor functional skills along with poor postdischarge support are usually admitted at a subacute level. If a patient, however, has decent postdischarge support as well as any hopeful neurologic signs, such as tracking and semipurposeful motor activity, an admission to the acute care setting should be considered.

It is very important to know in the beginning what type of rehabilitation benefits a patient has. Often, rehabilitation coverage is either minimal or absent. The families should know what the limitations are. An assigned case manager can be helpful. It is not wise to let payers force a patient into a category for which they will not pay. Admission should never be based on some arbitrary rating such as the functional level defined by the Rancho Los Amigos Scale (RLAS) level or a phrase such as "we do not cover cognitive retraining." It is frequently necessary to engender flexibility on the part of the payer. The physician has to explain to the payer how the parenchymal brain deficits respond to rehabilitative efforts. Usually, if both the payer and the physician are honest, a mutual trust can develop that in the long run can benefit all concerned. It is in the patient's best interests to have an opportunity for rehabilitation. Both the professionals and payers need to ensure that the patient has a safe discharge to a reasonable supervised environment. To ensure proper communication with the payer, a weekly team planning conference should be held that provides a synopsis of medical and functional progress as well as rationale for continuation in the rehabilitation program.

Acute Rehabilitation

The acute rehabilitation phase can consist of an inpatient stay as well as a community program. The seriously brain-injured person usually is transferred to another facility to begin an acute brain injury rehabilitation program. Occasionally, however, patients make a good enough recovery in the acute care setting and can go straight home or to an outpatient setting, or both. Even in patients who have had a fairly fast recovery, the next 6 months are classified as the acute rehabilitation phase.

The goals of the rehabilitation period are many. First, it is important to do follow-up neurologic reassessments, especially in patients who either are developing neurologic problems or are not showing signs of usual recovery. One needs to verify that all neurologic and functional impairments have been adequately identified. As one of the author's neurology professors used to say on a daily basis to remind his residents, "Be paranoid!" This is important because these patients are often cared for in centers via segmented care. The orthopedic surgeon looks at the bone injuries. The trauma surgeon keeps the patient's body functioning properly while the neurosurgeon looks over the brain injury, yet, often, no one has the time to adequately assess all conditions and what effect they have on function. Once these are identified, the physician guides the rehabilitation team via the weekly conference. This conference allows the weekly goals to be evaluated and the treatment to be modified. The actual length of stay is centered on both the extent of the injuries and the impairments as well as on the need for patient protection and support. Also, it is crucial that the family be integrally involved early in the care. They need to become part of the team and to learn about the medical, functional, and psychosocial effects of the injury. If discharge is forced too soon, the family is often unable to cope with the patient's condition, and this can be dangerous for all. An example of this is a man who experienced a serious brain injury and had significant problems with agitation. Because he was ambulatory, the insurance company deemed him able to be discharged home, and the physician did not fight the ruling. The early discharge did not leave enough time to train the patient's family, and they did not understand all the deficits. This was because the discharge was immediate and arbitrary. After going home, the patient was very difficult to handle, and the fact that he was ambulatory made the situation worse. One night he proceeded to leave his home and was involved in an altercation that caused further brain injury and rehospitalization. Such a situation could have been avoided.

An approximate length of stay for a patient with normal family support is 4 weeks for a confused, agitated, and inappropriate patient and 6 weeks for the same patient with the additional problem of poor mobility. Length of stay is usually less than 4 weeks for confused patients who do not demonstrate agitation. Length of stay for lower-level patients is harder to predict because some patients may progress more quickly than others. Usually, early progress correlates highly with continued recovery. A main source of variance is how the family copes with treatment.

The immediate goals on admission are centered on the patient's recovery as well as adaptation to injury. If a patient is showing adequate recovery with weakness, it is important not to waste time training the family about wheelchair mobility. Such a patient probably does not need a wheelchair. If the deficit does not appear to be resolving within the inpatient time frame, however, it is crucial to train the family in the aspects of wheelchair mobility. This type of prediction is crucial in holding down costs and keeping treatment effective. Not much room for errors can be allowed, and soon it may be the health care provider who pays the cost of an inappropriately ordered wheelchair.

Prediction of degree of recovery and assessment of adaptive skills required for home care identify the crucial education skills that should be taught to the family. The family must have knowledge about brain injury, be trained in working with their loved one, and emotionally adjust to the burdens that lie ahead. This is discussed in greater depth in the section Collaborative Care.

During this acute rehabilitation phase, most patients pass the stage of needing one-on-one therapy and learn to work with a greater number of people in more real-life surroundings. This phase is called the transitions program at the NRH. This program is very helpful for patients who have continuing rehabilitation goals that center on community and vocational reintegration. Candidates must have sufficient cognitive, physical, and behavioral abilities to participate in a 6- to 7-hour-a-day, 5-

days-a-week program. The major focus is on the use of groups rather than one-on-one therapy.

Such a program begins each day with an orientation session. All the clients discuss with the group how each can incorporate weekly goals into the day. Feedback from other group members is encouraged. These weekly goals include real-life activities of work, nutrition, exercise, and coping with others. Special group sessions, such as cognitive skills, coping skills, and substance abuse, help the client face the individual cognitive and behavioral deficits that are and will be a constant challenge.

Continuing Care

The third and final phase, chronic management or continuing care, lasts for the remainder of one's life. At this point, the patient is discharged from the formal outpatient therapy program. The insurance coverage has usually run out, and now the only help is through other federal, state, or private programs. Many patients disappear into their communities without ever wishing or knowing how to return. It is vital that the rehabilitation system try to contact them periodically to see how they are doing and what roadblocks they are confronting. Many times, patients and families require the greatest support during this period, but too often they are left alone to carry the burden of a permanently changed person in an unfriendly world.

At this point, patients are out of the rehabilitation setting and are either at home, in a residential facility, in a supported living facility, or in a nursing home. It is essential that one deal with the tendency of the brain injury network to fragment. Once the patient is discharged from the hospital or the transition program, he or she does not always have the means to stay involved in a rehabilitation program or may even wish to end participation in this program. The brain injury system, however, must allow for these patients to come in and out of the system at different times, depending on their needs. This allows those patients who have either voluntarily or involuntarily left the system to return at later periods of recovery. The overall goal of this period is to deal with the chronic impairment in such a way that the level of disability remains reduced or will be reduced even further. During this phase, the patient and family must deal with problems that may change from those that were experienced during the more intensive rehabilitation phase.

The role of the specialist, whether a neurologist, psychiatrist, or physiatrist, can be central as the principal physician. For example, for selected persons with brain injury and seizures, the principal physician has been a neurologist. For others with primary interpersonal issues, a psychiatrist could fulfill that role. To be effective, however, the physician should have a working knowledge of brain injury. Changes in the support structure that was originally established may be needed.

The following case illustrates the value of flexibility in treatment strategies. These strategies are in relation to the opportunity for re-entry to the rehabilitation system as appropriate. An 18-year-old young woman had been left comatose and on a respirator after a motor vehicle accident. She was initially turned down as an acute rehabilitation candidate because of her lack of responsiveness: no voluntary movement, no visual tracking, and only reflex movement, which is essentially a level II on the RLAS. This patient also was not breathing on her own and remained on a respirator for approximately 5 weeks after injury. The family was heartened and encouraged when they thought the patient seemed to respond to her name. Also, she possibly had a trace of voluntary movement. By the seventh week, the patient had finally been weaned from the respirator. None of the intensive care providers had seen similar motor or personal responses.

Nevertheless, this patient was accepted to the rehabilitation hospital for a 2-week evaluation because of ongoing medical concerns that could not be handled in a less intense care setting. During this trial, her neurologic and functional status was reassessed. She was found to have minimal voluntary movement and severely increased extremity tone. It was also discovered that the patient had an absence of responses to voice yet would react to visual stimuli. With visual information as a tool, it was found that the patient actually had better cognitive responses than originally thought. Still, her abnormal tone and severe weakness were quite limiting and consistent with the severe midbrain lesion that was found on MRI. She then went from being a patient who possibly was headed for a chronic vegetative state (as thought by experienced staff) to a patient who appeared to have significant potential for cognitive recovery despite being in a state of motor block quite similar to a locked-in state. During the next 2 weeks, it was thought imperative to get the patient in a seating system and to treat her tone. Because medications such as Valium and baclofen made her too drowsy, serial casts were done to try to reduce heel cord contraction, and range-of-motion exercises were aggressively performed to reduce the risk of contracture. The rate of recovery could not justify the intensity of an acute rehabilitation program any longer, but the goals of adequate assessment and treatment of tone and seating system allowed for a better chance that, when neurologic recovery occurred, she would not be saddled with untreatable contractures. She was then sent to a chronic facility until she had further improvement.

At the chronic care facility, she began to show more signs of life. At first, she would gaze toward her mother when she entered the room. She then began to use her legs, at first in an awkward, jerky way, then her arms. She clearly demonstrated a sleep-awake pattern. Time spent in a wheelchair lengthened. The crowning moment came when the mother visited, wanting to take her out on a summer day, and her daughter nodded her head and grabbed the visor! At this point, the patient was readmitted to an acute rehabilitation facility because she then met the criteria for admission to an acute inpatient program. At this time, she was fully awake but still confused. She could move all extremities but still could not stand or help with self-care or transfers. During a 3-month stay, the patient learned how to read lips to compensate for the deafness secondary to the midbrain injury. (This deafness was suspected during her initial stay but confirmed at the second admission.) She had regained some of her speech but continued to use an alphabet board. She also reached the point at which she was contributing approximately one-half of the effort needed for self-care and transfers but still could not stand. She was now able to go home and live with her mother. Training the mother was crucial at this point. Without her mother's support, she would have had to go to a chronic facility and possibly jeopardize her gains. This is true because many of these places are not staffed to take care of young patients with brain injury, and the tendency is to house them instead of rehabilitate them.

For 7 years, the patient's mother has taken care of her. For most of the time, the treatment has been primarily supportive, with the family trained to do all range-of-motion exercises as well as giving the needed cognitive training on a daily basis. They periodically would come to the clinic for reassessments, and the therapists would modify some of the treatments. The tone improved very, very slowly, and the patient became much more animated with a return of personality. She is accomplished at lip reading and has reached the point at which it is difficult to recognize that she is deaf.

Now, 7 years after injury, the patient has returned to the outpatient rehabilitation center to work on skills that "will let me walk." She is bright and funny and has an inordinate amount of willpower. Her mother and father have worked together, along with other relatives and friends, to support her efforts. Short-term memory loss, which had been an ongoing problem, has become less disabling with the increased use of an "orientation book."

This case also illustrates the role carried out by the patient and caregiver to participate in identifying the changes in status, which could then justify new goals. Particular value lies in the opportunity to maintain an ongoing relationship with the same physician to identify the opportunities for clear, specific goals along with the family and patient. The benefits of this long-standing physician-patient relationship are multiple. First, the family and patient do not have to be treated by physicians who do not know that a urinary tract infection may present with just a change in tone. Also, no physician would place the patient on highly potent major tranquilizers when she had several months of emotional outbursts and signs of depression. Furthermore, the family did not waste new resources in having their daughter re-evaluated because they were unhappy with their physician. Important to the brain injury physician is that he was able to see how an almost hopelessly impaired young woman made a tortuous and dramatic recovery. This relationship has given hope to all involved.

Comprehensive Care

The professional components of the treatment team vary depending on the phase and the range and intensity of the problems being faced. The ability to provide comprehensive care deals not only with the professionals who make up the treatment team but also with their expertise specific to treatment of brain injury. Coordination of a comprehensive range of interdisciplinary services would generally be required.

In the acute care setting, it is important to get a functional evaluation of the patient. This does not necessarily have to be performed by the rehabilitation physician. An experienced nurse reviewer can evaluate these patients and call in a physician as needed. The nurses should have a working knowledge of function, and a standardized way of measuring function should exist. The treating physicians should pay attention to the ratings and should re-evaluate if function either worsens or changes in an uncharacteristic way. Other members of this team can include a physical and occupational therapist as well as a social worker. Adequate observation then can be made regarding function, and the psychosocial situation can be assessed.

During the more intensive rehabilitation phase and the subsequent transition phase, one must deal with the entire spectrum of medical, neurologic, functional, and psychosocial sequelae. The team usually consists of a rehabilitation physician and a team of physical and occupational therapists, a speech therapist, a case manager, and a rehabilitation nurse. Within a 3-day period, an entire re-evaluation usually is done, and treatment intensity is chosen. For example, if a patient has primarily motor problems, then the day of therapy centers more on this aspect. If the problem is primarily cognitive, however, more time is spent with cognitive remediation via psychology and speech therapy, and less time is spent with motor training. At times, however, the physical therapist works on cognitive issues that surround motor functioning, and the speech therapist helps the physical therapist deal with communication issues that are hindering mobility.

Comprehensive care involves the need to look at ways of lessening the impairments of the patient as well as identifying, understanding, and, finally, repairing the roadblocks that the patient and family face once they are out of the hospital setting. Because of the myriad of different types of injuries, premorbid abilities, and different family styles and community support, one must have flexibility in the membership of the team at any given time. In addition to the professionals who work with the patient and family, a case manager is needed who can work with them and with the insurer or other payer to allow for an efficient use of resources.

The patient and the family are part of both the planning team and the treatment team. Eventually they will be trained to coordinate whatever needs to be done for the patient. If the patient can do a task independently, fine! Otherwise, the family member needs to learn the task. The physician remains the link to all the levels of brain injury treatment and recovery. Each person with brain injury is similar yet different from other persons. A personal relationship between the physician along with the patient and family is usually beneficial. This could possibly be a relationship developed over a life span.

Comprehensive care also includes a team of physicians consisting of neurologists, physiatrists, trauma surgeons, orthopedic surgeons, neurosurgeons, psychiatrists, and pulmonary specialists. The team needs to have expertise in brain injury. Not every physician feels comfortable working with brain injury, however, and therefore, many physicians tend to shy away from treating these patients.

The value of expert knowledge of the character of persons with brain injury is illustrated by the following case: A man with a very serious brain injury was approximately 2 years post brain injury. He had severe cognitive and communication deficits as well as increased tone and weakness. He never recovered to the point that he could do any self-care or mobility tasks independently. Because of his functional impairments, he had to be cared for in a nursing home setting that was primarily for the aged. His behavior had been fairly calm for several months until he became agitated over a period of 2 weeks. Also, during this same period, his gastrostomy site had begun to look inflamed, yet no one linked these two conditions together. A general surgeon was called in by the nursing home to evaluate the gastrostomy tube, but he did not seem to be concerned about the wound and never mentioned the patient's agitation. Another medical specialist was called, and a similar response was elicited. Finally, the patient's mother called the rehabilitation facility to have one of the general surgeons who was accustomed to taking care of persons with brain injury see the patient. This surgeon was able to recognize that the agitation was, in fact, related to the gastrostomy tube. He ordered an investigation via an abdominal CT scan, and a large abscess was found beneath the gastrostomy site. The abscess was drained, and the patient's agitation subsided. This case points out how comprehensive care is actually more cost-effective.

Also needed, besides experienced physicians, is a well-trained therapy staff that has expertise in brain injury. This includes all the common rehabilitation fields: physical therapy, occupational therapy, speech therapy, neuropsychologists, social workers, and vocational counselors. This group of professionals must learn to work as a team. The coordination of this large group of different therapists is particularly important in caring for persons with brain injury. In the midst of confusion on the part of the patient, the team must maintain a clear focus on priorities. Because of the patient's memory problems, the personnel of the team must be consistent over time. In the context of loss of executive functions on the part of the patient, the team must be clear in its own activities, maintaining the relationship between goals and their evaluation at specified times.

The team conference format with the team conference report performs many functions (Figure 6-2). First, it is a vehicle that improves team communication. It allows the different professionals to sit together in a room and understand the patient's impairments better in a total sense. Then this information can lead to a plan of treatment that is both objective and subjective. Objective information is demonstrated by marking the grids that standardize level of assistance and marking the grids concerning the need for cues or equipment. Then an area is left under the grid to give descriptive information about the patient. When the grid blocks do not show much change in function, the descriptive information can give other valuable data. These data add needed information concerning status and, it is hoped, can demonstrate proof of improvement. Finally, team goals are tracked week to week to demonstrate progress. This informational process forces the team to become aware of how the patient is doing overall and keeps them honest about progress or the lack thereof.

The conference also allows the team to become interdisciplinary in that members learn to feed off each other and give insight about the patient that cannot be learned alone. Just having all the different

professionals in the same room needs to be thought of as an advantage for the patient, not as the detriment many of us perceive when our turf is threatened. For example, at the NRH, we have a very good working relationship with the physiatrists, internists, neurologists, and various other specialties. In regard to the therapy staff, we have very few battles over who does what. We all must pitch in, and such an interdisciplinary atmosphere is catching. The team conference helps establish this atmosphere. The physician must be the leader, however, or it cannot work.

The interdisciplinary goals are tracked, and each service must update them weekly. What is nice about these kinds of goals is that they often must be achieved not by just the individual therapist but by the whole treating team. These goals also allow a chance to show meaningful progress when the grids are not sensitive enough to show functional improvement. Also, the family involvement is quite helpful when making up the new goals.

Such a team conference approach also allows the staff to get a better handle on the patient's caregivers' needs by understanding the individual nuances of each case. An example is an individual who was a total care patient. He experienced a severe SAH and was very confused, very weak, and totally incontinent. He also had ongoing medical problems. Individually, all members were certain that such a patient could never be cared for in the home. Yet the interdisciplinary team conference approach with the family allowed the team to understand that the family had no intention of sending this patient to the nursing home. The team then became united in trying to reduce the care load and spent less time trying to figure out why a family wanted to go through such work. The family was part of the decision-making process, and it was their voice that counted the most. Now, 2 years later, the family is still taking care of this man, and he has had very few complications at home.

Another function of the team conference format is to use the information obtained in a report format to update the payer on the plan of care. The tracking of function and goals is very helpful for the payer, and it keeps the team focused.

Once the team works as a functioning unit with regular team meetings and well-thought-out goals, it is amazing to watch the good consequences that come out of the process. The value of a comprehensive team is illustrated in the following case of a man whose problems relate to his continued employment.

An executive experienced a serious brain injury secondary to an AVM bleed. He was left with problems of language, as well as with poor attentional skills and increased emotional lability. He was unable to return to his previous level of functioning. After leaving the acute rehabilitation hospital, he entered the transitions program at the NRH. In this program the patient worked on all pre-vocational skills, learning to function in more real-life environments. He did well enough to be able to return home essentially independent and was able to go into the community with minimal help. Still, he had to think of how he could return to work. He owned a family business and was the only one who understood it, despite his impairments. His psyche was tied to his job, and he could not face the possibility that he could not work at the age of 50. After several months at home, he was able to work at the task of getting back to work.

The professionals involved included the physician, the vocational counselor, the speech therapist, the occupational therapist, the physical therapist, the psychologist, and the rehabilitation engineer. The vocational therapist took the lead role of this team. She first met with the patient and then with other employees at the business to identify the various goals to be achieved for the patient to return to work. Then the entire team met, and a plan was developed to achieve the goals. The patient was a vital part of the planning sessions because his contributions were necessary to achieve success. The vocational counselor functioned in coordination with the specific team members. (Sometimes it is easier to let the individual therapist work on the specific problems that must be mastered and to have the vocational therapist be the coordinator of the process.)

The following sections discuss major goals that were addressed.

How to Get to Work

The occupational and physical therapist had already trained the family and the patient on how to get in and out of his car. Because he still could not drive, his wife and daughter would take over that role. He also had to learn how to get in and out of his airplane. His son was planning these trips, so he was trained with his dad by the therapists.

How to Make the Workplace More Functional

The physical and occupational therapists worked with the rehabilitation engineer to pick out the best adaptive equipment that would allow the patient to use the phone and computer. His office had to have structural changes made so that it would be easier for him to move around the office.

How to Overcome His Cognitive Problems

The speech therapist worked with the patient on ways to maximize his language skills. It was believed that he could communicate best by using the computer, especially for questions that involved more than yes or no answers. The speech therapist also spent time with the patient's staff and educated them on how best to interact with him. They were taught how to handle his emotional swings by reducing the intensity and giving him more breaks from work. More one-on-one interactions were encouraged, and large group interactions were minimized.

How to Medically Optimize His Condition

Once in the workplace, it was found that the patient began to show some signs of poor cognitive endurance and even depression. The physician was alerted, and antidepressant medication was started. The first choice, trazodone, made him sleepy, but the second choice, sertraline hydrochloride (Zoloft), proved to be effective.

The psychologist also continued to work with the patient and the family. The entire family had to face changes in their lives, but because they all worked in the family business, it was vitally important that they make it work. Fortunately, the family was very dedicated to the patient and to getting him back to work. He was able to return to work as the executive who, although unable to do what he did before, could still impart his wise business acumen to his company while other coworkers, including family, developed ways to compensate in the areas in which he showed difficulties.

Three years later, the company continues to do well, and the patient and his family seem to be happy

Conference date:_____

Discharge date:_____

Medical, neurologic, musculoskeletal issues:_____

_____

_____

Restraints discussed____Y____N _____N/A   Continue as per order sheet

Nursing:

Bowel mgmt: _____	Bladder mgmt: _____
Swallowing: _____	Nutrition: _____
Tube feeding: _____	Skin status: _____
Tracheostomy: _____	Safety: _____

Psychosocial: _____

_____

Patient participation in therapy/team goal setting   Yes   No   _____
Family participation in team goal setting   Yes   No   _____
Therapist will discuss this week's goals with patient

Cognition/behavior:
Problem solving; memory; orientation; attention; participation; community; attention; social interaction; mood
Comments: _____

_____

_____

Communication/dysphagia:
Comprehension; expression; swallowing
Comments: _____

_____

_____

Functional mobility:

	Max 2/Dep.	Max	Mod	Min	C. G.	C. S.	D. S.	Ind. S/U	Cues	Equip
Rolling										
Bed mobility										
Sit to stand										
Bed, chair, wheelchair transfer										
Ambulation										
Wheelchair mobility										
Stairs										
Endurance										
Safety awareness										
Comments:										

Figure 6-2. National Rehabilitation Hospital Brain Injury Rehabilitation Program team conference report.

Functional mobility:

	Max 2/Dep.	Max 1	Mod	Min	C. G.	C. S.	D. S.	Ind. S/U	Cues	Equip
Feeding										
Grooming										
Bathing										
Toileting										
UE dressing										
LE dressing										
Toilet transfers										
Tub/shower transfers										
Home management										

Comments:

Previous short-term goals:
Achieved_____   Ongoing_____   Not achieved_____

Interdisciplinary short-term goals:
1._____
2._____
3._____
4._____
5._____

Individual therapy intensity (hours per week in addition to hours in groups):
PT_____   OT_____   SLP_____   SW/RCC_____
Psych_____   Acuity_____   _____   _____

Group treatments:

____ A. Motor	____ Aug. comm.	____ B. Motor
____ Breakfast	____ Cog. lang strategies	____ Cog. skills II
____ Community skills	____ Conversation group	____ Exercise
____ Life skills	____ Mobility	____ R.O.
____ Right CVA comm.	____ S.S.G.	____ Substance abuse
____ Upper extremity	_____	_____

Follow-up
Plan:_____
_____

Equipment:_____

Assessment:

Physician signature:_____   Date:_____

with the results. The business survived because of improvements on the patient's part as well as global adaptation to his deficits by his family and company.

In summary, comprehensive care does not need to be so much an expensive proposition as one that is well thought out. Large centers are probably better at handling brain injury by providing a number of different specialists who are needed to treat the condition. A cadre of different specialists can function under the direction of physicians who are particularly trained in dealing with brain injury. The organization of the treatment team is especially necessary to provide a clear model for the patient and family who must ultimately serve in the role of coordinators during the continuing care phase of life.

Some people question the need for such an expensive system of coordinated care. If the volume is relatively high, however, the costs can be controlled, and some savings could be achieved by identifying better ways to treat these patients. Also, it has been shown that such comprehensive coordinated care has better outcomes. A study in the United Kingdom in 1998 demonstrated better outcomes in patients enrolled in a coordinated multidisciplinary rehabilitation program, and they were better able to maintain the gains after input ended, when compared with the group that received single-service therapy in a less comprehensive program.[70]

Cost-Effective Care

The term *cost-effective* reflects the need to optimize the outcomes achieved in relation to costs. Brain injury has devastating economic consequences. Direct expenditures include acute hospitalization, acute rehabilitative services, chronic rehabilitative services, and possible institutional care. If the person is able to return home, some modifications may be needed to lessen the impact of the physical impairments. The inability of the person to return to the previous level as a family contributor also has an impact. Finally, there are economic consequences of not being able to return to the previous level of work or of simply being unemployed, perhaps for the remainder of a lifetime. Cost-effective care can be achieved by proper use of resources in centers with expertise, by flexibility in resource allocation, and by focus on the training and support of the family as integral members of the planning and treatment team.

Because the potential costs are so great, the opportunities for making a difference in long-term costs can be considerable. Each case of brain injury should be handled in a way that allows for best use of resources without compromising outcome. Efforts to reduce medical costs in acute care early in a patient's course can lead to long-term economic consequences that are far harsher to society than just the medical care costs. Expert care early can contribute to far better outcomes. Efforts invested to understand the patient in regard to the premorbid personal and family characteristics can aid in the proper use of resources during the rehabilitation phase with far-reaching consequences. Proper coordination of the rehabilitation in concert with the payer as well as the patient and family can optimize results ultimately lessening the individual patient's dependence on family and community.

Cost-effective care can consist of continuity in access to expert care. Too often, individual insurers try to lessen their own financial impact by refusing to pay for acute brain injury rehabilitation. Brain-injured persons are shunted into chronic care facilities without adequate medical follow-up. One example is the case of an 18-year-old young woman who was sent to a chronic care facility soon after her injury. Her mother contacted an acute rehabilitation facility approximately 1 year later. When doing the evaluation for admission, a follow-up CT scan was requested. It showed a severe obstructive hydrocephalus. Surgery was then done but was unsuccessful in the sense that valuable brain was permanently destroyed by the missed diagnosis for over a year. In the absence of any appreciable recovery, this young woman most likely will remain in a chronic facility for the remainder of her life instead of being home with her family. A potentially treatable problem was missed. The error was in sending this patient to a facility that had no expertise in brain injury.

Yet another case illustrating a more successful outcome is that of a 48-year-old man who had worked as a salesman. He was married with several children. After a car accident, he was comatose for 6 weeks. Because of his low-level state, he was sent to a chronic care facility that had little expertise in brain injury. The patient was very lethargic and akinetic. He remained totally dependent on others for mobility and self-care. After he had spent several months there, a re-evaluation was requested at an acute rehabilitation brain injury facility. A head CT and EEG were done and demonstrated CT findings consistent with a communicating hydrocephalus. The patient also demonstrated variability of performance, which is often seen in communicating hydrocephalus, and this improved markedly after serial lumbar punctures. The EEG showed active seizure spikes, and a seizure condition was diagnosed. With appropriate treatment, which included placement of a ventricular-peritoneal shunt to treat the hydrocephalus and Tegretol to treat the seizure disorder, the patient improved from his original bed-bound unaware condition to the point at which he was able to go home. He could walk with the aid of a cane. He did not need the thousands of dollars of modification in his home that had been requested by the staff of the chronic care facility. Although he still has poor memory and needs assistance from his wife, today he has a good quality of life with his wife and children.

The better results in this second case reflect an earlier review of neurologic status. An assumption can be made erroneously by well-meaning physicians that no hope of recovery exists because of lack of progress, but most good rehabilitation physicians always do follow-up brain CT scans on patients whose conditions do not improve. Certainly all potentially treatable conditions must be identified. The less expensive facility originally chosen did not necessarily lead to the lowest overall cost. With use of a facility with special expertise in brain injury, an even earlier identification of these treatable considerations could have led to an earlier discharge home with a lower overall cost.

The criteria for selecting those cases that can benefit from more intensive management are important to clarify, but such cases sometimes defy categorization. They are dynamic and unable to be explained in a critical pathway or in a flow chart. They require knowledgeable people doing a knowledgeable review. Even then, one may not judge accurately. The need for the physician to keep an open mind and to attend to all possible sources of information is illustrated by the following case.

A retired air force colonel had an SAH and went into a coma. Despite immediate heroic medical and surgical intervention including a shunt for hydrocephalus, he remained unaware, mute, and akinetic. After many weeks, all involved believed that he would not recover, and transfer was recommended to a nursing home. Before what seemed to be a decision of such finality, the family requested a review. On examination, no evidence of any response seemed to be present. The primary nurse who cared for him more than others, however, thought that at times he would respond to her. The family was adamant about this also.

The patient was admitted to acute rehabilitation. He began to respond after several weeks. Within 2 months, he was able to sit up and assist with transfers. He was then transferred to a less intensive transitional facility before going home some months later. Somehow his family and nurse knew something that was not evident in the routine examination by the house staff. Sometimes, one has to sense what persons appear to have the best observational skills.

Successful outcome is not just a function of the type and severity of impairment. As stated earlier in this chapter, patients who look very similar in regard to type of injury and level of unresponsiveness can have different hospital courses and outcomes. As in the above case, attention must be paid to the availability, adequate training, and maintenance of caregivers as integral members of the planning and treatment team. It also seems that, even if the costs to train an expert team are higher initially, the results justify them.

The following cases demonstrate the different outcomes in two patients with similar injuries. The first patient was the only daughter of a single mother and lived in a rural area. She was attending a community college at the time of an automobile injury and studying to be a paramedical technician. She was left comatose for a 5-week period and had no appreciable signs of recovery until the sixth week. At that time, she began to have some semipurposeful movement on one side and also began to show some visual tracking. From this point on, she began to make a slow, steady recovery. By the fourth month after the accident, she was able to ambulate with an assistive device and with a therapist giving her slight support. She went home approximately 4 months after injury. Her grandparents were willing to be her primary caregivers and spent several hours each day carrying out the recommended therapy in the home, leading to her further independence.

The second case was a young college student who came from a more urban area with both parents in the home, albeit working. She had many brothers and sisters. She also showed little functional cognitive and physical recovery and was an RLAS level II 3 weeks after her injury. Then she began to awaken and move the right side. Although she reached a similar level of function as the patient in the first case, her discharge was delayed a month further. Despite the apparent availability of a large number of potential caregivers, support was actually thin. All the family members who could care for her had to work, and no one was available to stay home with her. She therefore needed to reach a higher level of independent functioning before discharge.

The first patient, although seemingly in a more psychosocially precarious situation, was rescued by her grandparents and was able to return home sooner than the second. The second patient stayed longer despite the initial appearance of excellent family support. The family actually was superb, but the situation remained as it was: No extended family help was available, and the parents had to work.

An opportunity clearly exists in enlisting and enabling family members to be an integral part of the planning and treatment team, yet this opportunity is honored more in the breach than the observance, even when it is the stated principle. Implementation is not easily achieved. An example is a 22-year-old man who had an epidural clot after an assault during a robbery. Several years after his original injury, he had been living with his parents at their home. He continued to have residual difficulty with language and memory. He was enrolled in what was then one of the outstanding "re-entry" programs available. One of the stated precepts of this program was emphasis on family participation. The actual implementation consisted of a monthly meeting with the family. It was only at the start of the meeting that the opportunity to review the treatment plan for the next interval was given. The language used was technical and not clearly understandable even to these highly educated persons. Data derived from their son appeared inaccurate to them. They were not encouraged to contribute their own observations, and they felt intimidated in making any criticism of the procedures because of gratitude for the reduced fee they were being charged.

The opportunities for increasing the cost-effectiveness of care are substantial. Particularly untapped is the opportunity for enlisting the commitment of family members as personal therapists.

The methods for increasing participation are the subject of the next section.

Collaborative Care

Underlying the overall management plan is the development of the capability for self-management by the primary participants, that is, the patient and those closest to the patient. These individuals, whether family or significant others, can potentially be helpful in maintaining and aiding community life. The planning process must be a collaborative one, leading to conjoint contribution of both energy and ideas. Although the management of brain injury has similarities to that of other chronic neurologic illnesses, some attributes are unique to this particular disease process. The impact of the brain injury is sudden and goes beyond the devastating impact of the type of impairments, affecting not only motor actions but those that go to the depth of one's ability to act independently in our complex industrial society.

A fundamental impairment in the person's sense of self—in self-confidence and a sense of self-efficacy—can occur. This is the impact of the almost instantaneous nature of the transformation from an independent, free-thinking individual to someone who cannot care for him- or herself. One of the particular difficulties is the lack of memory for the accident so that the person can begin to account for the change in status. This problem in memory can lessen, but it is quite common for the patient to maintain a residual blank for the actual time of injury; therefore, no explanation exists for one's present status. The memory of one's status before the injury, however, is retained, and that memory of previous modes of action can be called on to good result. The drawback is that one cannot reconcile one's present status to that which had been true in the past. Major problems of anger and frustration in the context of present severe impairment are compounded by the sense of loss of previous status. The contrast is there, but the connection remains unclear. How one deals with this frustration and anger helps determine the outcome. Sometimes a patient may ignore it via denial mechanisms, but at other times he or she may work through it to achieve a level of self-awareness to a level that the brain injury allows. This process reoccurs with the caregivers' own struggle between denial and awareness. Thus, the rehabilitation team must be able to help the patient and the caregivers reach the awareness and to limit the denial.

The planning process, which underlies the development of alternative strategies for reducing the degree of disability, requires one to address the basic planning questions described in detail in Chapter 2. The measurement of the level of participation in answering any of those questions is the other variable described in Chapter 2. The first question deals with the existence of a problem. A scale described in Table 6-1 describes a modification of the basic scale described in Chapter 2 to reflect those with brain injury who are unwilling or unable to deal with the issue of acceptance or insight of a problem. Insight as to the existence of impairments and willingness to accept those impairments are prerequisites to the development of strategies for dealing with them. One study identified awareness of insight as a major factor in successful rehabilitation after brain injury.[71]

Most patients are much better at pointing out their mobility deficits than those related to cognition. A study in Australia[72] found that for a given level of cognitive function, the addition of a motor limitation results in a greater injury-related failure to return to work. One may also assume that the greater the physical deficits, the greater the burden of care for the family. Once the existence of a problem has been accepted at some level, such as in reference to the mobility issues, one can address the issue of alternative strategies. As an example, the 20-year-old man described earlier with marked problems in balance was nevertheless somehow able to call on the memory of previous motor systems to once again go down the ski slope. Moreover, attention to this as his priority area enabled him to have a meaningful success. Once he had seen that success could occur, he became more willing to begin to accept the existence of his other cognitive problems and to consider the possibility of seeking strategies for dealing with them.

It is thus desirable to focus on impairments that are easily identified and work up to the ones that are more difficult to grasp. Most young patients are much better at gaining insight into their mobility deficits than those of a cognitive nature early in the recovery process. These deficits are more amenable to treatment in the young, who make up a large percentage of those with brain injury. One can see that success can occur. The process of planning and evaluation can also serve as a prototype to address the other frequently less obvious cognitive issues. It may take years to gain enough insight into these areas and to come to some peaceful acceptance of the limitations that they have caused. Again, it is a stepwise process. Experience in addressing the questions as to goals and status and what actions one took in achieving those goals can help to address these questions once again in the cognitive areas.

Care may be comprehensive and continuous, yet not cost-effective if the family is left out. Care must be collaborative and centered on the patient and the patient's family. One of the most obvious goals for a patient and his or her family is to try to understand what they are up against, yet most families who go through this terrible experience often feel that "no one explained or included us in on the decisions." Hospital staff often talk to the families yet do not communicate with them. It is essential to identify, educate, train, and support family members in their ongoing activities. Quite often, they experience the worst consequences of the brain injury.

Most institutions are being asked to do more with a reduction in staff and to do it within a decreasing length of stay. In the pursuit of efficiency, deficiency in family training has increased. In the acute inpatient rehabilitation setting, more focus should be given to training these families in the collaborative sense that this book is trying to convey. Although resources are getting tighter for inpatient care, it is not wise to reduce family training. In fact, it makes more sense to make such training be more central and to devote attention to making such training more effective.

Table 6-1. Patient Participation Scale

1. Does not see problem (as reflected in LTG and status) and *does not* want to work on it
2. Does not see problem (as reflected in LTG and status) and is *willing* to work on it
3. Agrees (with LTG, status, STG)
4. Able to *restate* (LTG, status, STG) in own words
5. Appropriate (LTG, status, STG) *independently* developed/stated by patient

LTG = long-term goals; STG = short-term goals.

Table 6-2. Caregiver Training Module

	Day 1	Day 4	Week of Discharge	Postdischarge
Objectives	Identify concerns, priorities of inpatient CT plan: Medical Rehabilitation Psychological	1. Completion of caregiver plan (schedule, staff) 2. Integrate into overall inpatient interdisciplinary plan	1. Review inpatient CT plan 2. Establish community living CT plan	Review/revise community living CT plan
Activities	Family meeting	Initial team conference	Family meeting	—
Evaluation	Family needs questionnaire	Team conference report	Team conference report Family needs questionnaire	Family needs questionnaire

CT = caregiver training.

One method is via increased integration of family training at the various phases of acute care, rehabilitation care, and home care.[73] Increasing insight should be attained with each level as well as ways to deal with many of the facts that are quite unpleasant. It is hoped that a "buy-in" can occur that will lessen these unfortunate consequences. Insight cannot always occur immediately, nor should it, and it needs to be phased in.

At the NRH, a plan was made for improving the integration of the family members as a part of the planning and treatment team. A training program for the caregivers is established in the several areas (medical, rehabilitation, and psychosocial) by setting the goals and designing the activities that make those goals achievable (table 6-2). The goals will be dynamic and will differ from family to family. The rehabilitation team will ensure that an active process takes place in which these goals are identified and reviewed in concert with the family and the patient. One set of objectives will relate to the specific educational goals. Another set of objectives will include the ability of the family members to contribute increasingly to the planning process. The overall educational program must support the sense of competence and self-efficacy that the family needs to call on.

The activity to meet these goals is the family conference. At least two family conferences are held during the inpatient stay. The first conference occurs within the first week, and a list of potential problems will be reviewed with the family. Then the team will incorporate the family into the rehabilitation process to both teach and train them as well as to gain active insight into the issues that affect their lives. This involves having the family be active participants as much as they can be. This process will continue with a second family conference at discharge to again identify the problems that need to be confronted. It is hoped that this system of management will not only be beneficial to the family and patient but also to the staff so that they can be more effective in the treatment planning process. This process will not end with the discharge into the community. The team will continue to meet with the family at regular outpatient intervals to maintain the collaborative effort.

Once home, it is hoped that the patient and the family will have learned ways to increase insight and adaptation independent of the team. This is where the cost savings come in. The better the family is able to solve their own problems, the less likely that expensive intervention will be needed. Sometimes, it is how these relationships develop that determines the success or failure of the process. At this time, the collaboration of care is often pitted between the family as the supervisor and the person with the injury. It is quite common to encounter episodes of anger brought on by the realization of deficits. It is hoped that the patient can use this anger to improve insight and adaptation instead of falling into either denial or despair.

The awareness of the losses in cognitive function can lead to anger or depression, or both, and this is actually helpful if it ultimately leads to acceptance. The case described earlier of the 20-year-old man injured in the left parietotemporal area when assaulted illustrates this issue. One episode took place in a restaurant when he could not find the salt shaker he had just used. When confronted by his mother with the fact that he had a problem with memory, he became angry and verbally abusive to her. At other times, he would throw objects at himself in the mirror. He later described his feelings at the time as thinking that he was dead and that nothing would be lost if he jumped out of a window. He would say to his mother with anger and sadness, "You have a retarded son." Later, in a relationship with a speech therapist, he began to address the specific impairment in language and would accept strategies offered to compensate for his disabilities. He would call on the techniques he had used earlier in his life to deal with problems, namely, to set goals and develop alternative ways of doing things. For example, because he had difficulty in recalling nouns, he would write the word in the air or on his body and then say the word. The issue here is his increased readiness to accept and use the strategies offered. He was able to begin to deal with his depression by becoming increasingly aware of the strategies under his own control to regain function.

Still, the end result of understanding the deficits from brain injury is acceptance of the deficits, and that is not as easy to do. A case illustrating the severity of this impact is that of a father with two teenage sons who was injured in 1989. He was comatose for 4 weeks and then was in a controlled access brain injury unit for 5 weeks because of severe confusion, restlessness, and frequent emotional outbursts. He recovered to the point at which most people who met him would not notice any major problems aside from an adolescent type of demeanor. The recovery has been a grueling one for the whole family, however. His wife stayed at his side throughout the years despite her husband's inability to work full time and to sleep longer than 3 hours a night. He still has occasional emotional outbursts and becomes almost manic if he does not take lithium. His wife reports that they do very little with old friends and that taking care of her husband "is my second job after I come home from my first." She reports that they are no longer like husband and wife, "more like mother and teenage boy." Medication to control some of the inappropriate behavior has made the situation somewhat tolerable. The patient has never been able to achieve an adequate level of independence and autonomy and does not appear capable of ever being able to do so. Thus, it is his wife as the caregiver who carries out the work of caring for him and literally carrying him. Although this burden is quite frus-

trating, she has never once complained to her physician, but her strain is easily seen in her expressions and mannerisms. Still, she has never felt a need for counseling because she prefers working with the local brain injury society, and no resolution is possible. "This is my life," she states.

The following contrasting case shows that people sometimes are actually "better" after a brain injury. A 30-year-old former college athlete spent much too much time drinking and staying out late after his playing days were over. He drifted from job to job and, from family reports, had lost most of his good friends because of his drinking. He was involved in an accident and was knocked unconscious for 3 days. He gradually recovered over the next 6 months, but he has been left with a slight dystonia on the left side and has lost much of his high-level balance. Also, his personality changed, and he became much more subdued. The good news is, approximately 1 year after the injury, he found a full-time job coaching a sports team as an assistant, and he has given up alcohol. He is sad that he lost some of his previous physical and cognitive skills but is appreciative that he is alive and that he can work. His family also thinks that, in some ways, "he is a much nicer person now than before the accident."

In summary, collaboration of care requires active family involvement with the brain injury team. This type of treatment philosophy should result in measurable improvement in family satisfaction as well as improved independence and adaptation for the patient. The planning process remains collaborative with the family and is ongoing for as long as it continues to be effective. This enables the patient and the family to take ownership of the problems and allows the treating team to better identify the areas of emphasis for each patient and, it is hoped, to improve the efficiency of the treatment. It is hoped that this leads to a reduction both in wasted resources and in the overall costs both in human and monetary terms.

Measuring Effectiveness

Measurement of the effectiveness of treatment for persons with brain injury is crucial for many reasons. First, the treatment team needs to be able to demonstrate effectively the results of the rehabilitation process. This information is also needed to communicate to both the family of the patient and

Table 6-3. Glasgow Coma Scale*

Patient's Response	Score
Eye opening	
Eyes open spontaneously	4
Eyes open when spoken to	3
Eyes open to painful stimulation	2
Eyes do not open	1
Motor	
Follows commands	6
Makes localizing movement to pain	5
Makes withdrawal movements to pain	4
Flexor (decorticate) posturing to pain	3
Extensor (decerebrate) posturing to pain	2
No motor response to pain	1
Verbal	
Oriented to place and date	5
Converses but is disoriented	4
Utters inappropriate words, not conversing	3
Makes incomprehensible nonverbal sounds	2
Not vocalizing	1

*Instructions: Rate best response in the verbal and motor categories and the stimulus needed to elicit eye opening. Sum the three ratings to obtain the score.

the payer of the care. Finally, with effective measurement, some standards of treatment can be established between different facilities, programs, and hospitals. Caution should remain the key word, however. The most effective measurement tool remains elusive, and until it is found, we cannot allow measurement tools to be used in inappropriate ways that encourage denial of needed services.

An example of this is the RLAS. This scale is sometimes used inappropriately by payers to refuse needed rehabilitation care. Those in the industry use this tool only as a rough guideline for classification of brain injury and have been quite disturbed by its inappropriate use. Thus, it should remain a high priority of the brain injury rehabilitation providers to ensure that indicators of outcome are used appropriately and to continue to refine what is currently being used to improve the accuracy.

Measurement of Impairment

Impairment in acquired brain injury can be described as when a person experiences the loss or reduction of previous neurologic function. (This includes cognitive, behavioral, or neuromotor deficits.) For some functions, this is fairly straightforward and dichotomous. Some weakness that was not previously present may develop in an extremity. However, for many functions, primarily cognitive in nature, it is difficult to measure the degree of impairment. This is especially true when one tries to compare such functions in a normative group that has wide variations in normal functioning. Providers should emphasize individual mental functions such as functional memory and lack of awareness in the community rather than just to describe cognitive deficits. Also, the acuteness of the problem needs more emphasis, and the recovery curve must be emphasized.

The following scales are used fairly often in measuring impairment.

Glasgow Coma Scale

The GCS is the most commonly used scale to measure the initial severity of a brain injury (Table 6-3). It has excellent interobserver reliability and is used in the field by allied health workers to give a reliable initial assessment of neurologic injury.[74,75] It is based on three easily measured responses: eye opening, motor response, and verbal response. The lowest score that can be given is a 3, and it correlates with the least amount of neurologic activity possible; the highest score, 15, shows essentially normal gross responses. The GCS is an excellent triage tool that can separate out individuals who have a moderate to severe brain injury (3–12) from those who have a mild brain injury (13–15).

Because of its sensitivity in measuring unconsciousness, the GCS is also very helpful in making a general prediction of disability, because individuals who are comatose generally have worse outcomes than those who are not. Still, when used as an outcome predictor, the GCS is not always accurate. The author has seen many patients in a prolonged period of unconsciousness do quite well. Unconsciousness results from a diffuse bilateral hemispheric injury, a primary brain stem injury, or a combination of the two. They cannot be separated out accurately. One needs to wait and see which cause is responsible. The patients who make a sudden recovery to an almost normal state, compared with those who have more extensive damage, must have experienced a reversible brain stem injury without widespread cerebral involvement.

One study demonstrated that, when used alone, the GCS has limited value as a predictor of functional outcome.[76] Again, it is emphasized that this scale is helpful in categorizing the seriousness of the injury, but the recovery is dependent on many other factors.

Rancho Los Amigos Scale

The RLAS is used quite commonly in rehabilitation of acute brain injury (Table 6-4). It is very helpful in assessing moderate to severe brain injury but has little use in mild brain injury. The scale is broken into eight levels, but only seven categories actually are used in acute rehabilitation. The one category of little use is level I. The patients in this level have no responses at all, which is very rarely seen outside of an acute care hospital; very few patients do not have any responses after a period of time. Also, at the other end of the scale, levels VII and VIII describe individuals who have experienced a serious brain injury and have had lower original ratings. These categories should never be used when rating mild brain injury. These patients are also usually not treated in an acute brain injury unit. They do not have the level of confusion to warrant admission.

Levels II and III are helpful in categorizing bedbound patients, that is, the comatose, nearly comatose, and/or emerging comatose patient. Level II describes a person with generalized or reflex responses, or both. He or she has neither purposeful nor semipurposeful activity. Again, it is important to clinically evaluate the patient and not rely only on the rating. It is also important to evaluate the medical situation and the length of time in a level II state. Although this category would probably predict a poorer outcome, it is important not to let it cloud the treatment. All too often, a patient in this category is sent to a nursing home without a thorough neurologic and medical rehabilitation plan. A patient at level III almost always shows further recovery. The presence of even minimal purposeful activity implies that a real person may be lying semidormant behind the brain injury. Also, one cannot always guess at the level of cognitive impairment in these low-level patients. These levels are very motor response driven. Sometimes, a patient with severe motor impairment from a brain stem injury may have a fairly intact cerebrum. The RLAS rating of a

Table 6-4. Rancho Los Amigos Levels of Cognitive Function Scale

I. No response
II. Generalized response to stimulation
III. Localized response to stimulation
IV. Confused and agitated behavior
V. Confused with inappropriate behavior (nonagitated)
VI. Confused but appropriate behavior
VII. Automatic and appropriate behavior
VIII. Purposeful and appropriate behavior

Source: Reprinted with permission from C Hagen, D Malkmus, P Durham. Levels of Cognitive Functions. Communications Disorders Service, Rancho Los Amigos Hospital, 1972. Revised by D Malkmus, K Stenderup, 1974.

low-level state may also be misleading. One needs to be careful in assuming the worst. Time will tell the story, not the rating or the scale.

RLAS levels IV, V, and VI all represent patients who share the common trait of confusion. At level IV, the patient is confused, amnesic, and sometimes agitated. A level V patient is described as confused, inappropriate, and amnesic, but rarely agitated. A level VI patient is still confused and amnesic and lacks problem-solving skills. The behaviors are usually not inappropriate, and no severe level of agitation is generally present. Again, these scales are only helpful to screen patients into categories and should not be used in isolation. The rating helps the rehabilitation team do basic planning of care. The RLAS is especially helpful in determining where a patient should reside. It also helps in predicting length of stay, especially when combined with level of motor involvement.

Traditional Neurologic Evaluation

The clinical neurologic examination can contribute to the assessment of impairment. It requires a well-experienced practitioner to use the examination in the best manner possible. The following are parts of the examination that are more sensitive in prognostication.

Mental status. One needs to see how the patient responds to command and if premorbid personality or a pragmatic sign of communication is present. One needs to take into account when a patient is on sedating medications or is unable to communicate because of a tracheostomy, or both. Any positive nonreflex response to a command by a low-level patient is a meaningful sign for potential improvement and, sometimes, even recovery. A very bad sign is the absence of any meaningful motor response in combination with a distant blank stare. It is rare for patients to recover in a significant manner when they have had a prolonged period of that distant stare. It is difficult to describe and needs to be seen.

Cranial nerves. It is also a good sign if a patient shows any visual tracking of objects. It is important to assess the visual motor system before stating that no evidence of tracking exists. The presence of an oculomotor injury, especially to the third nerve, impairs this part of the evaluation. The presence or absence of the gag reflex and the absence of verbalization can also be misleading. The medical treatments or the tracheostomy, or both, can affect these functions. It is important to assess hearing, especially with patients who have had a midbrain injury, which can damage the central hearing pathways.

Motor system. Almost every serious brain injury case has an associated weakness. Often it is in a hemiparetic pattern or in a double hemiparetic pattern. Occasionally it may only be a monoparesis. The important thing to understand in assessing these patients is not to assume a direct link between motor function and cognitive function. On the positive side, any presence of a semipurposeful response is encouraging. This is true even if it is only seen in one limb. The cautionary side is when an unconscious or minimally responsive patient has tetraplegia, in which case one cannot assume that a similar amount of cerebral injury exists. These patients can sometimes look like "locked-in plus" patients once they recover (i.e., locked in by the brain stem injury yet with varying degrees of cognitive impairment).

These are the critical parts of the neurologic examination for assessment and prognostication. The evaluation of the reflexes, sensory system, and cerebellar systems are also helpful but not as crucial in making a prognostication. In a comatose patient or an emerging comatose patient, the neurologic evaluation is quite effective in measuring the degree of cognitive and motor impairment. It also can be a better predictor of recovery than either the GCS or the RLAS. Only the individual neurologic evaluation can report the specific nuances of a patient.

Two patients were seen on the same day several years ago. Both were RLAS level II cases and had identical GCS ratings on admission to the acute care hospital, yet one seemed to have more neurologic activity. Despite primarily decerebrate movement to voice or touch, one of the patients seemed to be able to move with some voluntary will. The patient with the lesser responses also seemed to have a distant stare. The patient who had more neurologic activity went on to wake up and go home with supervision. He had problems with weakness and tone but a surprisingly intact personality. Meanwhile, the other patient never recovered and ended up in a chronic care facility, only achieving the level of a minimally responsive state.

Measurement of Disability

Disability is related to the primary neurologic impairment. The ability to perform an activity that is within the range of normality for that specific patient is reduced or lost. This results in a decreased capacity to meet the demands seen in personal, social, or occupational activities. One must keep in mind that other impairments may be contributing to the overall disability. An amputee would have a much greater level of disability than a nonamputee with similar severity of brain injury.

Disability is related to impairment but is also affected by the environment in which the person must function. It is not always obvious if and when a brain-injured patient has a decreased capacity for an activity. Sometimes it may appear that the person only gets in trouble if the room is crowded or if he or she did not get a good night's sleep. Also, it may only occur if the person works on a task that is overly demanding. What really complicates the issue is that sometimes it is only the patient who feels the disability, and everyone else, including family, friends, and colleagues at the work site, think that everything is fine with the person. This invisible type of disability is quite daunting.

The following scales are commonly used in measuring disability in persons with brain injury.

Functional Independence Measure

The FIM is the most commonly used disability rating scale in brain injury. It is most helpful in the acute settings and starts to lose its effectiveness once the patient returns to the community.[77] This 18-item, seven-level scale has been shown to have high interobserver reliability.[78] It is a useful tool, especially for screening, monitoring, and assessment. However, it has its limitations. It does not measure cognitive disability very well, and it reaches its effectiveness as an indicator of disability at levels not sensitive enough to measure true community type of physical or cognitive burden, or both.[78] Still, it is easily done within a 20-minute period and is well accepted. The uniformity of the scale and its widespread use have allowed it to be the primarily used scale for research and clinical care. Nevertheless, it needs further refinement in the area of brain injury.

Functional Assessment Measure

The functional assessment measure (FAM) is a scale built onto the FIM to address some of its deficiencies. Areas of emphasis include cognitive, behavioral, communication, and community functioning in this 12-item scale. One of its drawbacks is that the cognitive ratings are a bit too abstract and can be difficult to complete.[79] Also, in the author's opinion, it separates many functions in a fairly artificial way. For example, social interaction and emotional status are two separate entities with two separate scores, yet they are interrelated. Further, although separated for the ease of the professional, they have no natural separation to the patient and are too artificial. This is true for many of the FAM items.

Another personal criticism concerning these two scales is the lack of environmental variability. A brain-injured person finds many challenges in varied environments, and no ordinal rating scale can accurately pick up on this with a gestalt rating system. It is hoped that improvements can be made to allow more sensitivity to environments and to accurately assess cognitive changes in those environments.

Glasgow Outcome Scale

The Glasgow Outcome Scale (GOS) is a global indicator of disability usually used at the time of discharge. The five original ordinal scales of the GOS are dead, vegetative, severely disabled, moderately disabled, and good recovery. The scale is not effective in measuring individual outcomes but better at looking at groups of patients. Because only one score is possible, it is impossible to really know finer discrimination.[80]

Disability Rating Scale

The Disability Rating Scale (DRS) is an extended ordinal scale based on the rating of arousal, awareness, and responsivity; cognitive ability for self-care activities; dependence on others; and psychosocial adaptability. The score of 0 is the one without disability, whereas the score of 29 would put a patient into the "extreme vegetative state" category. The same criticism of the GOS is true for the DRS. The level of disability remains a general single rating that tends to be more accurate at the lower functioning states. Further, human bias is built into this rating scale, as in most of the others, by assuming that the inability to move or talk is a more disabling condition than that of an ambulatory patient who has a great deal of amnesia and unawareness of deficits.

The author's personal bias is that these "disabilities" are just different and should not even be compared with each other. For example, a patient who is given a disability rating of "severely disabled" may in fact have a better QOL than many with a "good outcome" rating. Both the DRS and GOS have been proven reliable and valid.[81,82] One article showed that the GOS demonstrated a "more complete assessment" of disability than the DRS.[83]

Modified Rankin Scale

The modified Rankin scale is also an ordinal scale that is used primarily with stroke patients. It is divided into seven categories: 0, no symptoms at all; 1, no significant disabilities despite symptoms and individual is able to carry out usual duties and activities; 2, slight disability but can manage own affairs without assistance; 3, moderate disability in which individual requires some help but is able to walk without assistance; 4, moderately severe disability in which individual is unable to walk without assistance and unable to handle self-care without assistance; 5, severe disability in which individual is bedridden, requiring constant nursing care; 6, individual is dead. This scale is again biased toward stroke patients who are elderly. It does not give much input to cognitive issues other than saying that a patient needs assistance. It is not used frequently in brain injury but is mentioned because of its widespread use in stroke rehabilitation.

Supervision Rating Scale

The Supervision Rating Scale (SRS) simply measures the level of supervision that a patient receives from caregivers. It is based on a 13-point ordinal scale that can be ranked into five categories: independent, overnight supervision, part-time supervision, full-time indirect supervision, and full-time direct supervision. This scale has been shown to correlate well with the GOS and the DRS.[84] Good correlation has also been seen with independence of self-care. Further, because it is measured by observed behaviors, the scale may be less subjective. It is, nevertheless, dependent on certain characteristics of the patient and the caregiver. A more active caregiver could keep a patient from achieving a higher score because of an increased dependence. Also, certain cultures do not allow the impaired to do much for themselves, which could also skew the findings. The author likes this measure because it is a good yardstick to see how the patient and the caregiver are interacting, and this information can be most helpful once one delves into the context of the patient-caregiver relationship.

This is a sampling of some of the more commonly used disability rating scales. Criticisms can be leveled against all of them. First, they attempt to normalize activities when this is a difficult thing to do even in the well population. Second, many of the categories are artificial and can be biased by culture, economic status, and depth of motor impairment. Finally, all of these scales fail at the level of the high-functioning patient. They are not sensitive enough to pick up the finer details of disability and make it hard to plan ways to improve the treatment to reduce individual disability. Also, a high-level type of patient may be independent in terms of mobility and self-care and may be able to live by his- or herself, yet this person may lack certain executive brain functions and carry a higher risk of unemployment, drug abuse, and isolation because of the injury. These scales can be useful in research and in normative data yet not appropriate for the measurement of the individual. If they are left as the only criteria, treatable conditions or potentially salvageable environments could be missed.

Automated Neuropsychological Assessment Metrics

The ANAM is a computerized cognitive test battery designed for repeated use within the same person and is thus useful when multiple measurements are needed, such as in drug trials. After ANAM testing for a 4-day period, it was shown that the "normal" subjects displayed consistent improvement of performance whereas the "brain-injured" subjects showed erratic and inconsistent performance.[85] This type of information could be very helpful in identifying those individuals who have mild brain injury. Also, the ANAM can be used as a specific outcome measure for each individual patient when given medications to improve cognitive performance. For example, if a question arises regarding which stimulant will be most effective for a given patient, ANAM can be used to construct a simple yet objective double-blind placebo/stimulant A/stimulant B drug trial for that patient. It is this kind of outcome measure that should be a great help in really being able to monitor treatment and take into account the huge individual variability between patients.

Currently, the ANAM takes only 10–12 minutes and presents novel stimuli within five subtests. The ANAM yields measures of accuracy, lapses, reaction time, and standard deviation of reaction time. The five subtests include simple reaction time, running memory, memorization of letters (Sternberg), math processing, and spatial processing.[85] Some of ANAM's limitations primarily include the hardware, the computer, and the technical support. Efforts are being made to simplify the test and make it more accessible via telephone. This type of test will be quite helpful especially in optimizing late recovery by improving overall mental power via cognitive enhancement.

Measurement of Handicap

The definition of handicap as defined by the WHO is "a disadvantage for a given individual, resulting from an impairment or a disability, that limits or prevents the fulfillment of a role that is normal (depending on age, sex, and social and cultural factors) for that individual." The handicap involves the need to overcome obstacles by either compensation or accommodation.

Handicap is even more personal than disability. For example, if a 40-year-old neurologist were to sprain the right index finger, this would cause a certain amount of physiologic impairment and result in a disability due to loss of range of motion and decreased ability to use the finger. This would also be true if this happened to a 40-year-old ophthalmologist. The work handicap for the ophthalmologist, however, would be profound, whereas it might be only a minor handicap for the neurologist. This also helps in understanding the hardest part of a disability rating—cognitive functioning. It must be used in the context of premorbid functioning. In many instances, a person with a brain injury already has cognitive impairments either due to loss of brain power capacity, age, alcohol abuse, drug abuse, and so forth. This obviously complicates the measurement of the effects of the brain injury. The overall burden created by the brain injury is compounded by the presence of these other factors. Even a very mild brain injury can have very severe effects. It sometimes does not take more than a mild brain injury to completely disable a minimally functioning person in the premorbid state.

Most of the rating systems that take handicap into account involve the person in the community. The problems involving a comatose patient who emerges and returns to the community are profoundly different than those of a patient who has only a mild brain injury. For the emerging comatose patient, it is probable that the effects of the brain injury on the personality and the ability to move are still quite evident. For the patient with mild brain injury, however, the impairments that result from the injury may be invisible even to the patient. It may not be recognized that the problems at work and home are injury related; rather, they may easily be attributed to some character deficit. On the one hand, the severely injured person had the more serious injury, but the patient with mild brain injury may eventually face social isolation and unemployment as well.

A person with a brain injury who goes home is viewed as a success story. It is very important to track how a person is doing, however. How is the person doing at home? How is the person doing in the community? Has the person been able to find a job and, if not, why? Is it because of the person and his or her personal issues or is it because of the community and lack of resources? It is extremely difficult to arrive at successful scales that can be sensitive to all of these issues.

Community Integration Questionnaire

The Community Integration Questionnaire (CIQ) attempts to measure the degree to which a disadvantage is active in the life of a person with a brain injury. The 15 questions look at the areas of home life, social activities, and work-related activities. The CIQ has been found to be reliable and able to discriminate between persons with and without brain injury.[86] Also, the correlation of ratings between the person and the caregiver is high, which means that the individuals can do CIQ on their own without much difficulty.[87] Still, CIQ is primarily a scale that measures a general problem and cannot get too specific. This scale has a role as a screening tool. The scale has to be used by clinicians. Once a problem has been identified, the clinician can think of unique solutions to help alleviate the situation if possible.

Conclusion

The treatment of brain injury remains unique to each individual. With treatment, we can offer some promise of meaningful recovery. As we go forth and develop brain injury systems of the future, it is important to realize that knowledge does not always translate into wisdom, and it will remain wise to keep our eye on the person with the injury even as we track the population as a whole.

For instance, if we establish a prognostication system in the future that is 90% accurate, and we are able to estimate which individuals will do well and which will do badly, will that affect the way we treat these individuals as persons? Will we consider reducing the care of those who improve because they "already are expected to improve," and will we reduce the care of the more severely injured because our data determine a low probability of success?

The author's personal bias is that such a prognostication system is far off and that we need to give decent and humane care to all of these individuals no matter how serious the injury. With our knowledge and with time, we hope to come up with ways to improve the motor, cognitive, and behavioral skills, as well as the overall QOL for these individuals. Also, we need to raise the level of our teaching and treatment of the families and to improve the insight and QOL for the caregivers. Further, as we track outcome, we need to pay attention to the outcome of our society as a whole by meeting the huge challenges that this disease has placed on us.

The personal and monetary costs of brain injury will remain high. We need to inspire our community, medical, and business leaders to meet the challenges presented to us by this condition. Continued effort must be made to reduce the number of brain injuries and continued improvements in treating acutely brain-injured patients in a more effective and efficient, yet humane, manner. It is hoped that one day new treatments will be discovered that reduce the cascade of injury and result in a significant reduction in the neurologic impairments with which these patients and families are faced. We cannot, however, allow the rehabilitation period to be de-emphasized because of lack of knowledge or effort; it is the third leg of health care intervention (along with medical and surgical treatment). With this type of understanding, all insurance plans, both public and private, should develop payment plans that allow for wise and judicious treatment during all phases. A medical school teacher used to tell our class that a society is judged on how compassionately it treats its sick and infirm. This remains so. Our society must continue to shine such light on the condition of brain injury.

References

1. Kraus JF. Epidemiology of Head Injury. In PR Cooper (ed), Head Injury (3rd ed). Baltimore: Williams & Wilkins, 1993;1–25.
2. Thurman DJ, Jeppson L, Burnette CL, et al. Surveillance of traumatic brain injuries in Utah. West J Med 1996; 165:192.
3. Epidemiology of Traumatic Brain Injury in the United States. National Center for Injury Prevention and Control. June 1999 (http://www.cdc.gov/ncipc/cmprfact.htm).
4. Sosin DM, Sacks JJ, Smith SM. Head injury associated deaths in the United States from 1979–1986. JAMA 1989;262:2251.
5. Sosin DM, Sniezek JE, Waxweiler RJ. Trends in death associated with brain injury. JAMA 1995;278:1778.
6. Sosin DM, Nelson DE, Sacks JJ. Head injury deaths: the enormity of firearms. JAMA 1992;268:791.
7. Kraus JF. Injury to head and spinal cord. National Head and Spinal Cord Injury Survey. J Neurosurg 1980;53:S3.
8. Levin HS, Mattis S, Ruff RM, et al. Neurobehavioral outcome following minor head injury. A three center study. J Neurosurg 1987;66:234.
9. U.S. Department of Health and Human Services. Interagency Head Injury Task Force Report. Washington, DC: Department of Health and Human Services, 1989.
10. Tate RL, McDonald S, Lulham JM. Incidence of hospital-treated traumatic brain injury in an Australian community. Aust N Z Public Health 1998;22:419–423.
11. Guerrero JL, Leadbetter S, Thurman DJ, et al. A Method for Estimating the Prevalence of Disability from Traumatic Brain Injury. In Epidemiology of Traumatic Brain Injury in the United States. National Center for Injury Prevention and Control. June 1, 1999.
12. Kraus JF, Black MA, Hessol N, et al. The incidence of acute brain injury and serious impairment in a defined population. Am J Epidemiol 1984;119:186.
13. Kraus JF. Epidemiology of Head Injury. In PR Cooper (ed), Head Injury (3rd ed). Baltimore: Williams & Wilkins, 1993;10–11.
14. Kraus JF, Fife D, Ramstein K, et al. The relationship of family income to the incidence, external causes, and outcomes of serious brain injury, San Diego County, California. Am J Public Health 1986;11:1345.
15. Kraus JF. Epidemiology of Head Injury. In PR Cooper (ed), Head Injury (3rd ed). Baltimore: Williams & Wilkins, 1993;11–15.
16. Harrison-Felix C, Zafonte R, Mann N, et al. Brain injury as a result of violence: preliminary findings from the traumatic brain injury model systems. Arch Phys Med Rehabil 1998;79:730.
17. Hall KM, Karzmark P, Stevens M. Family stressors in traumatic brain injury: a two year followup. Arch Phys Med Rehabil 1994;75:876.
18. Max W, MacKenzie EJ, Rice DP. Head injuries: cost and consequences. J Head Trauma Rehabil 1991;6:76.
19. Bassuk EL, Melnik S, Browne A. Responding to the needs of low income and homeless women who are survivors of family violence. J Am Med Womens Assoc 1998;53:57.
20. Kelly MP, Johnson CT, Knoller N, et al. Substance abuse, traumatic brain injury and neuropsychological outcome. Brain Inj 1997;11:391.
21. McGuire LM, Burright RG, Williams R, Donovick PJ. Prevalence of traumatic brain injury in psychiatric and nonpsychiatric subjects. Brain Inj 1998;12:207.
22. Geddes JF, Vowles GH, Beer TW, Ellison DW. The diagnosis of diffuse axonal injury: implications for forensic practice. Neuropathol Appl Neurobiol 1997;23:339.
23. Jane JA, Steward O, Gennarelli TA. Axonal degeneration induced by experimental noninvasive head injury. J Neurosurg 1985;62:96.
24. Gram DI, Adams GH, Gennarelli TA. Pathology of Brain Damage in Head Injury. In PR Cooper (ed), Head Injury (3rd ed). Baltimore: Williams & Wilkins, 1993; 91–113.
25. Cope DN, Date ES, Mar EY. Serial computerized tomography evaluations in traumatic head injury. Arch Phys Rehabil 1988;69:483.

26. Gram DI. Hypoxia and Vascular Disorders. In JD Adams, LW Duchen (eds), Greenfield's Neuropathology (5th ed). New York: Oxford University Press, 1992;153–268.

27. Schneck SA. Cerebral Anoxia. In AB Baker, LH Baker (eds), Clinical Neurology. Philadelphia: Harper and Row, 1994;1–18.

28. Nagurney JT, Borczuk P, Thomas SH. Elder patients with closed head trauma: a comparison with nonelder patients. Acad Emerg Med 1998;5:678.

29. Hicks RR, Smith DH, Lowenstein DH, et al. Mild experimental brain injury in the rat induces cognitive deficits associated with regional neuronal loss in the hippocampus. J Neurotrauma 1993;10:405.

30. Kelly JP, Nicholes JS, Philley CM, et al. Concussion in sports. Guidelines for the prevention in catastrophic outcomes. JAMA 1991;266:2867.

31. Shimura T, Mukai T, Teramoto A, et al. Clinicopathological studies of craniocerebral gunshot injuries. No Shinkei Geka 1997;25:607.

32. Annegers JF, Hauser WA, Coan SP, Rocca WA. A population based study of seizures after traumatic brain injuries. N Engl J Med 1998;338:20.

33. Jennett B, Teather D, Bennie S. Epilepsy after head injury. Residual risk after varying fit-free intervals since injury. Lancet 1973;2:652.

34. Temkin NR, Dikmen SS, Wilensky AJ, ct al. A randomized, double-blind study of phenytoin for the prevention of post-traumatic seizures. N Engl J Med 1990; 323:497.

35. McLean MJ. Gabapentin. Epilepsia 1995;36(suppl 2); S73.

36. Massagli TL. Neurobehavioral effects of phenytoin, carbamazepine, and valproic acid: implications for use in traumatic brain injury. Arch Phys Med Rehabil 1991;72:219.

37. Wilson JE, McCarthy AD. Variability of functional performance as a clinical criteria in the diagnosis of normal pressure hydrocephalus in brain injured patients (abstract). Am J Phys Med Rehabil 1996;75:157.

38. Bradley WG Jr. Magnetic resonance imaging in the evaluation of cerebrospinal fluid flow abnormalities. Magn Reson Q 1992;8:169.

39. Marmarou A, Foda MA, Bandoh K, et al. Post-traumatic ventriculomegaly: hydrocephalus or atrophy? A new approach for diagnosis using CSF dynamics. J Neurosurg 1996;85:1026.

40. Gudeman SK, Kishore PRS, Becker DP, et al. Computed tomography in the evaluation of incidence and significance of post-traumatic hydrocephalus. Neuroradiology 1981;141:397.

41. Packard RC, Ham LP. Pathogenesis of post-traumatic headache and migraine: a common headache pathway? Headache 1997;37:142.

42. Schneider D, McCarthy AD. Undiagnosed cervical spine trauma on entry to a traumatic brain injury unit (abstract). Am J Phys Med Rehabil 1996;75:163.

43. Fitzgerald DC. Head trauma: hearing loss and dizziness. J Trauma 1996;40:488.

44. Fitzgerald DC. Persistent dizziness following head trauma and perilymphatic fistula. Arch Phys Med Rehabil 1995;76:1017.

45. Solomon S, Hotchkiss E, Saravay SM, et al. Impairment of memory function by antihypertensive medication. Arch Gen Psychiatry 1983;40:1109.

46. Smith KR Jr., Golding PM, Wilderman D, et al. Neurobehavioral effects of phenytoin and carbamazepine in patients recovering from brain trauma: a comparative study. Arch Neurol 1994;51:653.

47. Bowen JD, Larson EB. Drug-induced cognitive impairment. Defining the problem and finding solutions. Drugs Aging 1993;3:349.

48. Elitsur Y. Pameline (Cylert)–induced hepatotoxicity. J Pediatr Gastoenterol Nutr 1990;11:143.

49. Zasler N. Traumatic Brain Injury. In TR Dillingham, PV Belandres (eds), Rehabilitation of the Injured Combatant: Textbook of Military Medicine. Part IV, vol 1. Falls Church, VA: Office of the Surgeon General, 1998; 207–278.

50. Boyeson MG, Harmon RL, Jones JL. Comparative effects of fluoxetine, amitriptyline and serotonin on functional motor recovery after sensory motor cortex injury. Am J Phys Med Rehabil 1994;73:76.

51. Mysiw WJ, Jackson RD, Corrigan JD. Amitriptyline for post-traumatic agitation. Am J Phys Med Rehabil 1988; 67;29.

52. Jacobsen FM. Low-dose valproate: a new treatment for cyclothymia, mild rapid cycling disorders and premenstrual syndrome. J Clin Psychiatry 1993;54:229.

53. Small JG, Klapper MH, Milstein V, et al. Carbamazepine compared with lithium in the treatment of mania. Arch Gen Psychiatry 1991;48:915.

54. Bellus SB, Stewart D, Vergo JG, et al. The use of lithium in the treatment of aggressive behaviors with two brain-injured individuals in a state psychiatric hospital. Brain Inj 1996;10:849.

55. Levine AM. Buspirone and agitation in head injury. Brain Inj 1988;2:165.

56. Davidson JR. Use of benzodiazepine in panic disorder. J Clin Psychiatry 1997;58(suppl 2):26.

57. Erickson KR. Amnestic disorders. Pathophysiology and patterns of memory dysfunction. West J Med 1990; 152: 159.

58. Stanslav SW. Cognitive effects of antipsychotic agents in persons with traumatic brain injury. Brain Inj 1997; 11: 335.

59. Schreiber S, Klag E, Gross Y, et al. Beneficial effect of risperidone on sleep disturbance and psychosis following traumatic brain injury. Int Clin Psychopharmacol 1998; 13:273.

60. High WM Jr, Levin HS, Gary HE Jr. Recovery of orientation following post-head injury. J Clin Exp Neuropsychol 1990;12:703.

61. Kelly MP, Johnson CT, Knoller N, et al. Substance abuse, traumatic brain injury and neuropsychological outcome. Brain Inj 1997;11:391.

62. Yousem DM, Geckle RJ, Bilker WB, et al. Post-traumatic olfactory dysfunction: MR and clinical evaluation. Am J Neuroradiol 1996;17:1171.

63. Field LH, Yeiss CJ. Dysphagia with head injury. Brain Inj 1989;3:19.

64. Wood RL, Yurdakul LK. Change in relationship status following traumatic brain injury. Brain Inj 1997;11:491.

65. Mazaux JM, Masson F, Levin HS, et al. Long-term neuropsychological outcome and loss of social autonomy after traumatic brain injury. Arch Phys Med Rehabil 1997; 78:1316.

66. McCleary C, Satz P, Forney D. Depression after traumatic brain injury as a function of Glasgow Outcome Score. J Clin Exp Neuropsychol 1998;20:270.

67. Vieth AZ, Johnstone B, Dawson B. Extent of intellectual, cognitive and academic decline in adolescent traumatic brain injury. Brain Inj 1996;10:465.

68. Knight RG, Devereux R, Godfrey HP. Caring for a family member with a traumatic brain injury. Brain Inj 1998; 12:467.

69. Marsh MV, Kersel DA, Havill JH, et al. Caregiver burden at 1 year following severe traumatic brain injury. Brain Inj 1998; 12:1045.

70. Semlyen JK, Summers SJ, Barnes MP. Traumatic brain injury: efficacy of multidisciplinary rehabilitation. Arch Phys Med Rehabil 1998;79:678.

71. Sherer SM, Bergloff P, Levin E, et al. Impairment awareness and employment outcome after traumatic brain injury. J Head Trauma Rehabil 1998;13:52.

72. Hillier SL, Metzer J. Awareness and perceptions of outcomes after traumatic brain injury. Brain Inj 1997;11:525.

73. Holland D, Shigaki CL. Educating families and caretakers of traumatically injured patients in the new health care environment: a three phase model and bibliography. Brain Inj 1998;12:993.

74. Juarez VJ, Lyons M. Interrater reliability of the Glasgow coma scale. J Neurosci Nurs 1995;27:283.

75. Menegazzi JJ, Davis EA, Sucov AN, Paris PM. Reliability of the Glasgow coma scale when used by emergency physicians and paramedics. J Trauma 1993;34:46.

76. Zafonte RD, Hammond FM, Mann NR, et al. Relationship between Glasgow coma scale and functional outcome. Am J Phys Med Rehabil 1996;75:364.

77. Hall KM, Mann NIW, et al. Functional measures after traumatic brain injury: ceiling affects of the FIM, the FIM + FAM, DRS and CIQ. J Head Trauma Rehabil 1996; 11:27.

78. Hamilton BB, Laughlin JA, Granger CV, Kayton RM. Interrater agreement of the seven level functional independence measure (FIM) (abstract). Arch Phys Med Rehabil 1991;72:790.

79. Alcott D, Dixon K, Swann R. The reliability of the items of the functional assessment measure (FAM): differences in abstractness between FAM items. Disabil Rehabil 1997;19:355.

80. Bleiberg J, Cope DN, Spector J. Cognitive Assessment and Therapy in Traumatic Brain Injury. Phys Med Rehabil State Art Rev 1989;3;95–123.

81. Anderson SI, Hassley AM, et al. Glasgow outcome scale: an interrater reliability study. Brain Inj 1993;7:309.

82. Hall KN, Hamilton B, Gordon WA, et al. Characteristics and comparisons of functional assessment indices: disability rating scale, functional independence measure and functional assessment measure. J Head Trauma Rehabil 1993;8:60.

83. Pettigrew LE, Wilson JT, Teasdale GM. Assessing disability after head injury: improved use of the Glasgow outcome scales. J Neurosurg 1998;89:939.

84. Voc C. Supervision rating scale: a measure of functional outcome from brain injury. Arch Phys Med Rehabil 1996; 77:765.

85. Bleiberg J, Garmoe WS, Halpern EL, et al. Consistency of within-day and across-day performance after mild brain injury. Neuropsychol Behav Neurol 1997;10:247.

86. Dijkers M. Measuring the long-term outcomes of traumatic brain injury: a review of community integration questionnaire studies. J Head Trauma Rchabil 1997; 12:74.

87. Sander AN, Seel RT, Kreutzer JS, et al. Agreement between persons with traumatic brain injury and their relatives' psychosocial outcome using the community integration questionnaire. Arch Phys Med Rehabil 1997;78: 353.

Chapter 7

Management of Persons with Neuromuscular Disease

Susan M. Miller

Nature of the Problem

Extent of the Problem

Neuromuscular diseases (NMDs) are disorders caused by abnormalities in the motor neuron unit. The motor neuron unit is composed of the anterior horn cell in the spinal cord, the peripheral nerve, the neuromuscular junction, and the muscle. NMDs can affect one or multiple components of the motor neuron unit and may be acquired or hereditary (Table 7-1).

The general description of the comprehensive care of the patient with an NMD is difficult because the demonstrated demographics and types of complications in these disease processes can vary greatly between the many disease complexes within this category. Therefore, as a group, NMDs cannot be characterized in any general way in terms of age, gender, distribution of weakness, rate of progression, and so forth, as each disease process in and of itself is individual.

Nevertheless, NMDs do produce consequences to the patient's status that have commonalities throughout all individuals. The problems experienced in these particular disorders are those that affect the neuromuscular, musculoskeletal, cognitive, and cardiopulmonary systems of the body. Furthermore, many, if not most, of the NMDs are progressive in their course, thus causing a dynamic situation whereby patients must constantly adjust and then readjust again to an ever-changing bodily state. Such dynamics not only can place severe physical distress on one's bodily habitus but also are likely to cause significant psychological stress to patients and family that further complicates the physical consequences of disease.

No specific treatment is available for the pathophysiologic abnormality that occurs in NMDs; however, treatment of these diseases is not futile. Although it is not within the scope of this chapter to describe the medical regimens afforded to patients with NMD, the information presented here provides an overview of the management techniques that are appropriate to maintain the functional status of this patient population.

The goal of management in any patient is to provide that individual with a means to remain independent or at a level of maximal functioning for as long as possible, no matter what the disease process or course. Thus, such techniques can be considered for all patients with NMD. For any practitioner to appropriately provide treatment for such a population, however, the types of complications that are specific to these illnesses must be clearly understood.

The consequences of any disease process can be categorized in numerous ways. According to the model established by the WHO, diseases are subdivided into impairments, disabilities, and handicaps. Impairments are the signs and symptoms of the disease process, the abnormalities of the physiologic system that are out of the ordinary for the body as a whole. The disability is the func-

Table 7-1. Neuromuscular Disease Categories (with Examples)

I. Anterior horn cell disease
 Motor neuron disease
  Amyotrophic lateral sclerosis
  Spinal muscular atrophy
II. Disease of the neuromuscular junction
 Myasthenia gravis
 Eaton-Lambert syndrome
III. Neuropathies
 Charcot-Marie-Tooth disease
 Hereditary sensory and motor neuropathy
 Mononeuropathy (single or multiple)
 Recurrent polyneuropathy
IV. Myopathies
 Muscular dystrophy
  Duchenne's muscular dystrophy
  Becker's muscular dystrophy
  Facioscapulohumeral syndrome
  Limb-girdle syndrome
 Congenital structural myopathies
  Nemaline myopathy
  Central core disease
 Metabolic myopathies
  McArdle's disease (phosphorylase deficiency)
  Periodic paralysis
 Endocrine myopathies
  Hyperthyroid myopathy
  Hypothyroid myopathy
 Inflammatory myopathies
  Polymyositis (acute or chronic)
  Dermatomyositis
V. Hyperirritable syndrome
 Myokymia
VI. Degenerative disease of the cerebellum, brain stem, spinal cord
 Friedreich's ataxia

tional loss that the impairment causes. Weakened limbs, for example, can result in an inability to walk; weakened hands can cause an individual the inability to self-feed. The handicap is that which, from the patient's point of view, determines the true severity of the illness. It is the consequence of the disease to the individual that has its effects on a societal level. It can, for example, be the loss of a job, the loss of marital parity, or the loss of the feeling that the individual is truly participating in the role of a parent.[1]

Only the patient can determine how the disease has produced (or not produced) a handicapping effect on his or her life. If the health care team wishes to diminish the handicap as defined by the patient, they must understand the problems faced by the patient in daily life. To do so requires that the health care team, and specifically those who provide for rehabilitation management, focus on the patient and make him or her part of their treating unit, listening carefully to what the patient considers to have had a significant impact on his or her life.

An example is that of a 52-year-old retired clerk who had a 1-year history of progressive motor system involvement, diagnosed as ALS. He was impaired in both upper and lower extremities, with the left side more impaired than the right. No impairment in speech or swallowing was present. Fatigue was a major problem, as was pain in the area of fasciculation. When asked about his disabilities, he mentioned the expected problems with mobility: getting out of bed and self-feeding, particularly later in the day when his fatigue was more severe. What particularly troubled him was his isolation. He was unable to use the telephone to communicate with his friends. One of the priorities not necessarily identifiable was the need to select some technical aids by which he could once again communicate. Only by asking the patient about his disabilities could his problems be identified and a proper plan designed.

Thus, to successfully rehabilitate an individual with an NMD, a rehabilitation practitioner must understand the various problems faced by the patient. The first portion of this chapter therefore illustrates the nature of the difficulties experienced by patients with NMD. This is accomplished first by making the reader familiar with the clinical and physical manifestations of selected NMDs that affect adults. (Childhood conditions are not described in detail in this chapter.) The diseases that are discussed include ALS, the most common progressive motor neuron disease; the spinal muscular atrophies (SMA; often confused with ALS when they present in the young adult and adult form); and Becker's muscular dystrophy (BMD), a primary muscular disorder. ALS and the SMAs together demonstrate the medical problems that arise from injury to the proximal portion of the motor neuron unit, the anterior horn cell. BMD demonstrates the difficulties experienced by those who have a primary myopathy and thus represents pathology of the most distal component of the motor neuron unit. Viewed as a continuum, the symptoms of these disease complexes serve to illustrate to the reader the spectrum and diversity of problems presented by illness that affects the motor neuron unit. After the medical details of these specific NMD processes are summarized, the general consequences of NMD are detailed.

In the second portion of this chapter (Character of the Solution), the way in which the rehabilitation management team approach can be useful to a patient with NMD is demonstrated through actual case reports of patients with ALS, SMA, and BMD. In this way, the reader is able to see the link between the medical complications of these illnesses and their functional implications.

Finally, the means by which a patient's impairment, disabilities, and handicaps can be measured and followed is discussed in the final portion of this chapter, Measuring Effectiveness.

Nature of the Disease

Amyotrophic Lateral Sclerosis

ALS is a progressive neurologic disease that results from variable degeneration of both upper and lower motor neurons.[2] Overall, men are more often affected by this disease than are women (ratio, 1.5 to 1.0),[3] which commonly manifests itself between the ages of 40 and 60 years. Its worldwide prevalence is approximately five to seven cases per 100,000 persons, large enough to make it one of the more common NMDs found today. Overall, the median survival rate of this disorder is 2.5 years after the diagnosis is made. The main finding in ALS is its motor neuron symptom of skeletal muscle weakness.[4] Accompanying this symptom are other disorders of lower motor neuron disease, including atrophy, cramps, fatigue, fasciculation, dysarthria, and dysphagia. Additionally, in more than 80% of all individuals affected by ALS, the lower motor neuron disease is mixed with upper motor neuron findings of spasticity and hyperreflexia; at times severe.[2]

Adult ALS can be divided into three recognizable types: sporadic, familial, and Western Pacific. The majority of patients with ALS (approximately 65%) demonstrate the sporadic type of the disease, also known as *classic ALS*. In this form, features of upper motor neuron and lower neuron disease often combine in the patient's initial presentation. Weakness and atrophy of the arms and hands are usually more commonly seen at the initial evaluation than are symptoms in the lower extremities. Soon these symptoms are followed by bulbar and respiratory weakness in approximately 50% of patients. Spasticity occurs in about 50–75% of all patients. Extrapyramidal symptoms and dementia occur in fewer than 5% of these individuals.[2]

Several variants of sporadic ALS exist; of note is the progressive bulbar palsy type. Approximately 25% of patients with this variant demonstrate dysarthria and dysphagia at the onset of their disease, with variable involvement of the limbs. Pseudobulbar symptoms occur in up to 75% of these patients. In the variant of ALS known as progressive muscular atrophy, patients present only with lower motor neuron symptoms of weakness and atrophy in the limbs, but widespread involvement soon follows.[2] On the other hand, primary lateral sclerosis presents with the upper motor neuron symptoms of spastic weakness and increased reflexes.[3,5]

Familial ALS occurs in approximately 10% of patients, and approximately 2% are known to result from a specific chromosomal abnormality.[4] The disease is usually inherited as a dominant trait, with variable penetrance and expressivity. Men and women are equally affected; the mean age of onset is approximately 46 years. Clinically, the familial and sporadic types of ALS are similar. However, in the former process, lower extremity involvement at presentation is more commonly seen than in the sporadic type, and less mixture of upper motor neuron and lower motor neuron symptomatology is found. Moreover, dementia is more frequently found in familial ALS, as it is noted in approximately 15% of cases.[2]

Western Pacific ALS is endemic to Guam, Western New Guinea, and the Kii Peninsula. The onset of this disease occurs earlier than in sporadic cases, particularly in New Guinea, where the mean age of onset is 33 years. A slightly higher male to female ratio is also found in this disease than is found in classic ALS.[2]

In addition to the weakness of oral, pharyngeal, and skeletal muscles caused by all types of ALS, a weakness of respiratory muscles also occurs. At the onset of the disease, patients are frequently asymptomatic in this organ system; thus, pulmonary function tests must be used to confirm this impairment. As the disease progresses, so, too, does the weakness of the respiratory system, causing progressive shortness of breath, first on exertion, then while performing ADL, and finally at rest. Death in ALS usually results from respiratory failure.[6]

Spinal Muscular Atrophy

SMA is a disease complex characterized by degeneration of the motor neuron of the spinal cord. It can manifest itself with a spectrum of presentations, all of which have in common weakness and muscular atrophy due to the deterioration of the anterior horn cell. Sensory and sphincter involvement are usually absent in this process. Brain stem motor nuclei may also be affected in some of these disorders.[7]

Most commonly, SMA presents in one of three forms. SMA type I, also known as *Werdnig-Hoffmann syndrome*, accounts for approximately 25% of all presentations. It is inherited as an autosomal recessive pattern and occurs in approximately 1 in 25,000 live births of children born in England and 1 in 400 live births of children born to Karaite Jews in Israel. Mothers of affected babies can sometimes feel a decrease of fetal movement during their last trimester. Other children present as floppy infants at, or soon after, birth. These infants also demonstrate a poor suck and weak cry and are areflexic. Orthopedic abnormalities, such as congenital dislocation of the hips and flexion contracture of limbs, are not uncommon. The median survival age of a child with SMA type I is 7 months; only 5% of affected children live past the age of 18 months.[2]

SMA type II is otherwise known as *late infantile* or *juvenile-onset SMA*. It accounts for 45% of all cases. The clinical onset of this disease is variable (up to age 17 years) but usually occurs by age 5 years. Usually inherited as an autosomal recessive disorder, the disease presents with hypotonia and a delay in the normal developmental milestones of walking or climbing. Proximal weakness of the arms and legs along with atrophy of these same areas is very common. Scoliosis, muscular pseudohypertrophy, and chest deformities may also be seen. Mental retardation is occasionally associated with this condition, but, generally, the intelligence level of the affected child is measured to be above normal. Those children who manifest the disease early in life are more likely to experience severe functional consequences; those with late-onset disease (between 3 and 8 years) are usually still walking at age 10 years.[2] Respiratory compromise has been noted in affected individuals with SMA type II secondary to restrictive lung disease.[8] The median age of death in this process is greater than 12 years, with 15% of those affected still living at age 20 years.[2] Despite the usual autosomal recessive inheritance of SMA type II, approximately 10% of the affected individuals may have a disease that is due to a dominant mutation or is sex linked in nature.[2]

Type III SMA (adult-onset SMA), which accounts for 8% of all SMA cases, may be inherited in an autosomal dominant, autosomal recessive, or X-linked recessive pattern. The disease usually manifests between the ages of 20 and 50 years with symptoms of limb-girdle weakness and atrophy as the presenting complaints. Strength loss is slowly progressive over the years, and distal weakness can also eventually occur. Facial and tongue involvement is seen in up to 50% of individuals affected with this disease process.[2] Respiratory compromise is unusual, as is scoliosis. Intellectual functioning is usually within normal limits.[8]

Other forms of SMA include those with symptoms of significant dysarthria and dysphagia (bulbospinal muscular atrophy); significant weakness, atrophy, and hypotonia of the distal muscles of the arms and legs (distal spinal muscular atrophy); and pectoral-pelvic weakness that may or may not be associated with cardiomyopathy and a distal sensory neuropathy (scapuloperoneal SMA).[2]

Becker's Muscular Dystrophy

BMD is an X-linked, inherited progressive dystrophy of skeletal muscle that predominantly affects boys. This disease, caused by a mutation of a gene located on the X chromosome, produces an abnormality in the protein product known as *dystrophin*. As the component of muscle membrane, dystrophin contributes to plasma membrane stability. The defect in this protein product caused by BMD ultimately yields a chronic necrotizing myopathy.[7]

Overall prevalence of the disease is estimated at 3 to 6 per 100,000 male births.[9]

Approximately 10% of persons with BMD demonstrate a severe process of clinical signs and symptoms, including significant delay in motor milestones, with weakness appearing as early as ages 3–5 years. These same patients become wheelchair dependent for ambulation in their 20s.[7] The majority of individuals with BMD, however, show a milder course, with symptoms of the disease beginning around the age of 8–12 years and requiring the use of a wheelchair approximately 50–60 years later.[10]

Proximal lower extremity muscles are affected first in BMD; those involved most often and most severely are the hip and knee extensors, which experience progressive decline over the years. Proximal muscle weakness of the upper extremities occurs gradually over 10–20 years from disease onset. The neck flexors also seem to be affected early in the course of this disease, but their strength remains clinically stable as the rest of the disease progresses over the years. Severe contractures are not a general characteristic of BMD until wheelchair dependence occurs.[10]

Spinal deformity is present in BMD but is usually mild and rarely requires the need for surgical correction and stabilization. Similarly, respiratory compromise is usually mild in this disease process, with the percentage of predicted forced vital capacity (FVC) remaining essentially normal until the third or fourth decade.[10] Of serious concern, however, is the risk of significant life-threatening cardiac disease in BMD. The cardiac involvement of BMD does not necessarily follow the progression of skeletal muscle impairment. Life-threatening disease can occur in forms of this disease that present themselves with mild limb weakness. Electrocardiograms may demonstrate abnormal Q waves (correlating with localized areas of fibrosis on autopsy), right ventricular hypertrophy, right bundle branch block, and left ventricular hypertrophy.[11] Echocardiograms have been reported to demonstrate both left ventricular dilatation and global hypokinesia in BMD patients.[10]

Neurogenetics

Many NMDs have been found to be hereditary in nature. In some of these disorders, the chromosomal location of the abnormality is known and the causal gene has been identified.[12] Therefore, physicians are now able to rely on DNA testing to help diagnose some NMDs presymptomatically or to provide reproductive counseling to those who wish to have children, or both.[13]

The biomedical aspects of NMD are well beyond the scope of this chapter. However, because scientific advances have begun to place genomic medicine (the use of genotypic analysis or DNA testing) within the boundaries of routine clinical practice, the outcome of such scientific advances needs to be carefully considered by practitioners who care for those with NMDs.[13] With the rapidly accelerating growth of genomic medicine, the demands for genetic counseling are also increasing. Consumers with genetic concerns about their own risk for an inherited disorder or those concerned with the risk of passing on such a disease to their offspring freely question their physicians regarding DNA testing.[14] Although it may be true that direct DNA tests investigating neurogenic disorders can improve the power of diagnosis and lead to more accurate predictions of prognosis, this diagnostic procedure has numerous social, psychological, and ethical implications that need to be recognized and anticipated by those who use them.[15]

The practitioner needs to be aware that the benefits of genomic medicine can only be fully accessed by appreciating the effect that this type of information has on the patients' or family's knowledge base, mental well-being, and subsequent familial and societal interactions. Therefore, suitable counseling and guidance must be accessible to those affected by NMDs so that the feelings of anxiety, depression, shame, and guilt that accompany these illnesses can be addressed. Professionals must be available to aid in the development of an appropriate coping system to allow all those affected by these diseases to acknowledge the changes that are occurring in their lives and to learn to go forward in spite of them.[16–18]

Nature of the Impairments

Mobility Complications in Neuromuscular Disease

The weakness and spasticity caused by NMD are self-evident. These two qualities, however, are not solely responsible for the decrease in mobility and loss of ADL abilities witnessed in these patients.

Such disability secondary to NMD is also caused by contracture formation, spinal deformity, and entrapment neuropathies.

Contracture formation in those with NMD is caused by the interplay of structural changes intrinsic to the muscle itself as well as factors related to, but external to, the pathophysiology of the disease process. For example, in myopathies, abnormal muscle fibers are replaced with collagen and fatty tissue, resulting in muscle fibrosis and limited flexibility. (Neurogenic atrophy of muscle results in similar abnormal depositions, but usually in lesser amounts.) The clinical result of this abnormal process—limited strength and range of motion of the affected muscles—makes it difficult to achieve full, active movement of joints, particularly in the antigravity plane. This condition then produces as its detrimental consequence prolonged static posturing of a joint. Positioning of a joint so that muscles are placed in a shortened state for a long period can cause these structures to lose up to 40% of their sarcomeres and thus their potential for full range of motion. Muscle groups that cross more than one joint are at unique risk for contracture, because during the pursuit of normal activities, they are rarely in positions of maximal stretch. These muscles include the hamstrings, rectus femoris, gastrocnemius, tensor fasciae latae, iliopsoas, long finger flexors, biceps brachii, and pectoralis major. Their contractures lead to flexion deformities of the knees, hips, elbows, and ankles as well as the shoulder protraction and the hip abduction abnormalities that are so commonly seen in individuals with NMD.[19]

Some contractures, however, occur as compensatory mechanisms to maintain functional movement and as such can be considered postural substitutes that develop to maintain upright gait mechanics in the face of progressively weakening musculature. Haphazard attempts to correct these contractures could produce a functional decline in the status of the patient.

To understand this concept, it is necessary to know that standing is almost a completely passive activity as long as the upper segment of the body (head, trunk, arms) is properly aligned over the supporting limbs, allowing the line of gravity (or balance) through the body to fall behind the center of rotation of the hip, in front of the knees and ankles, and within the base of support created by the feet. This biomechanical arrangement maintains its stability by relying mostly on the restraining forces of the iliofemoral ligament of the pelvis and the posterior ligament and capsule of the knee, requiring only a minimum amount of active work by the gastrocnemius-soleus complex to create an erect, upright position.[20] Ambulation is an extension of this balancing act; it is a series of controlled falls followed by quick recoveries modulated by muscles that are all working in coordinated succession to move the body's center of gravity along a designated path, keeping a balance line within its base of support.[21]

In those with NMD, muscle weakness disturbs this series of coordinated events. Patients with Duchenne's muscular dystrophy (DMD) have lost approximately 45% of the body's total muscle mass by the age of 4 1/2. Weakness becomes most severe in the muscles that play a major role in maintaining upright posturing. Thus, the biomechanics of normal standing and walking must be altered to compensate.[21] For example, as the quadriceps muscle begins to weaken early in the course of the disease, an anterior pelvic tilt occurs to move the body's balance line in front of the knee joint to prevent falls. As time progresses, however, further decompensation of the quadriceps occurs, and this compensatory mechanism is no longer sufficient to stabilize the upright position. The patient therefore begins to use forceful contraction of the ankle plantar flexors to provide the motion that opposes knee flexion and again places the line of balance anterior to the knee joint. The individual thus begins to manifest an equinus posturing (tiptoe gait) to promote knee stability. Eventually, ankle plantar flexion contractures develop, but they do so, along with other postural changes, to keep the child with DMD upright and ambulatory.[22] Early interference with this contracture, without recognition or understanding of its integrative function to maintain proper body alignment, could be harmful to the patient's ambulatory status. However, when the practitioner views this mechanism as part of a larger series of adaptive effects of the body, he or she can treat this contracture appropriately via surgery or bracing, or both, as needed.[21,22]

Progressive NMD can also be associated with significantly deforming spinal disease. Such an abnormality may manifest itself as scoliosis, kyphoscoliosis, and hyperlordosis. In the most severe cases, scoliosis and its resultant pelvic obliquity can prevent functional upright sitting even in a wheelchair and thereby preclude the individual's accomplishment of normal seated ADL. In addition, spinal deformity can be painful, potentiate the development of skin breakdown, and may not only exacerbate the impairment caused by the pulmonary disorders of NMD but may prevent individuals from being fitted with the noninvasive bodily equipment designed to lessen the disability of their respiratory compromise.[23]

In the past, the rapid progression of spinal deformity in an individual with NMD was linked to the transition from two-leg ambulation to use of a wheelchair. This relationship, however, is no longer clear. More than likely, the development of spinal abnormalities in those with NMD is related to a combination of factors, including age at disease onset, progression of muscular weakness, and timing of the adolescent growth spurt. Whereas those with DMD are classically considered to be at risk for significant spinal deformity during the course of their disease, individuals with spinal muscular atrophy, facioscapulohumeral muscular dystrophy, Friedreich's ataxia, and congenital myotonic muscular dystrophy also frequently experience this abnormality.[23]

Patients who are immobilized for any reason or who use ambulatory aids, or both, are subject to entrapment neuropathies of the ulnar, median, radial, and peroneal nerves.[24–27] For example, in the upper extremity, high carpal canal pressures have been documented in the position of passive wrist extension, the posture frequently assumed by those who use wheelchairs, crutches, and canes.[24] Similarly, compression of the ulnar nerve is a documented phenomenon.[25] In those who use walkers, repetitive and strenuous contractions of the triceps muscles have been implicated in a mononeuropathy of the radial nerve.[26]

Although little research has been done on the topic, it appears that patients with NMD, and specifically those with ALS, share in this risk of entrapment neuropathies. Practitioners should not consider signs and symptoms of weakness and sensory loss over the pathway of isolated peripheral nerves to represent minor complaints in this patient population. Without appropriate interventional measures, the damage to these nerves could progress to unfavorably alter the function of an individual's hand grip or distal foot control, or both, and thus interfere with the ability to walk, use

an assistive device, and perform basic ADL. The diagnosis and treatment of an entrapment neuropathy in an individual with NMD can be managed by either a conservative or surgical approach as appropriate to maintain the highest level of function and QOL in the affected patient.[27]

Malnutrition

Chronic malnutrition is common in individuals with NMDs. Nutritional assessment is difficult in these patients; commonly used weight charts have little bearing in those who experience the symptoms of muscular atrophy, muscle replacement by fat, and growth retardation. Additionally, the muscular weakness imposed by the underlying disorder itself causes feeding problems in the preoral, oral, and pharyngeal stages of the alimentary process. For example, weakness in the skeletal muscles of the limb often makes it difficult for patients to have the strength necessary to bring hand to mouth to self-feed. Facial and oral muscular weakness presents difficulties in having the food remain in the mouth once it is placed there as well as in chewing and propelling the food from the lips to the pharynx. Pharyngeal muscle weakness can result in choking, nasal reflux, and aspiration.[28]

In one study of selected NMDs, an overall frequency of feeding complaints was noted in approximately 35% of polled individuals.[29] Few of the subjects reported eating difficulties in response to a global question on the subject; however, when asked specific questions pertaining to discrete symptoms related to eating, many more of these patients provided profiles indicative of nutritional or swallowing disorders, or both. Thus, a practitioner can easily miss the signs and symptoms that would provoke the necessary interventions to this important problem unless a detailed history is taken, actively searching for subtle signs of impairment.[29]

Cardiac Abnormalities

The NMDs are frequently associated with cardiac abnormalities, including cardiomyopathy, ventricular dilatation, and conduction defects. In some of these diseases, the extent of cardiac involvement is of little functional concern; in others, the demonstrated cardiac dysfunction has the potential to cause significant increases in morbidity and mortality. Examples of the latter include (1) DMD, in which heart failure may result in death in as many as 40% of the patients; (2) myotonic muscular dystrophy, in which cardiac abnormalities can provoke death in 4% of cases[30]; (3) BMD, in which clinically evident cardiomyopathy is found in 15% of patients younger than 16 years and 73% of patients older than 40 years, and may even be seen in those as young as 4 years; (4) Emery-Dreifuss muscular dystrophy, which can be associated with atrial paralysis and conduction block causing sudden death; and (5) Friedreich's ataxia, in which cardiac abnormalities are found in at least 90% of patients.[11]

The difficulty in recognizing a patient with the cardiac dysfunction of NMD is that, early on, related symptoms may be silent because of the relatively sedentary nature of the individual's lifestyle. Further along, symptoms of cardiac disease may be incorrectly attributed to respiratory decline. Thus, cardiac abnormality may not be appreciated until significant clinical progression is demonstrated or sudden unexpected death is reported.[31] It generally would seem prudent, therefore, to screen these patients with electrocardiography yearly. Particularly in those conditions in which significant consequences of cardiac disease are common, echocardiography should also be considered. These tests, and the judicious use of the cardiology consultation, may provide the appropriate avenues of preventative treatment of cardiac dysfunction in NMDs.[11]

Respiratory Complications

Breathing disorders are recognized as the leading cause of morbidity and mortality in NMD. Respiratory mechanics are impaired in these disease processes both by the increased loads on the muscles of breathing secondary to inadequate abilities to effectively clear airway secretions and by the changes in chest well compliance that accompany the spinal column deformity of scoliosis, kyphosis, and hyperlordosis. The obvious respiratory muscle weakness and fatigue that result from the primary disease itself, and the defects of central control mechanisms that result in both hypoxia and hypercapnia, also impair the respiratory mechanics of those with NMD.[32]

The ultimate failure of the respiratory system in this type of disease process can be acute in nature (or at least caused by an acute decompensation of the mechanical process, commonly by infection) or insidious in onset. The first condition is easily recognized by all physicians; the signs and symptoms of the latter condition may be missed by those who are unschooled in pulmonary medicine. They consist of sleep-related respiratory disorders demonstrated by morning headaches, nighttime nightmares, frequent arousals from sleep, daytime drowsiness, and occasional enuresis. Those symptoms more commonly appreciated by the general practitioner that demonstrate respiratory distress are orthopnea; dyspnea on exertion or at rest, or both; tachypnea; and paradoxical breathing patterns.[32–35]

The onset of respiratory failure signals the beginning of a deteriorating course for those with NMD. In most cases, mechanical ventilatory assistance is required to prevent death.[6] Exact numbers of individuals with NMD who require long-term ventilatory support are unknown. In the United States, this population has been estimated to be between 4,000 and 11,000 persons.[36] Both invasive and noninvasive means of part-time and continuous mechanical ventilatory support have been developed to help alleviate the respiratory dysfunction of the individual with NMD. Medical guidelines have been initiated for the use of these types of mechanical systems.[6,34] The decision as to whether to begin ventilatory support of a patient with NMD should not necessarily be reduced to mere consideration of laboratory-generated numbers on a chart. Instead, the burdens and rewards of this type of intervention to the patient, family, and primary support system must be weighed carefully, with balanced consideration given to the potential improvement in the quality of an individual's life through the use of this technology against the demands or prolongation of suffering, or both, that it may impose on the patient and the family.[36]

Both the law and medical ethics support a patient's right to decide how he or she wishes to be treated for any disease process. The difficult decisions that need to be made when one treats a patient in respiratory decline from NMD are best prepared for at the beginning of the disease process. At that point, the patient and those on whom he or she depends for important counsel have the time to consider their decisions carefully, and the patient retains the physical ability to communicate questions, desires, and decisions.[36]

The physician who is advising the patient on this matter must also carefully prepare him- or herself to approach this subject in a fair and open manner. Research notes that many health care providers do not make available to their patients full access to ventilatory support technology. The reasons for this are varied. Sometimes health care providers are not aware that a patient who initially refuses the concept of external ventilatory support early on in a disease process may reconsider this decision as the NMD progresses. Thus, if continued discussions are not actively pursued by a clinician who is comfortable in talking about this topic, a patient may essentially be denied mechanical respiratory support for the lack of an opening to this difficult subject. Patients particularly may respond to the concept of external ventilatory support if they are educated to the possibility of the use of noninvasive respiratory aids as opposed to the need for tracheostomy. Members of the treatment team must also consistently guard against well-meant but inappropriate evaluations of a patient's life satisfaction on ventilatory support. Health care providers may have the tendency to use their own personal experiences and cultural backgrounds to judge how a patient may accept life with the aid of a respirator. This may cause them to underestimate greatly the potential life satisfaction of their patients who are candidates to receive this type of technology. Studies have shown that patients with NMD have unusual capabilities to adapt to their life circumstances, and even with ventilatory support they have the ability to maintain a purpose and joy in life that confound their attendants. Health care providers must remain vigilant not to impose their personal biases onto the life circumstances of their patients.[36,37]

Ethics aside, inadequate community and financial resources also present a barrier to NMD patients who might require chronic mechanical respiratory support. Many assume that to maintain the "hardware" of prolonged ventilatory support, a patient must be institutionalized either in a hospital or in a long-term nursing facility; however, this assumption is false. Families can be trained to provide appropriate and adequate service to these patients in their homes. Estimates of the cost of care show that it can be delivered at anywhere from approximately one-tenth to one-third the cost of standard institutionalized inpatient care.[32,36]

The monetary outlay for ventilatory support may nevertheless be disruptive to the overall financial resources of the family. Even if this is not the case, the societal savings from treatment at home must not override the emotional issues that arise in this situation. Psychosocial support of the patient as well as the caregivers is of primary concern to the treatment team. Only by regular contact with those who provide care can the clinician assess the strengths and weaknesses of the patient and the home care providers and evaluate, intervene, and/or support the changing nature of the home and health environment.[36]

The decision to accept or reject prolonged ventilatory support is not an easy one for the patient, the caregivers, or the clinician. It is also not a singular decision, entered into completely and finally at one point in time. The dialogue between physician, patient, family, and care providers must be maintained on a long-term basis, with mutual respect and consideration afforded to all concerned.

Psychological Issues

The psychological stresses of NMD already have been mentioned. Little research is available to delineate the specifics of this problem or the treatment options. What is known, however, is what one might expect in understanding the disease processes themselves; that is, as those with NMD become more physically disabled, they may become uncomfortable with their appearance and handicaps and begin to isolate themselves socially from family and friends. This, coupled with the fears imposed by the threat of financial hardship and, in some cases, imminent death, may result in symptoms of anger, loneliness, anxiety, depression, and guilt for both patient and caregivers.[16,18,38,39]

It is easy for a clinician to stand aside from these issues and busy him- or herself in the physical problems presented by the disease process. It is important to remember, however, that health care providers treat not only disease, but also people. Based on research on patients with NMD as well as other debilitating and potentially terminal illnesses, several areas of psychological intervention have been recommended to the practitioners who care for these patients.

First, those who provide health care must supply a supportive relationship to the patient and the primary caretakers. The treating physician must be able to provide the patient with information regarding diagnosis, viable medical interventions, and realistic prognosis in a knowledgeable manner as well as understand how to offer this information in appropriate quantities that are timed to prevent the patient from becoming overwhelmed. The physician must also recognize the stages of denial, depression, anger, anxiety, and acceptance that patients go through in response to a devastating diagnosis and be able to guide and support all concerned wherever they may be within this continuum. Finally, the physician needs to recognize his or her own limitations in these areas and, when appropriate, direct and even encourage the patient and significant others to seek entrance into a support group or referral to a mental health specialist, or both, that can help them cope with the issues that surround NMD. Such interventions may help lessen the devastation of a disabling diagnosis and, therefore, help improve the quality of life.[39]

Employment

Employment for all, whether disabled or not, is an important factor in a feeling of well-being and satisfaction with life.[40] The employment characteristics of individuals with selective NMDs have been studied. Not surprisingly, those with NMDs who have obtained higher levels of education are more likely to be members of the work force then are those who have completed only lower levels of schooling. It also appears that obtaining advanced educational experience may be helpful in protecting individuals with NMD from dropping out of the work force as they age.[41]

Of perhaps more interest in these studies than the above, however, is the finding that individuals with NMD are given a low level of aid in their search for employment. This situation is found to result in part from the high percentage of rehabilitation counselors who readily self-acknowledge the lack of education and experience that they require to assess and advise individuals with NMD to evaluate appropriately their vocational potential. Moreover, it appears that physicians who treat individuals with NMD (physiatrists, orthopedic surgeons, pediatricians, and neurologists) also demonstrate a similar lack of appreciation for the potential vocational capabilities of their patients, and thus it is assumed that they make little to no effort to appropriately counsel or encourage interested individuals as to the resources that are available to help them achieve the goal of successful employment.[41] Finally, it appears that the lack of employers who either allow or offer work adaptations to reduce time and pressure demands on those with NMD is a strong factor that causes disabled workers to retire sooner than might be necessary.[40] These barriers of attitude, perception, and the inadequate experience of vocational rehabilitation personnel are perhaps more overwhelming than is the physical disability of NMD to those who seek to gain employment.

Summary

What has been described in this section represents a portion of the clinical spectrum of signs and symptoms that describe an NMD process. It is important to remember, however, that the medical characteristics of an illness do not necessarily define the consequences of disease. The manner in which any disease affects a given person is dependent on the perceptions of that individual as well as those who surround him or her. Thus, the reality of illness can differ radically between individuals with similar medical problems depending on personal characteristics and environmental and financial circumstances. For example, use of a wheelchair in some persons is a means to an end, a way to successfully mobilize the body to accomplish the tasks of a daily agenda. To other individuals, however, the use of a wheelchair is a jail sentence, a force that separates them from their normal routine, social interactions, and employment.

Management is a process whereby patients are asked to identify the problems that they face as a result of their disease process and are also encouraged to aid in the planning, prioritization, and evaluation of solutions offered to them by the professionals that they encounter. Thus, the process is unique to each patient who passes through it. The next section of this chapter illustrates this point by the use of case histories. Each has been chosen to demonstrate a different aspect of rehabilitation care available to a patient with NMD as well as to illustrate the method by which the patient was involved in his or her own clinical management and functional outcome.

Character of the Solution

Rehabilitation professionals are a different breed than most health care workers. They practice as a team, recognizing that multiple subspecialists, such as doctors, nurses, physical-occupational-speech-respiratory therapists, social-vocational counselors, and psychologists, among others, can contribute individual components of expertise, care, and concern to their patients that, together, offer the potential for a more favorable outcome than would be achieved by each professional on his or her own. They have been trained not only in treating disease processes but also in including their patients in these efforts; in doing so, they provide them the opportunity to identify and take control of those portions of their lives that have been stolen from them by their illness.

Toward this end, it is the author's belief that the evaluation of the patient with NMD should begin with a functionally driven history and physical examination, conducted not to evaluate a disease and its short-term treatment but instead to discover the means to lessen the restrictions that a disease process places on a patient's life. The author proposes an outline of a functional history (Table 7-2) that has been useful in this type of approach for the treatment of patients with NMD. This history-taking tool differs in subject and purpose from that which is usually taught in medical school. For example, the history of present illness concentrates on the patient's daily activities and how they are currently accomplished. The social history determines the systems of family and community support that may or may not exist for the patient and identifies the potential architectural and financial barriers that restrict the patient's lifestyle. The review of systems is used to assess comorbidities that may affect the patient's functional status. Although not part of the traditional teachings of medical school, this method of history taking has helped the author gather the necessary information to learn what her patients want to achieve from the management process. Organizing the information in the way that is shown further allows the author to partner with her patients and identify the treatment plan that can best allow them to accomplish their goals.

Likewise, the functional physical examination seeks out information that allows the patient to direct his or her plan of care. This examination is described in detail in this chapter because many believe that an office setting is not conducive to the performance of any kind of physical examination on a patient with moderate to severe NMD. It is true that, in an office setting, it may not be possible to transfer a patient from office chair or wheelchair to an examination area in a time-efficient manner with adequate attention being paid both to the safety of the patient and the medical personnel who are assisting in this maneuver. However, one can perform a physical examination with the patient seated that provides useful information in regard to function. This author has performed the examination described below on numerous patients and has found it to be efficient as well as comfortable for both patient and examiner. Moreover, combined with the functional history, it is very helpful in developing a global clinical picture that describes the needs of a patient with NMD.

Because vital signs usually are taken by a nurse before the physician's entrance into the room, the doctor's first encounter with the patient is to observe his or her posture during the history portion of the examination. Particular attention is paid to the positioning of the neck, noting whether the patient can maintain neutral extension without the use of a hand prop, collar, or high chair back.

The patient's formal physical examination can begin with a gross assessment of visual abilities. Such a maneuver indicates to the practitioner whether visual materials and cues can be used to enhance necessary rehabilitation attempts. This characteristic can be easily tested by holding objects or various numbers of fingers, or both, to be identified by the patient, approximately 18–24 in. from the face in the midline position. The patient's ability to follow general conversation in the examination room (assuming that no cognitive impairment exists) serves as a gross indication of hearing abilities. It must be remembered, however, that, particularly in the elderly, a single conversational voice might be well understood in a quiet room but not in a busy communal physical therapy gymnasium.

If the practitioner has any questions regarding a patient's cognitive capacity, a standard Mini-Mental

Table 7-2. Functional History of Present Illness

An answer of no requires further details.

Ask the patient: Can you, without help:

1. Get out of bed in the morning?
2. Perform normal sink hygiene (dental care, shaving, makeup application)?
3. Get on or off a toilet seat without using a push up from the sink, toilet, or nearby towel rack?
4. Get in or out of tub (tub shower, shower stall)?
5. Stand without support of the wall to take a shower?
6. Care for usual hairstyle?
7. Dry self after bath or shower?
8. Dress self (including bending over to pull on underwear, pants, socks, etc.)?
9. Successfully manipulate shoe ties, zippers, and buttons?
10. Successfully manipulate keys and doorknobs?
11. Successfully manipulate forks, knives, and spoons?
12. Bring food from plate to mouth?
13. Swallow without coughing, choking, or throat clearing?
14. Prepare a simple meal of soup, sandwich, and a cold beverage?
15. Arise from the sofa or kitchen chair?
16. Walk through the house without touching walls or furniture?
17. Walk up and down stairs?
18. Turn on lamps and TV or radio while standing?
19. Use a remote control?
20. Get in and out of a car?
21. Make pattern of speech that is understandable to clerks, waiters, and other persons outside the immediate family?

If applicable, ask the following questions also:

Can you, without help:

1. Use a keyboard in an efficient manner?
2. Dial a telephone for pleasure or emergency contact and express understandable desires and needs?
3. Drive a car or take public transportation as needed?
4. Walk in a mall or parking lot?
5. Perform usual household tasks such as grocery shopping and laundry?
6. Perform child care activities?

Functional social history:

1. Do you live with family, friends, or significant others?
2. Is someone at home all day who is capable of helping you if necessary?
3. Are there steps to get into your house from the outside?
4. Are a bathroom and bedroom located on the entrance level of your home? If not, how many steps does it take to get to the bathroom and bedroom?
5. Do you have any special equipment in your home for your convenience (e.g., toilet seat, bathtub, chair or benches)?
6. Do you walk with a cane, crutch, or walker or use a wheelchair?

Functional review of symptoms (an answer of yes requires further details as needed):

1. Do you experience chest pain, shortness of breath during rest or activity, or shortness of breath lying flat?
2. Can you easily read a newspaper as well as look outside a picture window with or without glasses?
3. Are you hard of hearing?
4. Do you have any joint pain at any time that makes you stop your usual activity?
5. Can you control your bowel and bladder without accidents?

State Examination can be administered. The author has not found this examination to be particularly useful, however, when investigating the functional capabilities of an individual and especially how well the individual may be able to respond to training techniques. Instead, after inquiries are made to denote the orientation of the patient to person, place, and time, problems of money management are presented consistent with the patient's educational level. The ability to follow single- versus multiple-step commands is tested, as is the ability to both read and interpret written and spoken words. Memory is checked not just for the ability to recall short-term and long-term thoughts but also for the ability to carry over instructions from one day to the next, a skill that might need repetitive examinations. Deductive reasoning is also challenged in this portion of the examination.

The proximal upper extremities are then examined both for active and passive range of motion of shoulder elevation and elbow and wrist flexion and extension. During this portion of the examination, the patient's strength can also be assessed in the traditional manner. It should be noted, however, that patients often may not have sufficient strength to manipulate their extremities against gravity; thus, to test only for the ability to "lift up the arm" does not demonstrate their full functional capability. For example, patients may not have the strength needed to lift a toothbrush to the mouth to perform their own oral hygiene. While seated at the bathroom sink, however, they may indeed have enough strength to slide the arms, supported by the counter top, toward the direction of the face and to place the toothbrush in their mouth while bending over, thus performing this basic task without help. At the very least, then, the strength examination should be broken down to evaluate whether any of the motions of the shoulder, elbow, or wrist can be accomplished against gravity, with gravity eliminated, or with the use of gravity. From this information, useful modifications can be suggested to enhance the patients' independence within their own environment.

After the more proximal joints of the upper extremity are examined, the range of motion, strength, and proprioception as well as positioning of the thumb and fingers can follow. The ability of the patient to actively extend and flex the fingers is noted, as is the patient's ability to place the thumb in opposition to the index or middle finger, or both.

Also assessed is the patient's ability to grip the examiner's two fingers in a cylindrical grasp. Both the strength of opposition and that of a cylindrical grasp can be qualitatively evaluated by the examiner without special equipment. Opposition strength can be judged by the patient's ability to maintain opposition of the thumb and the index or middle finger in an "OK sign" while the examiner attempts to break this positioning of the fingers; the qualitative level of functional strength of the cylindrical grasp can be judged by the examiner as the patient squeezes the two fingers. Further examination of the hand includes a determination of the patient's proprioceptive abilities at the distal interphalangeal and more proximal joints as necessary. This type of testing should also be performed at least at the interphalangeal joint of the thumb and again more proximally as needed.

Examination of the lower extremities, like the upper extremities, begins with the patient in the seated position. The examiner first assesses joint motion and muscular strength of the hip flexors, knee flexors, and extensors, as well as the ankle plantar flexors and dorsiflexors. Because of their gravity-dependent positioning while in the seated position, the knee flexors and the ankle plantar flexors can be evaluated qualitatively only for strength. The other muscles can be graded against gravity in the usual fashion; less than antigravity strength can be further assessed in a different position as required. While the patient is still seated, proprioception of the first toes and more proximal joints, as needed, can also be tested.

Once this examination of the extremities is accomplished, the examiner's attention can be turned to the patient's balance. It is recommended that balance be tested at least in the seated position. Static sitting balance can qualitatively be judged by asking the patient to come forward off the back of the wheelchair or office chair. It should be noted, however, that many patients "perch" in a single position but cannot maintain their balance while moving the trunk in space. Therefore, it is important to assess the dynamic sitting balance by once again pulling the patient off the back of the seat and requiring some spatial movement of the arms or trunk, or both, during the examination.

With the knowledge gained from the history and physical examination, the clinician has almost all the information needed to determine how well the patient can use the upper limbs and trunk to inter-act with the environment, as well as whether the patient can safely transfer or ambulate, or both, either with or without assistance. The one piece of important information not yet available concerns the status of the hip extensors.

In examining the patient in the seated position, examiners must remember that they deny them-selves the ability to fully assess strength and range of motion of the hip extensors, information that is important to note when predicting the patient's potential to achieve an erect, upright position or weight bear on the lower extremities, or both, during ambulation. This information, however, can be obtained during the observation of a change from a sitting to a standing position. Even if this position change needs to be assisted, examiners can evaluate the patient's use of the hip extensors versus lumbar-thoracic extensors to obtain the erect position. The patient's ability or inability to stand with locked knees can serve to indicate whether a hip flexion contracture exists and, if so, if it would interfere significantly with the upright position. While the patient is standing, both static and dynamic balance can also be assessed as applicable, and if possible, the patient's transfer and ambulation capabilities can be more fully evaluated.

At the end of the functional examination, the examiner can document how the patient can use his or her muscular strength, range of motion, endur-ance, balance, and proprioception in various func-tional tasks that combine all these individual skills into purposeful movement. This can be accom-plished by simply observing the patient reach for an item in space, put on or take off a jacket or sweater, or lean over to put on socks and shoes. Functional assessment of fine motor control of the upper extremities can be evaluated by asking a patient to manipulate coins or to turn single pages in a book or stack of papers.

The actual usefulness of this method of obtain-ing a history and physical examination is demon-strated in the three cases that follow. Each case highlights an individual with an NMD who comes to see a rehabilitation physician. These case presentations illustrate how the functionally oriented approach to the patient interview and physical examination can gather sufficient and appropriate information to allow the individual

patient and his or her practitioners to collaborate in a treatment plan that can diminish the obsta-cles that are considered by the patient to be most restrictive and handicapping to his or her life. The problems presented for illustration are geared toward rehabilitation intervention. Medi-cal and pharmaceutical therapies are also avail-able to those with NMD that can promote more functional living; it is, however, beyond the scope of this chapter to discuss these types of treatment. Suffice it to say that all clinicians must pursue the problems presented by their patients in a manner designed to provide comprehensive care along a continuum of clinical needs.

Case 1: Vague and Inappropriate Goal Setting

Individuals with NMDs are often referred to reha-bilitationists by well-meaning physicians of other specialties who have nothing of a pharmaceutical nature with which to treat patients but who still wish to provide them with some comfort and treat-ment. The patient is therefore sent for evaluation and treatment. On arrival to the rehabilitation spe-cialist, the patient often has no knowledge of why he or she has been sent there, and the chief com-plaint is, "My doctor wants me to see you." Such a new patient presentation often leaves rehabilitation specialists at a loss as to how to help the patient who sits before them, particularly one who is clearly physically and mentally overwhelmed by the frightening progressive deterioration of his or her bodily condition.

When faced with a global decline in function such as caused by a disease process like ALS, the clinician can use the functionally oriented history and physical examination to develop an inventory of patients' needs and desires during the course of an average day, even when the patients are not able to articulate this type of information themselves. By understanding the level of success or frustration that each activity causes the patient, and by listen-ing to the degree of importance assigned to each activity by the patient, the physician can then for-mulate an appropriately prioritized program that takes its direction from the patient's own goals.

Mrs. O is a 75-year-old right-handed woman who has been experiencing the symptoms of progressive weakness and spasticity of the arms and legs for the past 6 months. Recently, a diagnosis of ALS was made, and the patient was referred to a rehabilitation physician for therapy.

Through questioning, the physician found that the patient lived in her home along with her daughter (who worked) and her grandson (who attended school). A home health aide provided assistance to the patient for sponge bathing, dressing, and food preparation when family members were not present. The patient was able to self-feed, but only with her left hand, and was quite fearful of losing that skill, as she had recently lost the capability of grasp with the right hand. She wished that she could find a way to strengthen her right hand again because she thought it degrading to potentially have to rely on someone else to feed her like she was a baby.

The house in which the patient lived with her family was newly equipped with a stair glide chair. This chair was able to take her from her recreation area (where she was able to enter her house by climbing only one step) to the main floor (up a full flight of stairs), where she wished to spend most of her days. The patient required assistance to transfer. However, the accompanying family member who helped in this activity stated that transfers were frequently performed in an "off-balanced position." The patient also stated that she was capable of walking with a walker in her home for approximately 6–10 ft. To further questioning, however, she admitted that the distance ambulated was limited because of her severe unsteadiness. In fact, she noted that she frequently lost her balance and fell backward. Mrs. O felt that her transfers and her ambulation had become so unsafe in recent weeks that she had not left her house in the past month and a half except for doctors' appointments. This was particular concerning to her, as she had previously been quite active in her community of friends.

Mrs. O was being visited at home by occupational and physical therapists three times a week. The therapists' goals were to help the patient maintain range of motion, regain strength, and improve her kitchen-related activities.

Mrs. O's functional physical examination was performed as she sat in a wheelchair. Examination of the right upper extremity revealed no antigravity shoulder elevation. Passively, full range of motion was noted in this joint. The patient demonstrated barely antigravity flexion and extension of the elbow and wrist on the right. However, a weak, marginally functional two-finger cylindrical grasp was noted in the right hand. The tone of the right upper extremity was increased. Examination of the left upper extremity revealed antigravity shoulder elevation and elbow flexion and extension as well as wrist flexion and extension. A strong and functional two-finger cylindrical grasp was demonstrated on the left as well as opposition between rays 1 and 2. Bilaterally, the patient exhibited antigravity hip flexion as well as knee extension. Ankle dorsiflexion on the left was active against gravity; she had little movement of the right ankle dorsiflexors. Both lower extremities were noted to have markedly increased tone. Transfers from the sit to stand position assisted by the rehabilitation physician required moderate assistance. It was noted that the patient could use her hip extensors to stand erect. However, when the patient's daughter was asked to demonstrate how she helped her mother to stand, the maneuver was poorly performed, and both individuals were noted to be at risk for falls.

From evaluation of this case, the clinician was able to note that the occupational and physical therapy that the patient was receiving at home was purposeless. As the patient was experiencing a progressive deteriorating illness, therapy would never help her to "regain strength." Furthermore, she cared little (if at all) whether she possessed the ability to perform meal preparation in the kitchen. Given her disease process, she had only two primary goals that she desired to achieve: to maintain the ability to self-feed and to leave her home to attend family and community social events. In particular, the patient had a great need not to feel that she was a prisoner in her own home.

Based on this information, the physician suggested that the patient's therapists switch from their current home activities to initiate more functional therapeutic training for both the patient and her family. Specifically, occupational and physical therapists were asked to coordinate their efforts so that Mrs. O and her family members could be taught safe and efficient transfers between wheelchair and bed, commode, or car. Very importantly also, it was believed that the patient needed to learn to transfer from her wheelchair into her stair glider so that she could enjoy the main floor of her home as she desired and so that she could exit or enter her house from the recreational level. It was also necessary that Mrs. O's family members learn to handle her wheelchair outside of the home and in the community. They therefore required special training as to the use of a wheelchair on curb cuts, uneven surfaces, and so forth.

As the patient might not always have a wheelchair-accessible bathroom available to her in the community, techniques for family-assisted safe ambulation over short distances needed to be taught that could be used as long as her disease process allowed. Suggestions were made for the patient to attempt the use of a weighted wheeled walker set at a height slightly lower than normal that she could use to prevent backward falls. To accommodate the patient's weakened grasp in her right hand, built-up handles were ordered to be fashioned.

To help the patient maintain her goal of self-feeding, home therapists were instructed to modify the height of her kitchen table to facilitate a rocker motion of the elbow so that Mrs. O could take food from her plate to her mouth using the modified table height as a "pseudo-balanced forearm orthosis." If this technique (which the patient performed successfully during a mock-up situation in the clinician's office) did not prove feasible at home, then the patient's table height was to be modified to allow her to self-feed with her upper extremities using a gravity-eliminated (essentially horizontal) motion. The patient's weakened grasp on the right could be compensated for by using built-up handles on her utensils or, if necessary, a universal cuff.

The patient agreed to the logic of these suggestions, and appropriate orders were written for home therapy. It should be noted that this patient was surprised but quite pleased that such accommodations and functionally directed therapy sessions were available to her.

This case illustrates that the rehabilitationist, by obtaining a functional history and performing a limited but functionally oriented physical examination on this severely disabled women, was able to elicit her primary personal goals and to help her achieve them as long as she was able. Thus, the doctor helped Mrs. O to extend her current capabilities; not to limit them as had been done previously.

The case of Mrs. O soon became complicated, however, by socioeconomic factors beyond the control of all concerned. The physician and the treating therapists were members of two different health care systems. As such, no regular lines of direct communication were established between them. Rehabilitation is most beneficial when practiced as a team effort, not by specialists who are isolated from one another. In particular, efforts can be enhanced when the patient is made a member of the team and as such takes responsibility for his or her own care. This concept is well exemplified by the events that occurred next.

Approximately 3 weeks after the patient was seen by the rehabilitation specialist, her family called to inform the doctor that she had been discharged from her home physical and occupational therapy; yet she felt that none of her new goals had been accomplished. The physician called the home health agency that was providing the therapies and spoke to the administrator there, who stated that the patient's therapies were discontinued because Mrs. O was no longer making progress toward her goals. Specifically, it was explained that, because the agency's personnel did not believe that their efforts were useful in helping the patient increase her levels of strength, they had discontinued their services.

From further conversation with the administrator, the physician determined that the patient's therapists had never changed from their initial treatment approach, and, therefore, Mrs. O had had no therapy to address the functional goals that had been outlined. It was explained to the home health agency administrator that a patient with ALS is not expected to improve in strength and endurance; in fact, a deterioration of these physical characteristics can be expected. Thus, the previous therapy was without purpose. The real point of therapy should be to increase the patient's safety, ability, and function within the confines of her limits. The administrator acknowledged that she was unfamiliar with the usual symptoms and course of ALS and arranged for the patient to have the functionally ordered therapy provided to her. This was delivered over the next 4 weeks, and at the end of that time the patient's family was able to assist her in her transfers in a safe manner. Mrs. O had also accomplished her goal of returning to the community, as she was able to perform car transfers with her daughter and participate in weekend outings.

This case illustrates the importance of allowing the patient to participate on his or her own rehabilitation team. Because Mrs. O was made to appreciate the different forms of therapy available to her, she was able to realize that she had not received the particular training that would benefit her the most. This knowledge then allowed her to intervene for herself to obtain the appropriate services that were necessary to accomplish her own goals. To correct an inappropriately oriented therapeutic program, Mrs. O accessed her doctor, her "voice" in the rehabilitation process. Perhaps it would have been more satisfying if she had used her own voice to intervene with her therapists for appropriate treatment. However, her lack of ability to do so illustrates yet another point, that rehabilitation is best practiced in a collaborative manner. Members of the team advance a patient's goals most efficiently when they work together, not separately. Because of the constraints of our health care system, however, it is not always possible to have direct communication between all members of the rehabilitation team. Therefore, treating personnel must listen and hear what the patient has to say and use this valuable information as the blueprint to the overall therapeutic treatment plan.

Case 2: Durable Medical Equipment Prescription Goals

Few physicians outside the specialty of rehabilitation are trained in the use and delivery of durable medical equipment. Therefore, patients are frequently given general prescriptions for canes, crutches, wheelchairs, and so forth, and are sent to commercial venders of medical equipment for selection of these products.

Making the correct choice of assistive equipment is critical to any person with impaired ambulation. Such equipment, when appropriately chosen, can decrease the energy expenditure of this activity as well as improve balance and safety, thus maximizing an individual's level of independent functioning. However, mobility aids can also be quite dangerous. They can promote falls, pressure ulcers, joint contractures, peripheral nerve injuries, and scoliosis. Even appropriately prescribed equipment used incorrectly can be unsafe and unstable, establishing the conditions to further the patient's injuries due to the consequences of fractures and deep lacerations that result from serious falls. Moreover, mobility

aids are expensive. It is extremely important, therefore, that the aid of a rehabilitation professional be enlisted when assistive devices are needed. Decisions regarding these pieces of equipment can be critical to the functional level of the patient.

Mr. S is a 52-year-old man with BMD who consulted a rehabilitation physician to determine whether he could return to work. Approximately 6 months before his initial visit, the patient fell and sustained a left tibial plateau fracture. Before his fall, he was able to ambulate using a straight cane. After recovering from his tibial plateau fracture, Mr. S was no longer able to walk and therefore used a wheelchair. He found, however, that his maneuvering skills in the chair were poor, and thus he could not return to work in his former office.

The patient used a rented wheelchair obtained from a commercial vender who had chosen the particular model for him. The wheelchair had standard features with the addition of removable desk arms, swing-away elevated leg rests, and a sling-type seat. The patient stated that he propelled his wheelchair best when he removed the elevating leg rests and used his feet to push against the floor. Mr. S wished to continue to use a manual wheelchair and specifically did not want an electric-powered scooter device.

Further history revealed that the patient's transfers at home were assisted by a home health aide. The aide was not available to the patient if he returned to his office, however, and therefore he could not assist him in and out of a car.

On physical examination, the patient was noted to have active shoulder elevation of approximately 30 degrees bilaterally. Full passive range of motion of shoulder elevation was noted. Elbow flexors demonstrated 4/5 strength; elbow extensors lacked approximately 30 degrees of extension bilaterally but were graded as 4+/5 within their limited range of motion. Wrist flexion and extension were graded as 5/5 bilaterally; opposition between rays 1 and 2 as well as a two-finger cylindrical grasp was strong and functional bilaterally. In the seated position, the patient's hip flexors could not produce antigravity movement. His knee extension lacked approximately 60 degrees of full motion against gravity. Passively, however, the patient had full extension of the knees and at least 90 degrees of knee flexion. Ankle dorsiflexion was graded as 5/5 bilaterally, and plantar flexion was very strong. The patient's balance in his wheelchair (without back support) was determined to be good in both static and dynamic positions. To efficiently ambulate in his wheelchair, Mr. S removed his leg rests and primarily used his feet to maneuver. It was observed that only the patient's toes reached to the floor and that Mr. S. propelled himself backward much easier than forward.

It was believed that this patient's problem of decreased mobility in his wheelchair was partly caused by the standard chair prescribed by his vender, who did not observe his pattern of mobilization. Because the patient's wheelchair seat height was so high, he could not effectively use more than his toes to maneuver as desired. The clinician discussed with Mr. S the possibility of obtaining a hemiplegic wheelchair. The seat of a hemiplegic wheelchair is lower than that of a standard chair and is specifically adapted to allow a patient who has good use of at least one leg to "foot drive" a wheelchair. By making this simple substitution, the patient regained the ability to effectively ambulate in his wheelchair both inside and outside his home. This change allowed him to contract with a community-provided service that provided curb-to-curb wheelchair transportation between his home and his place of employment. The patient therefore had the means to pursue his former job at his workplace.

Mr. S remained independent in his wheelchair for approximately 1 year. At that time, he began to note that self-propelling his wheelchair for 9–10 hours a day was becoming an exhausting task. In fact, on certain days, Mr. S would go to bed earlier than normal because he could no longer function independently in his wheelchair. He also was inconsistently able to cross several 3/4-in. thresholds in his home due to his fatigue and thus was newly in need of assistance to enter his kitchen and his bathroom. At this time, the patient's functional history and physical examination supported the use of an electric wheelchair, to which Mr. S readily agreed.

In addition to the need for appropriate prescription of durable medical equipment, this case also illustrates the fact that NMDs are frequently progressive in nature. It is important that patients receive a continuum of care to address their changing needs. Appropriately timed interventions can promote independence in this population as long as feasibly possible.

Case 3: Quality of Lifestyle Goals

Many patients with NMDs are severely disabled and, through no fault of their own, tax the creative resources of their rehabilitation team, as all work together to solve the unique problems imposed by the disease process. Not all persons with NMD, however, require intensive evaluation and treatment to carry out the basic activities of their daily lives. Instead, these more able-bodied individuals are seeking means by which to maintain a "normal" lifestyle that allows them to participate in the world around them in an unlimited and uninhibited fashion. Such a goal as this, although not as fundamental to life support as other more basic goals, still demands a level of attention equal to that given to the most severely disabled patient so that those who are less disabled can participate in life as they want, within their family and community circles. In these instances, the physician should help the patient to obtain and maintain a desirable quality of lifestyle.

Mrs. T is a 31-year-old right-handed woman with the diagnosis of adult-onset SMA. She was referred to a rehabilitation physician for evaluation of her ambulatory capabilities. Functional history revealed that the patient sometimes had difficulty arising out of bed because of low back pain. However, three tablets of an over-the-counter nonsteroidal anti-inflammatory drug in the morning seemed to alleviate this problem. The patient further required a push-off to arise from the toilet seat, but perineal-perianal hygiene was accomplished without difficulty. Bathing both in a tub shower and at the sink was not a problem. Likewise, food preparation and the handling of pots, pans, stove knobs, faucets, and so forth was performed without any difficulty. The patient was able to drive without modifications to her car. She did, however, note some difficulty in getting out of the automobile. The patient ambulated without any mobility device but was able to do so for only 5 minutes before she required a rest period. Furthermore, she had numerous falls in the recent past secondary to tripping over small objects.

On functional physical examination, the patient demonstrated the ability to stand from a low chair but required a strong push-off from its seat. In the standing position, a static Trendelenburg sign was seen to be positive on the right and negative on the left. The patient's dynamic gait revealed her to be slightly forward flexed in the trunk while ambulating; otherwise, joint movement was smooth and without abnormality.

The patient's shoulder elevators and elbow flexors as well as her wrist flexors were graded as 5/5 in strength bilaterally. Elbow extension on the right was graded as 4/5, and on the left it was 3/5. Wrist extension was 3/5 bilaterally. Opposition of ray 1 to ray 2 was found to be functionally strong bilaterally, as was a two-finger cylindrical grasp. Hip flexion was graded as 2–/5 bilaterally, whereas knee extension and ankle dorsiflexion were graded as 5/5 bilaterally. Hip extension performed in the prone position was not antigravity. Proprioception was intact at the toes.

Because of her lower extremity weakness, this patient obtained a folding walker for short-distance ambulation and an electric scooter–type mobility aid for long-distance ambulation over the course of the next 2 years. With the use of these mobility aids, the patient's low back pain resolved. The only other significant aid obtained by the patient during this time was a riser cushion for her automobile that could boost her up 1–2 in. higher than the height of a normal car seat. She was still able to safely operate the foot controls of her car but found it easier to exit the automobile from the higher level.

After some time had passed and she began to feel comfortable with her physician, Mrs. T questioned this doctor regarding a means by which to accommodate the different capabilities demonstrated by herself and her able-bodied husband. The patient was married to a man who traveled frequently for his business. It was the husband's expectation that his wife would accompany him on his travels. Mrs. T expressed a fear of traveling because of her disability, her lack of knowledge regarding the accommodations that could be afforded to her, and her need for equipment as she pursued this goal. She felt that she was holding her husband back from an activity that he would enjoy and implied that she might be a burden to him and that this might even place her marriage in jeopardy. The clinician, who had traveled extensively around the world with disabled individuals, was able to provide the patient with general information on this subject. Furthermore, she found various resources that could supply the patient with written

material of practical suggestions and "how to" information on this subject. For example, the names of societies for the promotion of travel for those with disabilities were supplied to the patient. The location and telephone numbers of specialty shops where books, magazines, and other literature that discussed travel for those with disabilities were also given to her. Armed with this information, Mrs. T was able to successfully pursue the necessary travel arrangements to visit several cities within the United States. At the time of her last visit to her physician, she was making plans to travel overseas and felt so comfortable with her new-found abilities to investigate and request arrangements with airlines, hotels, and so forth that she declined her practitioner's offer to aid her in these endeavors. It was clear that the patient now felt comfortable that she and her husband could enjoy these activities together as a couple. Given the appropriate tools by which to educate herself, Mrs. T had achieved on her own terms a position of equality within her marriage and could take pleasure in the fact that her husband now viewed her as a true partner.

Of equal concern to this patient was her perceived inability to enjoy sexual relations with her husband. After detailed questioning, it was determined that her inability to participate in this activity was due to the fact that she and her husband always attempted to achieve sexual climax in the missionary position. The patient's pelvic musculature was too weak to perform the thrusting movement that she felt would make their lovemaking more fulfilling. The practitioner was able to advise the patient on several techniques that might solve this problem. In particular, several alternative positions were proposed as pleasurable substitutions for those that she and her husband usually assumed. Mrs. T, feeling that her concerns were being taken seriously, then began a frank and open discussion with her physician regarding the potential desire of herself and her husband to have children. Mrs. T voiced her concerns about the possibility of genetically transferring her disease to any potential offspring. She also was worried about whether her body could support the physical stresses caused by pregnancy and the early child care years. The physician was able to find information on genetic counseling, consultants who could advise and counsel disabled women on the medical and psychological aspects of pregnancy and parenting, and adaptive methods by which disabled parents could attend to their children's needs. When last seen, Mrs. T stated that she and her husband were newly enjoying the pleasures of a fulfilling sexual relationship. They were still undecided, however, about whether to attempt a pregnancy.

Although these concerns about sexuality, pregnancy, and travel may initially seem out of the realm of discussion during the usual medical follow-up appointment, they were clearly of high priority to the patient. It is therefore incumbent on the practitioner to address these subjects and to provide the appropriate resources to enhance the patient's QOL.

Measuring Effectiveness

As noted in the previous section, to provide adequate care to a patient with NMD, an appropriate assessment of the medical condition and its subsequent effects on the patient needs to be made. To do so, the provider must be able to find those measures of illness severity that adequately describe all the consequences of the disease process.

According to the WHO, disease can be defined at the levels of impairment, disability, and handicap. Impairments are the direct neurophysiologic characteristics of the underlying pathology of the illness. A patient usually visits a physician because of the characteristics that define impairment, otherwise known as the signs and symptoms of the disease. In NMDs, examples of impairment include contracture formation, muscular weakness, spinal deformity, and cardiopulmonary abnormalities. The means by which impairment can cause a loss of ability (for example, that muscle weakness can progress to a level severe enough to eventually interfere with ambulation) defines the functional consequences of the illness, otherwise known as its disability. The handicap of the disease process describes the societal consequences of the pathology and represents for the patient the choice, or lack thereof, to pursue those goals in the community that are otherwise taken for granted, that is, to pursue employment and the choice to live in any financially accessible housing that is available and to be considered the head of the household.[1] Various measurements are available to assess the impairment, disability, and handicap caused by NMDs.

Measurement of Impairments

Strength

Strength abnormalities and progressive loss of strength are major impairments in most NMDs. Manual muscle tests (MMT) are available to aid in the quantification of this measurement. In the United States, most orthopedic, neurologic, and physiatric literature agree on an MMT that ranks strength on a 0–5 scale. This scale uses the following definitions of muscle strength:

5: The muscle demonstrates range of motion against full resistance in the antigravity plane.
4: The muscle demonstrates complete range of motion against some resistance in the antigravity plane.
3: The muscle demonstrates full range of motion against gravity but takes no resistance.
2: The muscle demonstrates full range of motion in a gravity-eliminated position.
1: The muscle contracts, but no joint motion is noted.
0: No muscle movement is noted.[42]

The MMT is quite similar to the MRC scale, initially devised for patients with peripheral nerve injuries after war wounds. This scale defines muscular strength as follows:

5: The muscle demonstrates normal power.
4: The muscle demonstrates movement against resistance but is weaker than the contralateral side.
3: The muscle demonstrates movement against gravity.
2: The muscle demonstrates movement in the gravity-eliminated plane only.
1: The muscle demonstrates a palpable contraction but no visible movement of the joint.
0: The muscle demonstrates no movement.[43]

Both of these scales leave great room for the examiner's interpretation, particularly in the category of a "4" muscle. As a result, notations of strength designated 4+ and 4− have come into common use by both therapists and physicians, without objective basis.[44]

Brooke et al.[44] have developed a modified scale of muscle strength to overcome this problem. To rate strength in a category of 4, the scale depends on the choice of a reference muscle in both the upper and lower extremities. The other "4" muscles are then graded as stronger or weaker than the reference muscle to help encourage inter-rater reliability.[44] Further refinement of this scale has been performed by Kilmer et al.[45]

Strength can also be quantified in a static isometric mode. The Tufts Quantitative Neuromuscular Examination uses an electronic strain gauge tensiometer to measure maximal voluntary contraction of various muscle groups, such as the flexors and extensors of the shoulder, elbow, hip, and knee. In this particular testing scheme, the patient's position during measurement of strength is standardized for purposes of uniformity.[46] Dynamic tests of strength using isokinetic measurements are also available for selected muscle groups.[47]

Range of Motion

Joint contractures can be documented with a standard goniometer in the positions noted by Brooke et al.[44]

Spasticity

Spasticity can be measured by various means. Simply asking the patient to count the number of spasms experienced in any time period is but one measure of this problem. The clinician can also assess resting muscle tone by use of the Ashworth scale, an ordinal nonlinear measure that indicates resistance to passive stretch. A score of 0 records no increase in tone in the muscle groups tested; 1 reads a slight increase in tone; 2 indicates that the limb can be easily moved but that further tone is noted; 3 records difficulty in passive movement of the limb with a marked increase in tone; and 4 denotes a rigid limb.[48]

Muscle spasticity can also be measured by the Wartenberg pendulum test. During this test, the patient sits on the examination table with the legs hanging freely. The clinician lifts both legs simultaneously to the same horizontal level and then lets them go. Neither the table nor the patient should interfere with the free-swinging nature of the legs. In the person without a pathologic condition, the legs usually swing at least six to seven times, no matter what the initial height from which the test was started. The time of swing between the two legs can be compared; if one swings longer than the other, an abnormality is assumed. The quality of the swing can also be assessed. Normal movements are smooth and regular; abnormally increased muscle tone produces a jerky effect. Furthermore, if the muscle tone of the extensor muscles of the knee is greater than that of the flexors, the heel cannot swing back as far on the affected leg as on the normal leg.[49] The pendulum test is quite qualitative. It is, however, helpful in routine neurologic examination. It can also be quantified with an electrogoniometer or video motion analysis, or both.[50]

Scoliosis

The procedures by which x-rays are used to evaluate the progression of spinal deformity are standardized in the medical literature.[51]

Cardiopulmonary Functioning

The respiratory complications of NMD can be followed through serial examinations of total lung capacity (TLC), residual volume (RV), FVC, FVC at 1 second (FVC_1), forced expiratory volume in 1 second (FEV_1), and maximal voluntary ventilation (MVV). Maximal inspiratory-expiratory pressures can also be measured. Cardiac performance is measured by a standard 12-lead electrocardiogram and as needed by echocardiogram. Measurement of arterial blood gases or pulse oximetry, or both, can also be made.[6,11,35]

Measurement of Disabilities

The author believes it is necessary not only to perform the usual general medical-neurologic examinations as a means to measure impairment in those with NMD but also to use the functional history to learn how the patient's illness affects his or her ability to carry out normal ADL, that is, to learn of the patient's disability. Other authors offer various testing modalities to likewise accomplish this goal.

Functional Testing of Motor Skills and Timed Performance Tests

Several investigators have devised the means by which an individual's upper and lower extremities can be assessed not only in terms of impairment but function as well. This is accomplished through the actual observation of functional tasks. For example, in their evaluation scheme, Brooke et al.[44] note whether a patient can raise the arms above the head, place a weighted object on a shelf above eye level, raise an 8-oz glass of water to the lips, and pick up objects off a table. Furthermore, they note whether patients walk with the assistance of railings or orthotics, or both, or if a wheelchair is required.[44] Vignos et al.[52] have devised a system whereby the ability of a patient to arise from a chair or the floor is noted, as well as that individual's ability to climb stairs. Both of these testing schemes gather further information about patients' functional status by timing them during the performance of ADL.

The observation and timing of functional movements performed by a patient can provide a reproducible and semiquantitative basis by which to measure the performance capability of that individual. Such tests are relatively simple and are easily accomplished in the office. Although less precise in their measurements than some of the impairment evaluations noted previously, these methods of testing function produce an overall picture of capability or disability in the patient with NMD.

Measurement of Quality of Life

It is important to realize that, as time passes, the focus of attention in any degenerative illness shifts from pathology to handicap. Thus, NMDs have the potential to change from being a matter of science to an intensely personal series of lost choices, lost freedoms, and loss of control over one's life. Such is the measure of handicap: to quantify the societal consequences of disease that are personally relevant to the individual who is experiencing the illness. It is problematic to measure QOL in patients with NMD. However, scales do exist for this purpose.

Index of Domain Satisfaction Scale

The Index of Domain Satisfaction Scale has been used both in the general population and in those with NMDs (including those who require ventilator support for breathing). With this tool, participants are asked to rate their satisfaction of 15 life domains on a scale that ranges from very satisfied to very dis-

satisfied. The life domain areas include housing, family life, neighborhood, spiritual life, well-being, marriage, transportation, life as a whole, social life, employment, daily living tasks, money matters, general health, sexual life, and recreation.[53]

Medical Outcomes Study Short Form (SF-36)

The SF-36 was developed to represent the components of health that are commonly used in survey research. It is arranged in eight health domains, including physical functioning, role limitations due to physical problems, role limitations due to emotional problems, social functioning, bodily pain, general mental health, vitality, and general health perceptions. This assessment tool can be completed by any patient in only 5–10 minutes. Each domain is measured as a score of 0–10, with a higher score indicating better health.[54]

With the help of tools such as those mentioned here, studies have shown that the level of physical capacity at which an individual with NMD functions does not necessarily correlate well with the perceived QOL for that same individual.[55] In this author's opinion, what is more important than any measurement instrument found in the literature is the understanding that health care providers should not allow themselves to use their own standards and experiences to attempt to judge the lifestyle satisfaction of one who experiences an NMD. Such opinions are subjective and negate the values that each individual patient places on his or her own way of pursuing meaningful life. Instead, regardless of whether standardized measures of relative satisfaction of life situations are used, it is important—and even fundamental to the provision of patient care—to recognize that communication with patients in an honest and forthright manner is the key method by which to determine their satisfaction with the situation in which they find themselves. It is also the method that allows all individuals the opportunity to participate in the decisions that affect the way in which they choose to live their lives.

Acknowledgments

The author is deeply grateful to Ms. Sheila D. Dade and Ms. Natalie Speight for their extraordinary efforts on behalf of this chapter.

References

1. Wade DT. Measurement in Neurological Rehabilitation. Oxford: Oxford University Press, 1992;3–14.
2. Tandan R. Disorders of the Upper and Lower Motor Neurons. In WG Bradley, RB Daroff, GM Fenichel, et al. (eds), Neurology in Clinical Practice. Boston: Butterworth–Heinemann, 1996;1823–1852.
3. Ross MA. Acquired motor neuron disorders. Neurol Clin 1997;15:481–500.
4. Carter GT, Miller RG. Comprehensive management of amyotrophic lateral sclerosis. Phys Med Rehabil Clin North Am 1998;9:271–284.
5. Francis K. Rehabilitation of adult patients with amyotrophic lateral sclerosis. Kessler Physician's Quarterly, 1997.
6. Kaplan LM, Hollander D. Respiratory dysfunction in amyotrophic lateral sclerosis. Clin Chest Med 1994; 15: 675–681.
7. Chance PF, Ashizawa T, Hoffman EP, et al. Molecular basis of neuromuscular disease. Phys Med Rehabil Clin North Am 1998;9:49–81.
8. Carter GT, Abresch RT, Fowler WM, et al. Profiles of neuromuscular diseases: spinal muscular atrophy. Am J Phys Med Rehabil, 1995;74(suppl):S150–S159.
9. Adams RD, Victor M, Ropper AH (eds). Principles of Neurology. New York: McGraw-Hill 1997;1414–1431.
10. McDonald CM, Abresch RT, Carter GT, et al. Profiles of neuromuscular diseases: Becker's muscular dystrophy. Am J Phys Med Rehabil, 1995;74(suppl):S93–S103.
11. Lewis WR, Yadlapalli S. Management of cardiac complications in neuromuscular disease. Phys Med Rehabil Clin North Am 1998;9:145–166.
12. Martin JB, Longo FM. Molecular Diagnosis of Neurologic Disorders. In AS Fauci, JB Martin, E Braunwald, et al. (eds), Harrison's Principles of Internal Medicine. New York: McGraw-Hill, 1998;2293–2307.
13. Beaudet AL. Genetics and Disease. In AS Fauci, JB Martin, E Braunwald, et al. (eds), Harrison's Principles of Internal Medicine. New York: McGraw-Hill, 1998;365–395.
14. Valle D. Treatment and Prevention of Genetic Disease. In AS Fauci, JB Martin, E Braunwald, et al. (eds), Harrison's Principles of Internal Medicine. New York: McGraw-Hill, 1998;403–409.
15. Bird TD, Bennett RL. Why do DNA testing? Practical and ethical implications of new neurogenetic tests. Ann Neurol 1995;38:141–146.
16. Kessler S, Kessler H, Ward P. Psychological aspects of genetic counseling. III: Management of guilt and shame. Am J Med Genet 1984;17:673–697.
17. Bernhardt BA. Genetic counseling and patient education. Md Med J 1989;38:953–956.
18. Salkovskis PM, Rimes KA. Predictive genetic testing: psychological factors. J Psychosom Res 1997;43:477–487.
19. McDonald CM. Limb contractures in progressive neuromuscular disease and the role of stretching, orthotics and surgery. Phys Med Rehabil Clin North Am 1998;9:187–211.
20. Perry J. Normal and Pathological Gait. In American Academy of Orthopedic Surgeons (eds), Atlas of Orthotics. St. Louis: Mosby, 1985;76–111.
21. Siegel IM. Management of musculoskeletal complications in neuromuscular disease: enhancing mobility and the role of bracing and surgery. Phys Med Rehabil State Art Rev 1988;2:553–575.
22. Sutherland DH, Olshen R, Cooper L, et al. The pathomechanics of gait in Duchenne muscular dystrophy. Dev Med Child Neurol 1981;23:3–22.
23. Hart DA, McDonald CM. Spinal deformity in neuromuscular disease: natural history and management. Phys Med Rehabil Clin North Am 1998;9:213–232.
24. Werner R, Waring W, Davidoff, G. Risk factors for median mononeuropathy of the wrist in postpoliomyelitis patients. Arch Phys Med Rehabil 1989;70:464–467.
25. Davidoff G, Werner R, Waring W. Compressive mononeuropathies of the upper extremity in chronic paraplegia. Paraplegia 1991;29:17–24.
26. Ball NA, Stempien LM, Pasupuleti DV, et al. Radial nerve palsy: a complication of walker usage. Arch Phys Med Rehabil 1989;70:236–238.
27. Kothari MJ, Rutkove SB, Logigian EL, et al. Coexistent entrapment neuropathies in patients with amyotrophic lateral sclerosis. Arch Phys Med Rehabil 1996;77:1186–1188.
28. Willig TN, Bach JR, Venance V, et al. Nutritional rehabilitation in neuromuscular disorders. Semin Neurol 1995; 15:18–23.
29. Willig TN, Paulus J, Saint Guily JL, et al. Swallowing problems in neuromuscular disorders. Arch Phys Med Rehabil 1994;75:1175–1181.
30. Fowler WM, Johnson ER, Yang CCS. Management of medical complications in neuromuscular diseases. Phys Med Rehabil State Art Rev 1988;2:597–615.
31. McDonald CM, Abresch RT, Carter GT, et al. Profiles of neuromuscular disease: Duchenne muscular dystrophy. Am J Phys Med Rehabil 1995;74(suppl):S70–S92.
32. Benditt JO. Management of pulmonary complications in neuromuscular disease. Phys Med Rehabil Clin North Am 1998;9:167–185.
33. Howard RS, Wiles CM, Loh L. Respiratory complications and their management in motor neuron disease. Brain 1989;112:1155–1170.
34. Unterborn JN, Hill NS. Options for mechanical ventilation in neuromuscular diseases. Clin Chest Med 1994; 15:765–781.
35. Rochester DF, Esau SA. Assessment of ventilatory function in patients with neuromuscular disease. Clin Chest Med 1994;15:751–763.
36. Hotes LS, Johnson JA, Sicilian L. Long-term care, rehabilitation and legal and ethical considerations in the management of neuromuscular disease with respiratory dysfunction. Clin Chest Med 1994;15:783–795.
37. McDonald ER. Evaluation of the psychological status of ventilatory-supported patients with ALS/MND. Palliat Med 1996;10:35–41.
38. Delaporte C. Ways of announcing a late-onset, heritable, disabling disease and their psychological consequences. Genet Couns 1996;7:289–296.
39. Sigford BJ, Lanham RA. Cognitive, psychosocial and educational issues in neuromuscular disease. Phys Med Rehabil Clin North Am 1998;9:249–270.

40. Andries F, Wevers CWJ, Wintzen AR, et al. Vocational perspectives and neuromuscular disorders. Int J Rehabil Res 1997; 0:255–273.

41. Fowler WM, Abresch RT, Koch TR, et al. Employment profiles in neuromuscular diseases. Am J Phys Med Rehabil 1997;76:26–37.

42. Hoppenfeld S. Physical Examination of the Spine and Extremities. Norwalk: Appleton & Lange, 1976;26.

43. Wade DT. Measurement in Neurological Rehabilitation. Oxford: Oxford Medical Publications,1992;50–58.

44. Brooke MH, Griggs RC, Mendell JR, et al. Clinical trial in Duchenne dystrophy. I. The design of the protocol. Muscle Nerve 1981;4:186–197.

45. Kilmer DD, Abresch RT, Fowler WM. Serial manual muscle testing in Duchenne muscular dystrophy. Arch Phys Med Rehabil 1993;74:1168–1171.

46. Andres PL, Hedlund W, Finison L, et al. Quantitative motor assessment in amyotrophic lateral sclerosis. Neurology 1986;36:937–941.

47. Fowler WM, Carter GT, Kraft GH. The role of physiatry in the management of neuromuscular disease. Phys Med Rehabil Clin North Am 1998;9:1–8.

48. Nance PW, Bugaresti J, Shellenberger K, et al. Efficacy and safety of tizanidine in the treatment of spasticity in patients with spinal cord injury. Neurology 1994(suppl 9);44:S44–S52.

49. Wartenberg R. Pendulousness of the legs as a diagnostic test. Neurology 1951;1:18–24.

50. Nance PW. A comparison of clonidine, cyproheptadine and baclofen in spastic spinal cord injured patients. J Am Paraplegia Soc 1994;17:150–156.

51. Kittleson AC, Lim LW. Measurement of scoliosis. Am J Roentgenol Radium Ther Nucl Med 1970;108:775–777.

52. Vignos PJ, Spencer GE, Archibold KC. Management of progressive muscular dystrophy of childhood. JAMA 1963;184:103–110.

53. Abresch MS, Seyden NK, Wineinger MA. Quality of life: issues for persons with neuromuscular diseases. Phys Med Rehabil Clin North Am 1998;9:233–248.

54. Dijkers M. Measuring Quality of Life. In MJ Fuhrer (ed), Assessing Medical Rehabilitation Practices. Baltimore: Paul H. Brookes, 1997;153–179.

55. Shields RK, Ruhland JL, Ross MA, et al. Analysis of health-related quality of life and muscle impairment in individuals with amyotrophic lateral sclerosis using the medical outcome survey and the Tufts Quantitative Neuromuscular Exam. Arch Phys Med Rehabil 1998;79:855–861.

Chapter 8

Management of Persons with Multiple Sclerosis

Lauren B. Krupp

Nature of the Problem

Extent of the Problem

Multiple sclerosis is an inflammatory and demyelinating disease of the central nervous system (CNS). It frequently affects young adults in the prime of their life and often has an unpredictable and progressive course. MS typically affects individuals between the ages of 10 and 50 years, with a mean age of onset of 30 years. The ratio of women to men is 2 to 1. Men are more likely to have an older age of onset and more progressive course.[1] The average annual costs of MS exceed $34,000 per person. These costs are primarily due to lost wages and, to a lesser degree, health care costs.[2]

The prevalence of MS varies according to geographic area. Overall, a geographic gradient is seen, with decreasing incidence from north to south in North America and from south to north in South America. Similar gradients have been documented in other regions as well. The prevalence of MS varies from 10 to 100 per 100,000. Certain geographic areas have been reported to have clusters of MS, with rates as high as 300 per 100,000 or more, whereas MS is extremely rare in other areas.[1]

The role of environmental factors in the etiology of MS is supported by the geographic distribution and the clustering of MS in certain areas. In addition, migrational studies have suggested that the risk of MS associated with a geographic region is determined by where an individual lives until the age of 14 years. In other words, no matter where an individual lives in later years, geographic risk is determined by the region in which he or she lived during the first 14 years of life. No single environmental agent has been identified.[1]

Evidence has also been found for genetic predisposition to the development of MS. Population-based studies of monozygotic twins indicate an overall concordance that ranges from 20% to 40%. Among dizygotic twins, concordance ranges from 3% to 4%. Among females with MS, the lifetime risk is 5% for their female siblings and 2% for their male siblings. Among males with MS, the lifetime risk is 3.5% for their female siblings and 4% for their male siblings.[3,4]

Nature of the Disease

Pathogenesis

MS is characterized by multifocal white matter disease in which areas of demyelination develop after bouts of inflammation.[5] The pathogenesis of MS has not been clearly defined. Most evidence suggests that immunologic, genetic, and environmental factors contribute to the etiology, but no one factor fully accounts for the disorder. An immune etiology is suggested by the histopathology of MS plaques within the CNS, which are characterized by inflammatory cell infiltrates that are characteristic of autoimmune disorders. During acute exacerbations multifocal perivascular mononuclear infiltrates and demyelination of the axonal white matter are seen. With repeated inflammatory attacks, oligodendrocytes are lost and astrocytic gliosis occurs.

The T cells that react to antigens of the myelin sheath can be retrieved from the blood and CSF of MS patients and otherwise healthy volunteers. In MS patients, however, the T cells react with specific immunodominant antigenic fragments (epitopes) in the context of HLA markers and specific T-cell receptor chains. Another feature of an exacerbation is the activation of autoreactive T cells in the blood with impaired T-cell suppressor cell function. Up-regulation in the expression of adhesion molecules on the endothelial cell layers of the blood-brain barrier and on activated T cells permits passage of the T cells into the CNS. As a result, local T cells within the CNS are activated, and macrophages, microglia, and proinflammatory cytokines are increased.

These changes, in association with myelin-associated antibodies and complement activation, lead to axonal demyelination. Research on the animal model of MS, experimental allergic encephalomyelitis, has enhanced our understanding of the immunopathogenesis of MS.[5] Further observations suggestive of an autoimmune basis of MS include the higher frequency of females affected (a trend across most autoimmune disorders), the association of certain major histocompatibility complex antigens (DR2), and a favorable response of the disorder to immunosuppressive or immunomodulatory therapies.

The current treatments available for improving the disease course are based on an autoimmune etiology for the disease. The interferon-β medications function as immune modifiers and have multiple potentially beneficial effects on the immune system in MS. These effects include down-regulation of proinflammatory cytokines (which enhance CNS inflammation), inhibition of lymphocyte trafficking across the blood-brain barrier, enhancement of suppressor cell activity, and decreased HLA expression on antigen-presenting cells. These actions result in decreased T-cell activation and less disease activity. Other treatments are based on a competitive inhibition with myelin basis protein within the trimolecular complex. This complex is associated with T-cell activation, proliferation, and enhancement of the immune response.

Most investigators believe that the etiology of MS is multifactorial. Multiple predisposing genes and infectious triggers interacting with the immune system are thought to be important contributing factors.

Diagnosis

The key to establishing an accurate diagnosis of MS is recognizing that the disease manifestations are extremely variable and occur over time. It is helpful to determine whether symptoms and signs of CNS dysfunction are separated in time and space,[6,7] as this is a hallmark feature of MS. Symptoms such as weakness, numbness, loss of coordination, and vision loss (i.e., variations in CNS localization or space) can occur at different points in the course of the disorder. These are referred to as attacks. The most common initial presentations in MS are loss of sensation, vision loss, motor symptoms, double vision, and gait disturbance. Difficulty in balance, vertigo, bladder symptoms, pain, fatigue, cognitive dysfunction, and affective disturbances are less common but not rare. Seizures, aphasia, and movement disorders can also occur but are less characteristic.

Diagnosis is based on a thorough history and medical evaluation. Evidence must be present of CNS involvement and more than one relapse attack separated by at least 1 month. A relapse is an episode of neurologic dysfunction that lasts a minimum of 24–48 hours. Alternatively, another presentation pattern can be a gradual progression over at least 6 months that involves more than one area of the CNS. Diagnosis further requires that no other clinical explanation can account for the neurologic symptoms and signs.

The diagnosis should preferably be established by a specialist such as a neurologist. Objective abnormalities that reflect white matter involvement must be seen on examination. In addition, other etiologies should be thoroughly ruled out. For example, individuals with multiple white matter abnormalities but with normal CSF should be evaluated for conditions such as vasculitis, mitochondrial encephalomyelopathy with lactic acidosis and strokelike episodes, multiple ischemic lesions, or Lyme disease. Diagnostic workup should also include routine laboratory tests, including B_{12}, folate, venereal disease research laboratory test, and Lyme titers. Individuals from certain geographic areas (e.g., the Caribbean islands or Japan) should also be tested for human T-cell lymphotropic virus type I infection. Individuals with risk factors for human immunodeficiency virus should be tested as well.

Lumbar puncture is useful for determining whether oligoclonal bands or elevated immunoglobulin G index are present to confirm the diagnosis. CSF examination may also help exclude other infectious or inflammatory etiologies. Visual and somatosensory evoked potentials may aid in identifying additional or subclinical lesions, or both.

MRI of the CNS has several roles in the diagnosis. Findings can be used to exclude other etiologies of neurologic dysfunction and identify involvement of the cerebral white matter beyond what is apparent on clinical examination. The characteristic finding in MS is at least three to four white matter lesions. Lesions that are periventricular, infratentorial, or larger than 6 mm are most characteristic. New lesions can be seen on MRI. Because of inflammation, they typically enhance with contrast administration. Altered vascular permeability of the cerebral white matter is also apparent with gadolinium enhancement and focal vasogenic edema. MRI is useful in monitoring disease activity and progression as well.

The diagnosis of MS should not be rendered over the telephone. It also is not a diagnosis made solely on the basis of MRI findings. It is a clinical diagnosis that should be conveyed in person. Typically, individuals become overwhelmed on hearing this diagnosis for the first time. They may require an additional follow-up evaluation to answer subsequent questions. It is also helpful to provide them with a brief, understandable description of the disorder as well as referral information to local chapters of the National MS Society.

MS is currently divided into four types, which are determined by the history of the disease course (Figure 8-1). Relapsing-remitting MS refers to individuals who develop attacks (relapses) that have no interval progression between them. Secondary progressive MS refers to individuals who initially have a relapsing course and then develop interval progression between attacks or a gradual progressive course without additional attacks. Primary progressive MS is characterized by a gradual progressive course without attacks. Progressive-relapsing MS is a rare form and the least common.

It is characterized by a progressive course at onset followed by superimposed attacks.

Most individuals with MS initially experience a relapsing-remitting course (75–85%), and between 10% and 15% experience a progressive course at onset. Approximately 40% of individuals with a relapsing disease develop a progressive form, usually within 15 years of initial diagnosis.[8]

Although it is impossible to predict any individual's disease course at onset, certain characteristics are associated with more or less favorable outcomes. Individuals with primarily sensory symptoms or optic neuritis who experience few attacks and whose attacks are followed by full recovery have a more favorable outcome. Other positive prognostic factors include female sex, younger age of onset, and minimal disease burden on MRI. Areas of decreased signal intensity on T1-weighted images are associated with axonal injury, gliosis, and increased neurologic and cognitive impairment. Brain stem and cerebellar involvement, high frequency of attack early in the course of the disease, and multisystem involvement (e.g., sensory, motor, visual) within one attack are less favorable predictors of disease course.[9]

Treatments That Alter Disease Course

The advent of treatments for altering the disease course is relatively recent.[10–12] The first drug approved by the Food and Drug Administration for relapsing-remitting MS was interferon-β lb (Betaseron) in 1993. Interferon-β 1a (Avonex) subsequently became available, and in 1997, glatiramir acetate (Copaxone) was approved. Individuals with relapsing MS who decide to begin treatment for altering the disease course thus have three drugs from which to choose.

In clinical trials these treatments have been demonstrated to decrease the frequency of MS attacks, lessen the severity of attacks, increase the interval between attacks, and decrease the number of enhancing lesions on MRI. With Betaseron, the clinical trials showed an overall decrease in lesion burden over time. Clinical trials with Avonex demonstrated that disease progression, as measured by the expanded disability status scale (EDSS), was slowed. Copaxone significantly decreases the severity and frequency of attacks with minimal side effects. It appears to help mildly impaired individuals more

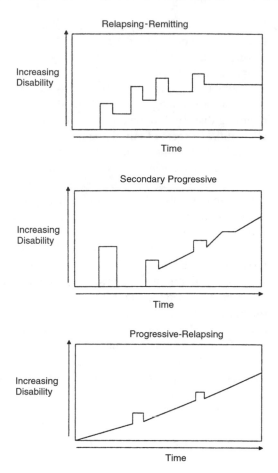

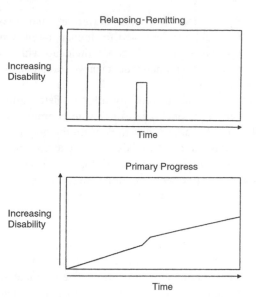

Figure 8-1. Clinical patterns of multiple sclerosis.

than those who are more severely impaired, however, and the MRI data are less compelling.

The availability of these agents raises a number of issues for individuals and their physicians. All the drugs require parenteral administration. Betaseron requires a subcutaneous injection every other day, Avonex requires a once-weekly intramuscular injection, and Copaxone requires a daily subcutaneous injection. One of the most important issues for individuals with MS is the decision whether to initiate therapy. These drug treatments do not alleviate symptoms, and individuals usually do not feel better while on them. However, they are the one form of intervention available that is most likely to alter the disease course and increase hope for the future. Many individuals are energized by the opportunity to be proactive. These treatments can also be viewed as a form of insurance. They are designed for the future in the event that progression occurs.

All of these agents have some side effects. Compared with the types of immuosuppressive agents previously used in MS, such as cyclophosphamide, the side effects are mild; however, they are still a potential concern. The most common side effects associated with interferon-β medications are flulike symptoms such as muscle aches, low-grade fever, fatigue, and headache. Injection site reactions involving erythema are not uncommon with Betaseron, and the patient may experience discomfort at the injection site with Avonex. Some individuals become depressed, and rare reports of seizure have been described. Copaxone has fewer side effects but can be associated with injection site reactions, and a subset of individuals develop noncardiac symptoms of chest tightness and anxiety with one or two injections. Most of the side effects subside after several months, and a variety of techniques are available for modifying their severity, including administering prophylaxis with nonsteroidal anti-inflammatory agents, taking the dose at bedtime, and icing the injection site.

Despite the potential of these drugs to modify the disease course, individuals with MS are often reluctant to get frequent injections. For some, understanding the need for medication designed to improve the future disease course but not to provide an immediate benefit can be difficult. Further, some physicians have been slow to recognize the proven efficacy of these agents, possibly due to a long history of failed treatments for MS. Patient education that includes a summary of the results of clinical trials with the different agents and the natural history of the disease is important before either Betaseron, Avonex, or Copaxone is prescribed, and explanation of the disease and the clinical trials to date is important.

During an attack, if an individual with MS experiences abrupt changes in vision, balance, or strength, glucocorticoid treatment can shorten the duration of the bout and decrease short-term disability. Glucocorticoids have anti-inflammatory and immunosuppressive effects and reduce the number of gadolinium-enhancing lesions on MRI. The radiologic and clinical benefits have been most clearly demonstrated with high doses of intravenous methylprednisolone given as 1 g per day for 3–5 days.[13,14] Oral administration is associated with variable absorption, and lower doses may not be as effective.

MS is characterized by a highly unpredictable course with a variety of specific symptoms. The nature of impairment in MS results from the neurologic effects of acute relapses and the increasing dysfunction associated with the progressive phases of the disease. Treatment of MS consists of therapies designed to alter the natural history of the disease, treatments for acute exacerbations, and therapies that are designed to provide relief of symptoms.

In summary, MS is a disorder that predominantly affects young adults. Its course can be difficult to predict, and it is characterized by multiple relapses and remission and steady progression. Women are affected more often than men and symptoms reflect a wide range of possible CNS involvement. The management of persons with MS must be responsive to these characteristics.

Nature of the Impairments

Impairments are viewed as the direct consequences of the underlying pathology. The type and extent of the impairments are a result of the character of the disease process and the distribution of lesions in any particular instance. They are the symptoms or signs that one would assess in the course of the medical-neurologic examination. Normal medical practice is to use the type and distribution of the impairments to deduce the underlying disease process. In the case of MS, the aim is to establish a diagnosis on the basis of multisystem involvement. It is useful here to consider the WHO terminology and to distinguish between the presence of impairments and the consequent disabilities. Impairment has been defined as "any loss or abnormality of psychological, physiological, or anatomic structure or function."[15] It thus can be considered to be at the organ level. A disability exists at the multiorgan level of function.

Given the progressive quality of the disease and the limited effects of treatments designed to alter the course of disease, the other primary treatment approach consists of symptomatic therapies.[16,17] Each of the major MS symptoms can be treated with a combination of nonpharmacologic and pharmacologic strategies (Table 8-1).

Motor Symptoms

Gait disturbance is present in the majority of individuals with MS either due to weakness, spasticity, or impaired balance. Ambulatory aids can prevent falls and provide needed stability. Weakness is best treated with physical therapy and exercise. In many instances individuals with footdrop can benefit from orthotic devices, such as an ankle-foot orthosis, regular cane, four-pronged cane, or walker. However, individual acceptance may be slow. Discussions with the physician, evaluation by a physical therapist and orthotist, and follow-up assessments often can convince otherwise reluctant individuals of the benefits of such devices. These may significantly enhance ambulation and balance.

Stiffness and spasticity often respond favorably to physical therapy. Medication is also frequently necessary. Baclofen and tizanidine are the two most widely used agents for spasticity.

Table 8-1. Commonly Used Medications for Symptoms of Multiple Sclerosis

Symptom	Medication
Spasticity	Baclofen (Lioresal), 10–60 mg; tizanidine (Zanaflex), 4–32 mg; intrathecal baclofen, 50–200 µg
Tremor	Clonazepam (Klonopin), 0.5–2.0 mg BID
Pain/paresthesia	Amitriptyline (Elavil, Endep), 75–150 mg QHS; gabapentin (Neurontin), 300–1,800 mg
Neuralgia	Carbamazepine (Tegretol), 200–1,200 mg
Fatigue	Amantadine (Symmetrel), 100 mg BID; pemoline (Cylert), 18.75–75.00 mg
Spastic bladder	Oxybutynin (Ditropan), 5 mg QD–QID; hyoscyamine sulfate (Levsinex)

Individuals who do not respond to one may benefit from the other, and in some cases combination therapy is helpful. Benzodiazepines may complement these agents. Dantrolene has been reported to be helpful but has limiting side effects. For individuals with severe spasticity that does not respond to oral therapy or for those who experience unacceptable side effects (such as confusion, lethargy, or increased weakness) from oral agents, intrathecal administration of baclofen via a baclofen pump can be extremely rewarding. This can significantly lessen pain and enhance QOL even for the severely impaired, wheelchair-dependent individual. Focal spasticity may respond to nerve blocks and surgical procedures. The management of spasticity and spasms is described in greater detail in Chapter 5 in the context of involvement of the spinal cord.

Tremor is a very difficult symptom to treat. Sometimes it can be managed by attaching small passive weights to the wrist. Medications are often ineffective. Benzodiazepines may help. Other agents with anecdotal reported benefit include primidone, carbamezpine, and isoniazid. Newer approaches under investigation include intravenous ondansetron (a serotonin antagonist) and, in specialized centers, thalamic surgery involving either sterotactic thalamotomy or thalamic electrostimulation.

Sensory Problems

Paresthesias, or numbness in one or more limbs, is the most common initial symptom of MS. Changes in the quality of sensation on various parts of the body may affect the person's ability to experience sexual intimacy. Tricylics or anticonvulsants can often provide relief. Vision disturbances such as diplopia are also common and reflect brain stem involvement. Optic neuritis should be aggressively treated with steroids if vision is significantly impaired.

Pain can be acute or chronic in MS. Examples of paroxsymal pain include trigeminal neuralgia, painful tonic spasms, radicular pains, and dysesthesias. Chronic pain includes dysesthetic extremities, back and shoulder pain, and pain secondary to spasticity. Medications include tricyclic antidepressants such as amitriptyline or nortriptyline, anticonvulsants such as gabapentin, carbamazepine, benzodiazepines, and nonsteroidal anti-inflammatory agents. Physical therapy is often effective. Evaluation for frozen shoulder, aseptic necrosis of the hip, osteoporosis, and compression fractures should also be considered. The overall management of persons with chronic pain is described in greater detail in Chapter 11.

Fatigue

Fatigue is a key clinical feature of MS. It is reported by as many as 87% of individuals with MS, and approximately 20% list it as their most disabling symptom.[18,19] Individuals with MS distinguish between physical and mental fatigue and report experiencing both. MS fatigue is significantly worsened by heat in more than 90% of cases.

Fatigue overlaps with depressive symptoms and is associated with mental well-being and global health status. However, it is also a distinct problem that needs individualized attention. Fatigue treatment requires a multidisciplinary approach. Education and reassurance are very helpful. In addition to reassurance, other nonpharmacologic treatment measures for fatigue include a graded exercise program, behavioral modification structured in a format analogous to chronic pain treatment groups, avoidance of heat, and rest periods. Exercise is a powerful means to combat deconditioning and enhance self-esteem, but overexertion can be detrimental. For some, reductions in selected activities should be considered. When depression coexists with fatigue it must be aggressively treated. Counseling and anti-depressant therapy are often critical. Some of the treatment procedures overlap with those described in detail in Chapter 11 in the context of the management of persons with fibromyalgia.

Often, nonpharmacologic measures for fatigue must be supplemented with drug therapy. Amantadine (Symmetrel) is the treatment of choice, followed by pemoline (Cylert). Both have been shown to be effective in controlled trials. Other options include CNS stimulants such as methylphenidate and dextroamphetamine.

Poor sleep can contribute to fatigue. In MS, a variety of factors negatively affect sleep, including nocturia, nocturnal spasms, pain, and, less commonly, sleep disorder. Nocturia can be treated with oxybutrin or intranasal vasopressins. Nocturnal spasms respond to baclofen, carbamazepine, gabapentin, or benzodiazepine. Suspicion of an underlying sleep disorder should be investigated with polysomnography.

Urinary, Bowel, or Sexual Dysfunction

Among the most distressing symptoms is loss of bladder and bowel control, which is mainly associated with involvement of the spinal cord. Such accidents are often humiliating and embarrassing. Therefore, the goal of symptom management is to provide control. The two major problems involving bladder function in MS are failure to empty (a flaccid bladder) and failure to store (a neurogenic spastic bladder). Individuals with emptying problems find that they cannot void despite the urge to urinate and are prone to large postvoid residuals. This is a setup for infection and dribbling. Treatments for this problem include bethanechol and intermittent self-catheterization. Individuals can empty the bladder in the privacy of a bathroom and resume daily activities without fear of an accident. Sometimes after following a self-catheterization program for several weeks, self-catheterizing is no longer necessary, and normal bladder function is restored.

A hyperactive bladder is able to store only small amounts of urine. This results in the sense of urinary urgency and frequency. Typically, individuals state that the first thing they look for when entering a new building is the bathroom. Medication can successfully "tone down" the bladder. This includes oxybutynin (Ditropan), propantheline, and hyoscyamine sulfate (Levsinex). Anticholinergic drugs, including tricyclic antidepressants, can also be helpful.

Bowel problems can be very difficult and include constipation, fecal urgency, and fecal incontinence. Constipation can be treated with a combination of stool softeners, peristaltic stimulants, increased fluid intake, and dietary manipulation, including increased fiber content. Fecal incontinence may require disimpaction and enemas. The management of such problems both in bladder and bowel control is described more completely in Chapter 5, which deals with the effects of SCI.

Sexual dysfunction is another frequent problem in men and women. In men, erectile dysfunction is not uncommon and usually is associated with neurogenic as well as psychological factors. Pharmacologic approaches include oral medications (yohimbine, sildenafil, clomipramine), topical drugs (nitroglycerin, minoxidil, papaverine), and intracavernosal self-injection (papaverine, phentolamine, alprostadil). In women, decreased libido, decreased sensation, and decreased arousal and lubrication can all contribute to sexual dysfunction. Evaluation of sexual dysfunction should include a comprehensive physical assessment and frank discussion with partners. Psychosocial factors, fatigue, decreased libido, and symptoms of depression should be addressed. Referral to a urologist with expertise in issues of sexual dysfunction is usually most helpful. This problem is also described in detail in Chapter 5.

Cognitive and Psychiatric Problems

Cognitive loss is a particularly disabling symptom of MS. Neuropsychological studies from outpatient and community samples have varied widely in their estimates of the frequency of cognitive impairment in MS (e.g., from 30% to 70%). The most common areas of cognitive impairment are memory, visuoperceptual ability, conceptual reasoning, and cognitive processing speed.[20] Consultation with a neuropsychologist is useful to establish a baseline cognitive profile for reference and to assist with cognitive rehabilitative strategies.

Psychiatric disturbances can also occur in MS. Mood disorders and depression in particular have been recognized in MS for more than 70 years. Although depression can understandably occur as a reaction to living with the disorder, most studies suggest that individuals with MS have a higher frequency of depression compared with other neurologically impaired groups. The prevalence of depression in MS varies from 22% to 50% across studies.[21,22] Of perhaps the greatest concern is the elevated risk of suicide, reported to be up to 7.5 times the risk of the general population, with a cumulative risk of 2%. Other psychiatric complications of MS include bipolar disorder, which has been associated with neuroimaging abnormalities, and anxiety disorders.

The issue of depression in MS is particularly important given that two of the drugs currently in use as prophylactics for relapses and disease progression, interferon-β 1a and interferon-β 1b, have been shown to increase risk of depression. In addition, rehabilitative interventions can be hampered by the adverse impact of depression and anxiety on QOL and motivation. Management of affective disorders in MS requires a multidisciplinary approach. Individuals should understand that depression is a possible manifestation of the disease itself as well as an understandable reaction to living with the illness. A variety of treatment approaches, including biofeedback, educational counseling, cognitive-behavioral therapy, and supportive psychotherapy, can help individuals with MS. Antidepressants are frequently appropriate.

Symptoms reflect a wide range of possible CNS involvement. The most frequent impairments are those that relate to the motor system, including fatigue as well as disturbances of motor control. Crucial to the maintenance of QOL is a commitment to compensate for the ongoing and progressive impairments.

Nature of the Disabilities

Disability refers to the functional (behavioral) consequences of the varying impairments. WHO[15] has defined disability as "any restriction or lack, resulting from impairment, of the ability to perform an activity within the range considered normal . . . for a human being." The disabilities refer to the effects of the impairments in the life of the person. They are a result not only of the type and extent of the impairments but also of their interaction with the person who is experiencing them. As such, the functional disabilities cannot be deduced merely from the medical neurologic examination. Input from the person who is experiencing the impairments helps to define the disabilities that are predominant in the life of that person. The specific disabilities to be ameliorated vary with the goals and the characteristics of the person. Normal rehabilitation practice deals with this level of analysis. One of its aims is to reduce the degree to which the impairments disrupt the life of the person by training the actions that remain unaffected and the use of various assistive devices to compensate for the functional problems.

Although the disabilities are ultimately determined by the individual's idiosyncratic characteristics, the nature of the disease and the persons who are most likely to be affected determine the overall pattern of disabilities. The usually progressive quality of the disease process and the remittent and frequently unpredictable nature of the "attacks" can affect the person's ability to cope with the effects. In addition, the multiple impairments inherent in the nature of the disease add to the burden of disability.

The relief of suffering must be one of the primary ends of the treatment of persons with a chronic illness such as MS. The distinction is made between chronic disease and chronic illness.[23] Disease is defined as "specific entities characterized by disturbances in structure or function of . . . any part of the body. Illnesses . . . affect whole persons and are the set of disordered functions, body sensations and feelings by which persons feel themselves to be unwell."

Cassell[23] eloquently describes how suffering, although generally coupled with pain, need not be synonymous with it. Pain is only one of the sources of suffering. The element of suffering can also include fears of what tomorrow will bring. In the context of MS as a progressive disease, each tomorrow can be seen as worse than today, as heralding increased disability, and never as the beginning of better times. In the context of MS as a disease subject to unpredictable relapses, one can perceive oneself to be subject to forces beyond one's control. The body is not only untrustworthy in its performance, but it does not even misbehave consistently. One could suffer from the immediate effects of the disease, but one could also suffer even more from the perception of the future.

The nature of MS is like that of any chronic neurologic illness that affects the ability of the person to use the body. A woman with MS describes the objectification of the body in illness that forces attention to the body as a daily occurrence[24]:

> I must overtly take [my physical disabilities] into account as I go about my world. I must be aware of my dysfunctional body as both physical encumbrance and as malfunctioning physiological organism. . . . The "diseased body" with its ongoing demands necessarily stands in opposition to the self. . . .With chronic illness, one perceives one's body as permanently impaired. Consequently . . . alienation from, and unwilling identification with, the body is particularly profound.

Because chronic illness is defined in terms of the person rather than the disease alone, the person finds him- or herself "inescapably embodied, irrevocably attached to an essentially malfunctioning bodily organism which promises to disrupt all their involvements in the world. Such disorders are consequently experienced as world threatening."[24]

The relative young age of the persons affected and their gender create specific problems in relation to the effects of the bodily impairments caused by the MS. Because the demographics of MS lead younger women to be the most affected, issues of family planning are often at the forefront of concern. Women with MS have two primary concerns: first, that their MS will worsen during pregnancy. The current opinion based on data from prospective and retrospective studies is that no worsening occurs during pregnancy. In fact, some studies have indicated a tendency toward a decreased frequency of exacerbation. In the postpartum period, however, the risk of exacerbation is slightly increased. However, the overall course of MS does not appear to be significantly altered by pregnancy. A second concern women with MS have is the risk of passing on the disorder to their children. Although studies suggest that genetic factors contribute to the development of MS, multiple genes are likely involved. In addition to the concordance rates discussed previously, daughters of a parent with MS have a 2–5% risk, whereas the risk for sons is somewhat less.

Given the unpredictable nature of the disorder, planning can help an individual with MS gain a sense of control and minimize the distress and psychosocial impact during times of acute illness. It is advisable to choose a time when the symptoms are minimal to make long-term plans for all aspects of the future. These plans should include contingent conditions to deal with both the case of a mild disease course as well as the case of progressive disability that results in loss of wages and loss of ability to perform ADL. Finances, child care, and other aspects of living should be considered and decided on in detail.

Another aspect of dealing with the disorder is educating the patient to learn to recognize early signs of an impending attack. This enables the patient to seek medical intervention earlier and to refrain from activities that can exacerbate symptoms. One woman with long-standing, relapsing MS has dealt with her sense of loss of control by becoming aware of the early signals of relapse. With notification of her physician, immediate treatment is administered by her husband at home.

Certain losses or injuries are likely to cause suffering. The sense of powerlessness and hopelessness that can arise in a person with MS can almost invariably cause suffering. Alienation from one's body, which is seen as untrustworthy, can lead to suffering. The only way to learn whether suffering is present is to ask the individual. Although each person's response to impairment touches features that are common to us all, the response of each contains features that must be defined in terms of a specific person at a specific time. The character of the solution in the management of persons with MS must be responsive to the need to relieve this sense of suffering that is unique to the individual. MS presents many challenges; however, patients now have many options for improving their sense of well-being, minimizing symptoms, and possibly altering the disease course.

Character of the Solution

Overall Plan

Individuals with MS are best served by a comprehensive treatment approach that includes continuity of care and places the patient at the core of the treatment team. Due to the possibility of disease progression and the unpredictability of the disease course, continuity of care is essential. Coordinated treatment may include an interdisciplinary treatment team that consists of the neurologist or other primary health care provider, physical therapist, and social worker. Ultimately, a central role for the individual with MS for all treatment decisions can lead to a sense of empowerment and control. A generic model for doing so is described in detail in Chapter 2. The application of a similar model to the management of persons with MS, called a *psychoeducational approach*, seeks to develop patient self-responsibility and self-monitoring as means of increasing adherence to regimens.[25]

Living with MS is difficult on many levels. First, it has no cure. Second, the nature of the disorder is not predictable, and, therefore, individuals can never be certain when and if another attack will occur. With an attack, individuals with MS may lose control of their functioning (e.g., motor, bladder, coordination, cognitive). Although attacks usually occur without any identifiable trigger, patients tend to blame themselves or attribute causal factors that may not be relevant. Stress may contribute to increased disease activity, but it is an unavoidable part of life (although it can be minimized). Particularly early in the disease course, individuals with MS experience fatigue, cognitive disruptions (e.g., decreased concentration and memory difficulties), paresthesias, and other unpleasant symptoms that can be quite unsettling. Further, these symptoms are not readily apparent, and, therefore, family, friends, and coworkers may have difficulty in understanding the person's discomfort and limits in functioning. A videotape provided to individuals with MS by the National MS Society, entitled "Yet You Look So Well," encapsulates the frustrations that many individuals with seemingly mild MS experience.

Certain personal decisions can have a dramatic effect for the individual with MS. It is critical to maintain a positive attitude, avoid denial, and keep communication open with all family members. For many people, participation in self-help support groups, as well as support groups for partners and children, may be particularly rewarding. Being proactive about one's overall health is another important self-empowering step. Being as physically fit as possible, taking steps such as getting a flu vaccine to avoid infection, and maintaining a regular sleep pattern and well-balanced diet as much as possible are all good health habits that are important for living with MS.

The following cases exemplify a variety of patterns of the disease as well as the age and gender of the persons in whom MS tends to occur. These cases illustrate the value of continuity of care incorporating medical and nonmedical care that is responsive to the patient or family, or both. It is important to encourage these primary participants to articulate their needs and take part in their own care.

A Young Woman Newly Diagnosed

Carly is a 28-year-old woman with relapsing-remitting MS that was diagnosed when she was 27. Her initial symptoms occurred at her job as a clerk for an insurance company, when she noticed that she had trouble tapping the keys of her computer and was making numerous errors. She was also unsteady when standing and walking. Additional history revealed a prior episode of bilateral leg numbness, which had occurred 3 years earlier. Her examination revealed a mild intranuclear ophthalmoparesis, ataxia of gait, right upper extremity dysmetria, and sensory loss to vibration in the distal lower extremities.

The possibility that she had MS was discussed, and literature was provided describing the disease. Another visit after diagnostic testing was scheduled 2 days later. An MRI scan revealed multiple lesions in the periventricular white matter and the right cerebellar peduncle on T2-weighted MRI. Blood tests for Lyme disease, B_{12} deficiency, anemia, and thyroid disease were negative. The patient was eager to return to her previous level of normal balance and dexterity. She stated that her primary goal was to be able to return to work as soon as possible and to recover as much neurologic function as she could. She was started on a course of parenteral solumedrol (1 g/day) for 5 days as an outpatient, and a program of outpatient physical therapy was arranged to focus on balance and fine finger movements.

At the next follow-up visit 4 weeks later, her balance and sensory findings were improved but not fully back to baseline. The diagnosis was further discussed with her and her husband. She chose to continue physical therapy. The couple was counseled and referred to patient support groups through the local MS chapter for individuals with newly diagnosed MS. At a later visit with the social worker, family planning issues were discussed. Her main goal was to continue to work and to begin planning a family. She chose not to go on prophylactic medication and later became pregnant. During the postpartum period, she had transient sensory loss that resolved spontaneously. She continued to work and care for her daughter. The need to recognize an attack so that she could get treatment quickly was reviewed, and it was also pointed out that if attacks continued she should strongly consider prophylactic medication.

One year later, after an attack associated with increased ataxia and tremors, Carly was ready to consider further treatment. She now asked for help in managing the effects of her disease, particularly her increased fatigue and tremor as well as dealing with the possibility of further attacks. Her examination showed dysmetria and mild ataxia. She was having increasing difficulty performing household chores, was no longer able to function at work (because of excessive typing errors), and was frequently exhausted. A meeting was scheduled with her and her husband, during which her new goals were articulated. She wished to better conserve her energy, decrease the time spent outside the home at work, and take whatever measures were necessary to prevent her MS from worsening.

Carly changed to a part-time position that required less typing and took several steps to improve her fatigue. These included inserting a rest period in the afternoon and modifying the home by making appliances more accessible so that she did not have to walk up and down the stairs while doing housework. The advantages and disadvantages of the different prophylactic therapies were reviewed, and she chose to go on an interferon-β form of therapy. She has continued on this treatment and has not had any further attacks in the subsequent year.

A comprehensive patient-oriented approach including articulation of changing goals as they developed over time led to successful symptom management and treatments directed toward the future. Both patient and spouse received educational materials and were directly involved in all treatment decisions.

A Middle-Aged Man with Progressive Disease

James is a 50-year-old man who recently moved into the area and carries a diagnosis of secondary progressive MS. Six years ago, he had an episode of optic neuritis that resolved. Four years ago, progressive gait difficulty developed. An MRI evaluation of the cervical spine showed an area of increased signal intensity in the C3 region on T2-weighted imaging. A CSF study was positive for oligoclonal bands. A diagnosis of MS was made at that time.

At the time of his evaluation, he was divorced but had made some new friends. He complained of severe leg stiffness, difficulty with sleep due to pain, weakness, and a tendency to fall. Neurologic examination was notable for bilateral leg weakness, increased muscle tone, and inability to walk more than 40 meters without holding on to a side rail. His goals were reviewed. His primary goals were to decrease his pain, improve his sleep, and use as little medication as possible.

Various treatment options were discussed, including physical therapy, muscle relaxation exercises to combat insomnia, and medication for spasticity. James chose physical therapy. At a follow-up visit, however, he agreed to try medication for his spasticity, as he was still having pain and insomnia. Options for taking the medication during the day or exclusively at night were reviewed. He found that the antispasticity medication, when taken at night, relieved his pain and helped him sleep, but, if he took the medication during the day, he became sleepy. By taking his medication at night and using relaxation exercises and physical therapy, he was able to accomplish his major goals.

At a follow-up visit 3 years later, James could no longer ambulate independently and was experiencing episodes of loss of bladder control, which caused him embarrassment at work. He stated that his goal was to continue to work while not being a burden to his employer or coworkers. Job modifications had been made, such as moving his office closer to the elevator and bathroom so that the distance he needed to walk was decreased. He continued to be self-conscious and worried. He expressed a lack of interest in his job (which he had previously enjoyed) and showed increased irritability. An interview with the social worker after his visit with the doctor confirmed the diagnostic impression of major depression.

James chose not to go on antidepressant medication. He did agree, however, to an evaluation regarding his bladder function. A postvoid residual was performed in the office and was in the normal range. He was prescribed anticholinergic medication for the bladder (oxybutynin), and he noticed improvement. At a subsequent visit, he agreed to enter counseling with the social worker. His motor skills have continued to decline, but he has adapted to using a wheelchair and is coping well.

Continuity of care was critical in helping James deal over time with the different stages of his disorder. He had choices throughout in making decisions about his treatment. As an example, his observations about the effects of the antispasticity medication were instrumental in maintaining QOL. His participation in monitoring the effects of the medication made it more cost-effective. As a further example, his initial decision about the management of his depression was honored but could be modified in light of ongoing follow-up.

*A Woman with Long-Term Disease
but Short-Term Needs*

Alice is a 58-year-old woman who has had MS for more than 25 years. She first noticed a problem when she dropped her plate at a birthday party for her young daughter. Several days later, she noticed that her left hand was numb and weak. She never saw a physician, and her symptoms resolved spontaneously. However, 5 years later, she had an episode of vision loss in the right eye. She saw an ophthalmologist, who made the diagnosis of optic neuritis and referred her for a neurologic evaluation. The neurologist performed a lumbar puncture and informed her that she had MS. She initially had a relapsing-remitting course. She was able to continue to work full time due to the support of her supervisor.

By age 49, however, her course became progressive and was characterized by increasing gait impairment. She went from using a cane to a walker and has been in a wheelchair for the past 3 years. She stopped working after she lost ambulatory function. At present, her primary problems are difficulty in drinking from a cup due to hand weakness and pain and stiffness in her legs. Her goal is to maintain self-care activities, including the ability to feed herself and perform self-hygiene. Her husband continues to work

and is not at home during the day. Her children have moved out and are living in another state.

She was referred to an occupational therapist. A device was provided that enabled her to hold a cup more effectively. With physical therapy and use of baclofen for spasticity, her stiffness and pain improved. Referral to a social worker provided assistance in obtaining a home aide for several hours each weekday. Both the patient and her husband felt better about their situation and thought they had more options.

A multidisciplinary approach led to improved QOL for this neurologically impaired woman. Her disease process had been slowly progressive. Despite her ongoing impairments, she managed to carry on her life without the help of physicians. By defining her needs at this time, she was able to get the help she needed in learning about some specific assistive aids. Cost-effective treatment need not be long term if it is properly focused.

The development of any treatment plan requires a definition of the outcomes and their ongoing review and revision. Health outcomes must be jointly derived and meet the needs of both the physician and patient. A multidisciplinary treatment program for achieving goals can be developed as needed for each individual patient. Ultimately, the measurement of effectiveness must be an integral part of any interaction between the professional and the persons most involved. The ongoing relationship between the professional and the patient must lead to increased self-management by the patient. Contribution to the planning and treatment process can be empowering. Particularly helpful in creating a sense of self-efficacy is the review of the ideas that worked in the context of monitoring progress in relation to the goals originally set. The aim must be to enable patients to measure outcomes that are meaningful to them and clear enough so that they can develop a sense of hope in their capability in managing their own life.

Measuring Effectiveness

Measurement of Impairments and Disease Status

The most frequently studied outcomes of impairment and disease activity are MRI, the EDSS by Kurtzke,[26] and relapse rate. Areas of demyelination on MRI can be quantified according to number and volume. These measurements are used to determine the lesion load and are helpful for assessing the disease activity. Increased disease activity can also be identified with gadolinium-enhanced images during periods in which individuals are asymptomatic. In most of the major clinical trials demonstrating the benefits of prophylactic therapy, changes on MRI were key outcome measures. A reduction in lesion load and number of new gadolinium-enhancing lesions were signs of drug efficacy for Betaseron and Avonex.

The EDSS, developed by Kurtzke, is rated by the neurologist and grades impairment along a scale from 0 (normal) to 10 (death) in 20 steps. Grades 1–4 assess increasing levels of impairment according to functional systems that encompass pyramidal, cerebellar, brain stem, sensory, bowel and bladder, visual, mental, and other systems. Grade 4.5 and above relate to dysfunction in ambulation. This is the most widely used outcome measure in clinical trials. In all the major clinical trials that led to the U.S. Food and Drug Administration approval of Betaseron, Avonex, and Copaxone, the EDSS was a major outcome measure.

The EDSS has a number of limitations. One problem is that the functional systems are not anatomically independent. Another is that the scale can be insensitive to important deficits such as severe dementia or blindness if no associated gait impairment is present. (An individual with legal blindness, urinary incontinence, and dementia who can ambulate 500 m would score only a 4.0, whereas someone who is less neurologically impaired with full cognition, normal vision, and bowel and bladder function but who requires a cane to ambulate would have a worse score [6.0].) The scale also has poor reliability. For example, the correlation among independent neurologic examiners using the scale is a kappa of only 6.0. Despite these problems, the EDSS is still used in clinical trials and is applied by many neurologists in the routine follow-up of patients who attend MS comprehensive care centers. Modifications in the instructions for its use have improved inter-rater reliability.

An alternative is Scripps Neurologic Rating Scale,[27] which grades the extent of neurologic involvement from 0 (maximum) to 100 (normal). It may be somewhat more reliable but has problems of insensitivity.

Another means of assessing disease activity is to measure relapse rate. Most clinical trials for relapsing-remitting MS used annual relapse rate as a primary or secondary outcome measure. Although measuring relapse rate appears to be straightforward, the severity of each relapse is difficult to quantify. Further, relapses are appropriate measures for patients in the early phases of the disease, but they do not apply to those who are in a progressive stage.

Measurement of Quality of Life

Patient-based, health-related QOL measurements in MS include generic health status inventories and MS-specific measures. The Medical Outcomes Study Short Form (SF-36) health survey[28] is a widely used instrument that has been applied to patients with MS. It includes measures of physical functioning, role functioning, social functioning, mental health, vitality and energy, and general health perception. The results are transformed into scale scores that range from 0 to 100, with higher scores indicating better QOL. In a study of 97 participants with MS using the SF-36, MS subjects scored lower in physical functioning, role functioning due to physical activity, and energy and vitality compared with the general population.[29] In advanced cases of MS, however, the SF-36 shows a lack of sensitivity and has floor effects.[30]

An MS-specific health status measure that is gaining use is the Functional Assessment of Multiple Sclerosis.[31] This inventory covers a range of ADL. It is administered by self-report and contains 44 items that are divided into six subscales: mobility, symptoms, emotional well-being, general contentment, thinking and fatigue, and family and social well-being. The mobility subscale was strongly predictive of the EDSS. The scale appears reliable and has good internal consistency, ranging from 0.82 to 0.96.

A subcommittee of the Consortium of Multiple Sclerosis Centers has developed a comprehensive manual for the most appropriate measures of symptoms that directly affect QOL in individuals with MS.[32] This collection of measures includes modifications of the SF-36, measures adapted from the shortened versions of other established scales. A QOL measure that is comprehensive but not too lengthy or exhausting for individuals with MS to complete is critical for evaluating individual responses as well as assessing the efficacy of interventions.

Ultimately, the most important outcomes are those that are specific to the individual patient. During the disease course, setting specific goals, such as reducing the number of nocturnal awakenings due to painful spasms or urinary urgency and improving ambulation by reducing falls either through physical therapy or use of ambulation aids, is useful for addressing the effect of MS on QOL.

References

1. Sadovick AD, Baird PA, Ward RH. Multiple sclerosis: updated risks for relatives. Am J Med Genet 1988;29: 533–541.
2. Whetten-Goldstein K, Sloan FA, Goldstein LB, Kulas ED. A comprehensive assessment of the cost of multiple sclerosis in the United States. Mult Scler 1998;4:419–425.
3. Sadovnick AD, Ebers GC. Epidemiology of multiple sclerosis: a critical overview. Can J Neurol Sci 1993;20:17–29.
4. Paty DW, Ebers GC. Multiple Sclerosis. Philadelphia: Davis, 1998.
5. Martin R, McFarland HF. Immunological aspects of experimental allergic encephalomyelitis and multiple sclerosis. Clin Rev Clin Lab Sci 1995;32:121–182.
6. Schumacher GA, Beebe G, Kibler RE, et al. Problems of experimental trials of therapy in multiple sclerosis: report by the panel on evaluation of experimental trials of therapy in multiple sclerosis. Ann N Y Acad Sci 1965;122: 552–568.
7. Poser CM, Paty DW, Scheinberg L, et al. New diagnosis criteria for multiple sclerosis: guidelines for research protocols. Ann Neurol 1983;13:2227–2231.
8. Weinshenker GB, Bass B, Rice GP, et al. The natural history of multiple sclerosis: a geographically based study. I. Clinical course and disability. Brain 1989;112:133–146.
9. Weinshenker GB, Rice GPA, Noseworthy JH, et al. The natural history of multiple sclerosis: a geographically based study. III. Multivariate analysis of predictive factors and models of outcome. Brain 1991;1:114:1045–1056.
10. IFNB Multiple Sclerosis Study Group. Interferon beta-1b is effective in relapsing-remitting multiple sclerosis. I. Clinical results of a multicenter, randomized, double-blind, placebo controlled trial. Neurology 1993;43: 655–661.
11. Jacobs LD, Cookfair DL, Rudick RA, et al. Intramuscular interferon beta-1a for disease progression in relapsing-remitting multiple sclerosis. Ann Neurol 1996;39: 285–294.
12. Johnson KP, Brooks BR, Cohen JA, et al. Copolymer 1 Multiple Sclerosis Study Group. Extended use of glatiramer acetate (Copaxone) is well tolerated and maintains its clinical effect on multiple sclerosis relapse rate and degree of disability. Neurology 1998;50:701–708.
13. Durelli L, Baggio GF, Bergamasco B, et al. Early immunosuppressive effect of parenteral methylprednisolone in the treatment of multiple sclerosis. Acta Neurol (Napoli) 1985;7:338–344.
14. Milligan NM, Newcombe R, Compston DAS. A double-blind controlled trial of high dose methylprednisolone in patients with multiple sclerosis. J Neurol Neurosurg Psychiatry 1987;50:511–516.
15. World Health Organization. The International Classification of Impairments, Disabilities and Handicaps. Geneva: World Health Organization, 1980.
16. Anderson PB, Goodkin DE. Current pharmacologic treatment of multiple sclerosis symptoms. West J Med 1996; 165:313–317.
17. Clanet MG, Azais-Vuillemin C. What is New in the Symptomatic Management of Multiple Sclerosis. In AJ Thompson, C Polman, R Hohlfeld (eds), Multiple Sclerosis: Clinical Challenges and Controversies. London: Martin Dunitz, 1997.
18. Krupp LB, Alvarez LA, LaRocca NG, Scheinberg L. Clinical characteristics of fatigue in multiple sclerosis. Arch Neurol 1988;45:435–437.
19. Fisk JD, Pontefract A, Ritvo PG, et al. The impact of fatigue on patients with multiple sclerosis. Can J Neurol Sci 1994;21:9–14.
20. Rao SM. Neuropsychology of multiple sclerosis: a critical review. J Clin Neuropsychol 1986;8:504–542.
21. Schiffer RB. The spectrum of depression in multiple sclerosis: an approach for clinical management. Arch Neurol 1987;44:596–599.
22. Remick RA, Sadovnick AD. Depression and Suicide in Multiple Sclerosis. In AJ Thompson, C Polman, R Hohlfeld (eds), Multiple Sclerosis: Clinical Challenges and Controversies. London: Martin Dunitz, 1997.
23. Cassell EJ. The Nature of Suffering and the Goals of Medicine. New York: Oxford University Press, 1991;49.
24. Toombs SK. The Meaning of Illness. Boston: Kluwer Academic, 1993;75.
25. Halper J. The psychoeducational approach to complex protocols in neurorehabilitation. J Neurol Rehabil 1997; 11:149–154.
26. Kurtzke JF. Rating neurologic impairment in multiple sclerosis: an expanded disability status scale (EDSS). Neurology 1983;33:1444–1452.
27. Sipe JC, Knobler RL, Braheny SL. A neurological rating scale (NRS) for multiple sclerosis 1984;34:1368–1372.
28. Ware JE. SF-36 Health Survey Manual and Interpretation Guide. Boston: Nimrod, 1993.
29. Brunet DG, Hopan WM, Singer MA, et al. Measurement of health related quality of life in multiple sclerosis patients. Can J Neurol Sci 1996;23:99–103.
30. Freeman JA, Langdon DW, Hobart JC, et al. Health related quality of life in people with multiple sclerosis undergoing inpatient rehabilitation. J Neurol Rehabil 1996;10:185–194.
31. Cella DF, Dineen K, Arnason B, et al. Validation of the functional assessment of multiple sclerosis quality of life instrument. Neurology 1996;47:129–139.
32. Rivito PG, Fischer JS, Miller DM, et al. Multiple Sclerosis Quality of Life Inventory: A User's Manual. New York: Consortium of Multiple Sclerosis Centers Health Services Research Subcommittee, 1997.

Chapter 9

Management of Persons with Parkinson's Disease

Jonathan H. Pincus

Nature of the Problem

Extent of the Problem

PD is a progressive illness. The nerve cells that produce dopamine in the substantia nigra degenerate for reasons that are unknown. If the degenerative process remains confined to dopaminergic cells, the therapeutic problem posed by PD is straightforward: Replace dopamine. If the degenerative process consumes neurons other than dopaminergic cells, the therapeutic problem is much more difficult to solve.

Incidence and Prevalence

Mostly sporadic, PD rarely can be inherited as an autosomal dominant disorder. When this is the case, the onset of the disease can be quite early, in the second or third decade. Ordinarily, PD begins at age 59 years on the average, and it affects approximately 1% of the population older than 60 years. According to most estimates, approximately 1 million persons are living with PD in the United States.

Parkinsonlike symptoms have many causes other than dopamine deficiency. For example, cerebrovascular disease and primary degenerative disorders can produce bradykinesia, postural instability, and rigidity. However, the resting tremor that is improved by voluntary movement is pathognomonic of dopamine deficiency or dopamine receptor blockade. In addition, it is generally a good prognostic sign.

The definition of PD has been somewhat imprecise. The term is directed at both those patients with pure dopamine deficiency and those who have more complicated parkinsonism. Sometimes the latter is referred to as Parkinson's plus. The word plus indicates the involvement of nerve cells outside the dopaminergic system. Many degenerative diseases primarily affect portions of the nervous system that lie outside the dopaminergic system. Such diseases can also cause some degree of dopamine deficiency. The symptoms that result from dopamine deficiency can be treated, but the symptoms that arise from degeneration outside the dopamine system are usually untreatable.

Striatonigral degeneration, olivopontocerebellar atrophy, progressive supranuclear palsy (PSP), multisystem atrophy, corticobasilar dementia, and Lewy body dementia (LBD) are all diseases that result from the degeneration of neurons that are outside the dopamine system. In each of these diseases, some degree of dopamine deficiency is present as well as symptoms of parkinsonism that derive from it. Only the symptoms that are the result of dopamine deficiency can be treated with dopamine replacement. Until we know the actual pathogenesis of each of these diseases, we cannot determine if they and PD are separate entities or if they are all different points in the same spectrum.

This confusion has muddied the understanding of the impact of PD on the lives of patients and how they can be treated. For example, the term end-stage PD has developed two meanings. One use of the term describes a patient with widespread disease of the nervous system who is curled into a little ball in flexion, helpless and demented. Dopamine replacement therapy has no beneficial effect and only makes the patient hallucinate more. The other use of the term describes a patient who has no dopaminergic neurons left but no other brain involvement. Properly treated for dopamine deficiency, he or she functions normally, both motorically and intellectually. To add complexity, a patient may at first have symptoms that respond fully to dopamine replacement and then, in time, develop other symptoms that do not.

Burden

Costs, including the costs of medication and the burden of care for medical expenses and so forth, should be discussed. The progressive quality of the disease process and its relatively frequent relationship to other disease processes associated with dementia and nonresponsiveness to dopamine are also characteristics that can add to its burden. The elderly age of onset is another factor in that the availability of caregivers is a problem because the mates are themselves elderly.

Movement disorders are a significant problem, particularly in the elderly. The prevalence of this problem is likely to increase with the increase of individuals in the older age group of the population. The availability of a treatment and the possibility of continued good function make management of movement disorders particularly important. The continued use of the eponym for the description of the major type of movement disorder reflects our limited knowledge of its etiology.

Nature of the Disease

Spectrum of Disease

The relationship of PD to other more malignant, untreatable brain degenerations has been elucidated. PD and other degenerative diseases of the nervous system may be similar in relation to the basic defect that is present in each.

Many of these degenerative conditions are sporadic, but when they are genetic, they are transmitted as autosomal dominant diseases. These include AD, frontotemporal atrophy (Pick's disease), Creutzfeldt-Jakob disease, ALS, spinocerebellar atrophies, and Huntington's disease. Each of these diseases seems to have an abnormality of one protein. The protein is a normal constituent of nerve cells, but it contains a subtle abnormality; sometimes only a single amino acid is out of place.

Genes direct protein synthesis and determine the number of amino acids that comprise a protein and the order in which they appear. Each gene uses the nucleic acids of its DNA to direct the manufacture of a protein. Each amino acid that comprises a protein has a genetic code. The trinucleotide sequence, cytosine-arginine-guanidine (CAG), codes for the amino acid glutamine. If the sequence, CAG, repeats with too great a frequency in the DNA, the resultant protein will have too many glutamine molecules. The location of the gene that contains these trinucleotide repeats determines the disease. The number of CAG repeats determines the severity of the illness. The abnormal deposition of protein filaments in Huntington's disease and some spinocerebellar atrophies is the result of trinucleotide CAG repeats in a gene.

According to a modern theory, in each of the other degenerative disorders mentioned previously the accumulation of a different abnormal protein from the one in Huntington's disease occurs. This protein is deposited in filaments that collect within the nerve cells and, ultimately, causes the nerve cells in which it is deposited to degenerate. In AD, Pick's disease, PD, and other disorders, the filaments involved have been shown to consist either of the microtubule-associated protein, tau, or alpha-synuclein.

Mutations in the gene for tau have been identified as the genetic causes of some cases of AD and frontotemporal dementia (Pick's disease). Deposition of alpha-synuclein has been described in PD and several diseases in the Parkinson's spectrum. The discovery in 1998 of neuronal intranuclear inclusions in Huntington's disease and other disorders with expanded glutamine repeats, along with the data on tau and synuclein accumulation, has suggested a unifying mechanism underlying the pathogenesis of all the neurodegenerative diseases that can be inherited as autosomal dominants.[1]

If a protein looked like a string of pearls, perfect except for one imperfect amino acid, the problem would be relatively minor. However, proteins are constructed more like a Slinky toy. If a middle portion were twisted, the whole toy would become useless. Proteins are usually tightly wound and exist in a three-dimensional structure. Because of its abnormal shape, the abnormal protein cannot be broken down by the usual enzymes, and parts of the protein accumulate within the cell. The accumulation of the abnormal bits of protein leads to the death of the cell.

In PD, an abnormal form of a normally occurring intracellular protein, alpha-synuclein, has been demonstrated in the dying dopaminergic neurons in the substantia nigra. The intracytoplasmic inclusions that characterize degenerating nerve cells in PD (Lewy bodies) are loaded with the abnormal synuclein. An abnormal gene for the manufacture of alpha-synuclein appears to be responsible for the rare cases of genetic PD that are transmitted in autosomal dominant fashion. The gene in this disorder has been identified, and the abnormal protein product of that gene has been characterized. Fluorescent antibody techniques have identified the abnormal alpha-synuclein microscopically in brain tissue.

Using the fluorescent antibody technique, scientists have found that the abnormal form of alpha-synuclein is not only present in patients with the genetic form of PD but also in the Lewy bodies in the brains of patients with ordinary, sporadic PD. In this "garden variety" PD, patients have a normal gene for the production of alpha-synuclein. How the brain cells of genetically normal patients can make the abnormal form of alpha-synuclein is a puzzling subject of current research and thinking, and the hypothesis has been put forward that a form of prion disorder akin to Creutzfeldt-Jakob and mad cow disease may be responsible.

The fluorescent antibody technique has also identified the abnormal alpha-synuclein in the Lewy bodies of the cerebral cortex in LBD and in the hypothalamic nuclei of patients with multiple-system atrophy.[2] Fragments of this protein also exist in the plaque of patients with AD.[3]

LBD is characterized by progressive cognitive impairment with prominent parkinsonian features. Identified only in the last decade as a "new" degenerative dementia, LBD overlaps AD and PD clinically, pathologically, and genetically. Clinically, typical parkinsonian motor features are tremor, bradykinesia, and postural instability, but with a relatively rapid progression. The motor symptoms become dominated by postural instability and bradykinesia, the treatment of which does not relieve the motor symptoms satisfactorily but instead leads to worsening of hallucinations and confusion. Psychosis is a prominent feature, with recurrent complicated visual hallucinations and rapid fluctuations in alertness.

The neuropathologic hallmark of LBD is the widespread presence of intracytoplasmic inclusions and Lewy bodies, identical to the inclusions that are typically seen in PD. The distribution of these Lewy bodies, unlike that in typical PD in which they are limited to the substantia nigra, is widespread throughout the neocortical and paralimbic regions. In LBD, the Lewy bodies often coexist with plaques that are typical of AD.

It is not yet clear whether all these diseases have a similar, or indeed an identical, pathogenesis, but the idea that PD and certain syndromes related to PD may have a similar etiology, in the sense that they are caused by the accumulation of the same abnormal protein, might explain the large overlap among these conditions and the fact that typical PD with dopamine deficiency alone can evolve into one or more of the other clinical types. Is PD a different disorder from Parkinson's plus, LBD, and multiple-system atrophy, or is the same basic biochemical defect common to all, with the clinical syndromes distinguished only by where the abnormal protein is deposited? These questions cannot be answered at present.

Pathogenesis

The first symptoms of PD do not appear until at least 80% of the dopaminergic neurons have been lost. Individuals who have sustained a 75% loss appear normal. PD is a progressive disease, and the symptoms worsen with the passage of time. Not all parts of the dopaminergic system are equally affected, which accounts for the existence of unilateral PD symptoms or regional symptoms of PD and the only occasional impairment of cognition. Biologically, the difference between 80% depletion and 75% depletion is not significant, but clinically, it makes the difference between illness and the appearance of normality.

Dopamine is stored in small vesicles within the axon terminals. At least two presynaptic pools of dopamine exist: those that are immediately adjacent to the axon terminal membrane and those that are further away. With stimulation of the nerves, the vesicles that touch the axon terminal membrane release their contents into the synaptic cleft. The majority of the vesicles are located some distance from the membrane and are not available for release when the nerve is stimulated; their contents remain stored and, hence, inactive.

Once released, dopamine acts on postsynaptic receptors. The reuptake mechanism quickly terminates the postsynaptic action of dopamine. Once it has been taken back into the dopaminergic nerve terminal, dopamine is repackaged in vesicles and stored, mostly in the inactive pool. Hence, reuptake means inactivation. Some dopamine is not repackaged and is degraded by the enzymes monoamine oxidase and catechol-o-methyltransferase. The products of enzymatic degradation are cleared by the circulation.

The geometry of the dopaminergic neurons is like a tree. The trunk is the cell body, the root system comprises the dendrites that receive impulses from other neurons, and the leaves are the axon terminals through which each dopaminergic nerve cell communicates its messages to other nerve cells. Each nerve cell has approximately 10,000 connections with other cells. The dopaminergic axons project from the substantia nigra in the midbrain up to the caudate, putamen, and globus pallidus to portions of the frontal lobe and to the limbic system. Dopamine is synthesized, stored, released, and taken up again by the same dopaminergic axon terminal that released it.

Dopamine in the caudate, putamen, and globus pallidus modifies movement, although it is not the primary mover. Its action can be likened to that of oil in the engine of a car. Gas moves the car; however, even a perfect engine with a full tank of gas does not respond in the absence of oil. A fraction of the full capacity of oil is all that is necessary for normal movement of the car. Although it is not a lubricant, dopamine allows the motor system of the brain to work. Even if all else is perfect, the motor system does not work in the absence of dopamine. Without any dopamine, the individual is immobilized. Adding a little restores the appearance of normality.

The analogy does not hold in the case of overdosage. If one adds too much oil, the automobile engine does not race. However, too much dopamine acutely results in an excessive racing of the motor system of the brain, with too much movement that has been drug induced. This movement is called dyskinesia, which means chorea that has been caused by a drug.

To treat dopamine deficiency, one would hope to use dopamine, but dopamine cannot pass through the blood-brain barrier. Its immediate metabolic precursor, dopa, does pass through the blood-brain barrier, and in the brain it is decarboxylated to dopamine. Dopa is administered orally in the levo form as levodopa, or L-dopa. We can reduce the amount of L-dopa needed to provide a good therapeutic response by combining it with another drug called carbidopa. This is a dopa decarboxylase inhibitor that reduces the decarboxylation of L-dopa to dopamine before dopa can reach the brain, thus permitting more of the administered dose of L-dopa to enter the brain.

The effect of L-dopa on end-stage PD patients is remarkable. When it was first introduced in the 1960s, totally incapacitated patients who had been in nursing homes for years could rise again and resume normal motor function. L-Dopa is one of the most dramatically effective medications in the history of medicine.

It is curious that dopamine can be generated from dopa in severe PD to provide even a short period of normal functioning. After all, the dopamine neurons have died. Where does dopamine synthesis occur? The answer is not known, but presumably dopamine is generated elsewhere and diffuses to its postsynaptic receptors. The generation sites may be serotonergic terminals or interneurons containing a decarboxylase enzyme that can convert L-dopa to dopamine. Any neuron that contains decarboxylase enzymes that can decarboxylate L-dopa can generate dopamine from L-dopa. Apparently, many such neurons exist in the brain that are not primarily devoted to making dopamine but that can do so when loaded with L-dopa.

The loss of presynaptic dopaminergic nerve terminals challenges the brain's capacity to generate dopamine. This part of the therapeutic problem can be easily solved by the administration of L-dopa, but the synthesis of dopamine in a brain that has no dopaminergic neurons creates another problem: how to inactivate used dopamine after it has acted on the postsynaptic dopamine receptor. Normally, the inactivation of dopamine depends on reuptake and storage by the dopaminergic neurons. The loss of dopaminergic neurons reduces the brain's capacity to inactivate and store dopamine. The loss of the inactivation mechanism allows higher and more prolonged elevations of dopamine in the immediate vicinity of the dopaminergic receptors after administration of L-dopa. This predisposes to toxicity manifested as dyskinesia and hallucinations.

Stages

Dopamine deficiency has several stages that can be differentiated by the patient's response to administered L-dopa.

Stage I. Stage I is mildly symptomatic, with just over 80% reduction of dopaminergic cells and considerable storage capacity left, enough storage capacity that a patient might be given a dose of replacement dopa three times a day, once a day, or even every other day with good effect and without causing much variation in the patient's good motor response. Once dopamine is released, the remaining dopaminergic neurons can take it up, thereby inactivating it. Extra dopamine can be stored within the dopaminergic neurons. Such patients cannot tell when a particular dose of L-dopa begins to work or how long the good effect of the L-dopa lasts. Their symptoms of parkinsonism may not recur until they have ceased taking L-dopa for 2–3 days. Because most doctors prescribe L-dopa on a three-doses-per-day schedule, compliant patients in this stage of illness experience a smooth response to L-dopa that is not linked to the timing of the doses.

This state lasts for 5–10 years. PD advances more quickly when it begins early (fourth or fifth decade) than if it begins in the seventh or eighth decade. In general, the older the patient at the onset of symptoms, the longer the mildly symptomatic stage lasts.

Little clinical evidence has been found that treatment with L-dopa hastens the degenerative process in PD, but much has been made of this possibility. Explanations of how L-dopa–accelerated degeneration could occur have substituted for evidence that this happens. For fear of doing harm, many neurologists prefer not to use L-dopa, the most effective antiparkinsonian agent, until it is absolutely necessary or try to use as little as possible, substituting other less effective drugs.

The premise of withholding L-dopa is the mistaken belief that it harms the brain and that the neu-

rologist can pick the "good" years of smooth response to L-dopa when he or she wants them. This theory has been encouraged by drug companies, which want neurologists to prescribe their expensive, less effective products.

We agree that the patient may have only a few years of smooth response to L-dopa, but we believe that they occur early in the illness, and waiting a few years before using the drug loses them forever. No convincing clinical evidence has been found that L-dopa does harm to the brain or accelerates the course of PD. Further, no compound has been found superior to L-dopa in slowing the course of PD. L-Dopa has dramatically reduced the death rate in PD, and its use early in the course of PD may actually lengthen patients' lives.

Overwhelming evidence has shown that the diminished storage capacity of dopaminergic neurons, not receptor down-regulation, is responsible for "wearing off." This evidence is summarized as follows: (1) Patients with the wearing-off phenomenon retain the capacity to respond clinically to L-dopa. (2) More frequent dosing of L-dopa is effective in controlling the wearing-off phenomenon. (3) After discontinuation of an intravenous L-dopa infusion, fluctuating patients sustain the anti-parkinsonian effect of the medication for a shorter time than do stable patients. (4) PET studies with (F)-6-fluorodopa in patients with PD have shown less of an accumulation of fluorodopa and its metabolites in the striata of fluctuating patients than in the striata of stable patients. (5) Rat striata deprived of dopaminergic afferents exhibit a diminished capacity to store dopamine. (6) During "off" periods, patients retain the capacity to respond to injections of apomorphine, a dopamine agonist. This indicates that the dopamine receptors are functioning normally. (7) Normal to increased levels of dopamine receptor binding sites are present in the striata of patients with PD.

These facts indicate that postsynaptic receptors are available for dopaminergic stimulation but that the presynaptic storage of dopamine is defective. In other words, when patients run out of dopamine, they become bradykinetic until the next dose of L-dopa arrives.

Stage II. Stage II is moderate PD. This phase is characterized by the wearing-off phenomenon. Wearing off describes motor fluctuations that are closely related to the timing of L-dopa administration. The wearing-off phenomenon is probably a reflection of disease progression, with an attendant decrease in the brain's ability to store dopamine. Much evidence supports the hypothesis that presynaptic failure of dopamine storage explains this phenomenon and that it is not the result of progressive insensitivity of dopamine receptors (down-regulation).

The hallmark of the wearing-off effect is the patient's capacity to tell how long it takes from the time he or she swallows a dose of L-dopa to the time that the dose becomes effective in relieving symptoms (usually approximately 30 minutes). The patient can also tell how long the therapeutic effect of a particular dose lasts (usually approximately 3 hours).

Stage III. Stage III, the end stage of PD, is characterized by the "on-off" phenomenon. This is the final phase, in which the patient has virtually no dopamine storage capacity. A constant delivery of L-dopa to the striatum is essential to support continuous dopamine synthesis in the brain. The normal brain and even the moderately affected parkinsonian brain have an excess of dopamine stored in the presynaptic neurons that is available for release should the delivery of L-dopa to the brain be interrupted for any reason. The stores of dopamine can support movement for a little while if the next L-dopa dose is delayed in entering the brain. No dopamine storage is found in stage III PD, and the only dopamine in the brain is generated from the administered L-dopa. If L-dopa fails to enter the brain or is delayed in crossing the blood-brain barrier, no dopamine is present in the brain to facilitate movement and bradykinesia, or freezing (off) periods occur abruptly.

Strong evidence has been shown that peripheral pharmacokinetic factors contribute to or cause the complex fluctuations in patients with severe depletion of dopamine storage that are called on-off. Even a minor delay in the entry of L-dopa into a brain that is totally depleted of its dopamine neurons can cause the patient to become abruptly parkinsonian. This delay can result from a delay in gastric emptying (L-dopa is absorbed in the small intestine) or blockage to the entry of dopa across the blood-brain barrier.

The most important cause of reduced L-dopa movement into the brain is a high level of circulating, large neutral amino acids (LNAA) in the plasma. These amino acids are derived from dietary protein, and they compete with L-dopa for the carrier that brings both L-dopa and LNAA into the brain. The deleterious effect of dietary protein on movement is only experienced in stage III PD, even though elevated plasma levels of LNAA at any stage of PD slow the entry of L-dopa into the brain. Because no dopamine is stored in the brain in stage III PD, the patient experiences apparently unpredictable episodes of L-dopa–resistant bradykinesia whenever the plasma LNAA concentration rises above the level that prevents L-dopa from crossing into the brain. Freezing of motor functions can be sudden. Patients are like cars that have just run out of gas: They stop moving.

It is seldom possible to raise the blood levels of L-dopa high enough to overcome the effect of elevated plasma concentrations of LNAAs. The combination of high plasma concentrations of both L-dopa and LNAA is responsible for the phenomenon called peak dose bradykinesia.

The stage III parkinsonian patient also experiences episodes of severe dyskinesia. The complete loss of the presynaptic dopaminergic cells in the patient with stage III results in the loss of the dopamine-inactivating reuptake mechanism. This makes it difficult to provide just the right concentration of dopamine at the postsynaptic receptor.

Dopamine's duration of action at the receptor is normally very short. Without the inactivating reuptake mechanism, dopamine may remain too long at the receptor. This causes an unmodulated increase in dopamine concentration at the postsynaptic receptors that can result in symptoms of overdosage, excessive motor movement, and/or hallucinations. The absence of any dopamine storage capacity aggravates the tendency to dyskinesia and hallucinations.

Therefore, as the disease gets worse, patients may experience alternating periods of being off (parkinsonian) and on (mobile or dyskinetic). It is somewhat counterintuitive but true that patients seem to become more sensitive to L-dopa as their disease gets worse, responding to slight overdosage with marked dyskinesia and hallucinations. At other times, patients experience periods of apparent unresponsiveness to L-dopa. The therapeutic window between underdosage and overdosage in stage III is very narrow, and the threshold dose to produce dyskinesias is much lower in patients with end-stage PD than it is in those with stable early PD.

In summary, the progressive nature of the disease process is reflected in the gradual lack of responsiveness to dopamine replacement alone. Management becomes increasingly difficult in the later stages with the narrowness of the therapeutic window. Patients have problems with fluctuating drug levels leading to dyskinesias and rigidity, and that makes their lives unpredictable. It becomes necessary to develop alternative treatments including modification in diet that require a greater degree of patient self-management.

Nature of the Impairments

The WHO model[4] developed to describe rehabilitation can be used to clarify the various aspects of treatment in the management of persons with chronic neurologic illness. The main pathway in the disablement process is as follows: Pathology (the presence of disease) leads to impairments (anatomic and structural abnormalities), which in turn can lead to functional limitations. Impairments are the direct consequences of the underlying pathology. They are the symptoms or signs that one would assess in the course of the medical-neurologic examination. The aim in normal medical-neurologic practice is to reduce the degree of impairment with the use of medication. PD provides one of the major opportunities to modify the impairments found in the management of persons with chronic disease. Dopamine replacement has been one of the outstanding success stories of modern medicine. However, some of the impairments are a result of the improper application of the replacement medication in interaction with the later stages in the disease process. The difference between underdosage and overdosage is so small that impairments such as dyskinesias can be superimposed that limit the effectiveness of treatment with medication alone.

Motor Impairments

The major impairments in PD are those that relate to the motor system. PD has three major symptoms: tremor, bradykinesia, and postural instability. Rigidity, a physical sign, is also characteristic.

The tremor of parkinsonism occurs mainly when the patient is resting or holding sustained postures. It is dampened during voluntary movements. For this reason, of the three cardinal symptoms, tremor interferes least with normal motor functioning. The tremor of PD is absolutely characteristic, and only one other condition can be confused with it: the extrapyramidal side effects of dopamine receptor blocking drugs. Most of these are neuroleptics, but metaclopramide and prochlorperazine (Compazine), common remedies for nausea, also can produce all the symptoms of PD, including resting tremor.

Bradykinesia is best defined as slowness in carrying out motor acts, in initiating and sometimes arresting movements. It can seriously impair functioning and makes it difficult for a patient to be dexterous both in fine and gross motor acts. When it is mild, the disability it imposes can be misunderstood by patients and physicians as the result of normal aging or arthritis. Bradykinesia causes parkinsonian patients to delay a few seconds before they can begin walking. This is especially noticeable when they first rise from a seated position or when they change the direction of their gait. Sometimes freezing occurs under these circumstances. Some patients experience freezing in open doorways. This feature, really a form of gait apraxia, is also seen in patients with frontal lobe dysfunction who do not have dopamine deficiency. Patients with PD lose associated or spontaneous movements, such as swinging the arms while walking. The gait of the typical parkinsonian patient is narrow based. Patients with degeneration of nerve cells that are outside the dopamine system tend to have a broad-based gait.

Postural instability can be the most disabling of these common symptoms. An inability to adjust rapidly to postural changes can result in frequent falling and serious injury. Sometimes patients take several short, hesitant "stuttering" steps (marche à petits pas, festinating) when they start walking or when they turn. The falls that this symptom causes can result in serious injuries. This is particularly a problem in elderly persons who might need to get up at night to urinate. It illustrates the confluence of impairments that might occur given the nature of the disease and the nature of the person who experiences it.

Other clinical features of parkinsonism affecting the motor system that relate to the three cardinal symptoms are expressionless features, a feeling of weakness and of being slowed down, flattening and weakness of the voice, diminished dexterity, micrographia, and cogwheel rigidity.

Patients may have tremor without the other symptoms or bradykinesia or postural instability without tremor, or both. Symptoms can be unilateral, confined to the arms or to the legs without involvement of the rest of the body, or generalized. Patients whose symptoms commence with tremor have the best prognosis; 80% do not become demented. Dementia occurs in two-thirds of patients without tremor.

Another motor symptom is dystonic cramps. Dystonia refers to an abnormality of posture caused by an abnormal involuntary contraction of a skeletal muscle. A writhing, athetoid component is often present and sometimes an action tremor. It is not always painful, but dystonia occasionally causes a painful cramp. This symptom reflects deficiency of brain dopamine levels. Dystonia develops in approximately 25% of PD patients who are in the second or third stages of disease.

The cramp often occurs as the previous dose of L-dopa is wearing off and the dose that has just been taken has not yet taken effect, in other words, just after the patient takes the medication. These have been called beginning-of-dose and end-of-dose dystonia. Because of this sequence, many patients feel that L-dopa has caused the cramp. Unsophisticated medical personnel can be fooled by this report. It is the lack of L-dopa, not its use, that is the problem.

Dystonia can occur at night when the patient awakens in a relatively unmedicated state. Nighttime does not lessen a patient's need for dopamine. Dystonic symptoms should be treated by instructing the patient to take L-dopa throughout the night on a regular schedule. More frequent dosing and sometimes increments in doses of L-dopa usually control it.

All odd pains in patients with PD who are being treated with L-dopa are possible examples of dystonia because any skeletal muscle in the body can be affected. Normal gastrointestinal series and other negative investigations to determine the origin of pains can lead to a mistaken psychiatric diagnosis.

Because it is often manifested by involuntary movements, dystonia can be confused with dyskinesia. The distinction is important, as the treatment of dystonia requires more L-dopa and dyskinesia requires less. Dystonia is often associated with akathisia. It is painful, maximal at the time of dosing when L-dopa levels are low, interferes seriously with motor functioning, and is more apparent to the patient than to the caregiver. Dyskinesia is not painful, is maximal approximately 1 hour after dosing when L-dopa levels are at peak, does not interfere much with motor function, and is not as bothersome to the patient as to the caretaker.

Mental Impairments

Insufficient dopamine cannot only cause slow movement but also slowness of thinking (bradyphrenia). Excessive dopamine can cause racing thoughts, mania, delusions, confusion, and visual hallucinations. Presumably the cognitive manifestations of dopamine deficiency and overdosage are mediated through dopaminergic projections to the frontal lobe and the limbic system.

Several behavioral concomitants of PD may easily be misinterpreted as psychiatric. These are depression, anxiety attacks, odd pains and cramps, periods of weakness, and psychosis with delusions, visual hallucinations, and manic excitement.

The coexistence of depression and PD is very common but clearly does not reflect the severity of PD. Depression is not a simple reaction to having PD. Some PD patients can be very mildly affected motorically but have severe depression, and patients with severe PD may have no depression at all. Probably the majority of patients with PD do have depression at some point during the course of their illness, and generally, the depression can be very effectively relieved by antidepressant medication.

Depression is thought to be the result of the inadequacy of the neurotransmitters serotonin or norepinephrine. Indeed, the original papers that described the brain neurochemical abnormalities in PD found 50% depletions of norepinephrine and serotonin as well as 90% or more reduction in the brain dopamine level. Therefore, depression in PD may be the result of serotonin or norepinephrine deficiency, or both. This neurotransmitter deficiency, like that of dopamine, is the direct consequence of the same degenerative neuropathologic process that causes PD. It is not attributable to psychological factors.

Depression in PD is probably a reflection of disease of the brain that lies outside of the dopaminergic system. In other words, it is a manifestation of

Parkinson's plus. It seems likely that depression in PD is the result of a more widespread neuronal degeneration. In support of this concept is the observation that depression in PD is related to dementia. Dementia predicts depression in PD patients. A Mini-Mental State Examination score below 24 increases the probability of major depression by a factor of 6.6.[5]

It is important to know that both underdosage with akathisia and overdosage with dyskinesia can cause unbearable anxiety. The first requires more L-dopa, and the second requires less. Anxiety attacks in PD usually represent episodes of akathisia and reflect inadequate amounts of dopamine in the brain. Patients complain of shakiness that is internal and cannot be seen by other observers. They want to move but either cannot or fear that soon they will not be able to move. Sometimes they ask family members to move their extremities, lest they become frozen. The patients are gripped by fear that they find difficult to express and appear to be agitated and unreasonable. They cannot be calmed by the verbal reassurances of caretakers. It is easy to misunderstand these symptoms, and not a few patients have been mistakenly and ineffectively treated with antianxiety drugs to relieve such episodes. If the patient is consistently treated inadequately with L-dopa, he or she may have constant "anxiety," really akathisia. This can be debilitating to the patient and to the caregiver.

Undiagnosed, akathisia may seem to the family and the physician to represent excessively dependent, neurotic, annoying, attention-seeking behavior in a patient who is very anxious and prone to unreasonable fears. Some of the author's patients have been referred to psychiatrists who specialize in the emotional problems of the elderly. Although most psychiatrists are very familiar with the akathisia induced by neuroleptic drugs such as haloperidol (Haldol) that block the action of dopamine, they have no idea that akathisia can occur in inadequately treated parkinsonians whose dopamine deficiency does the same. It is not clear why all parkinsonian patients and all those treated with neuroleptics do not develop akathisia, but many do. The increased intake of L-dopa alleviates the akathisia of PD.

Symptomatically similar to the anxiety of akathisia is the opposite, the agitation of dyskinesia. Dyskinesia is the result of L-dopa overdosage. Patients may be in constant motion, crossing and uncrossing their legs, inverting and everting their feet, drumming their fingers, bobbing their heads, writhing, twitching, grimacing, thrusting their tongues, grunting, and, in general, projecting the picture of physical discomfort.

Many patients do not experience discomfort during periods of dyskinesia even though they look uncomfortable. Most much prefer dyskinesia to the symptoms of underdosage. Some patients are not even aware that they are dyskinetic. Yet a few individuals experience a loosening of the coherence of their thought processes during dyskinesia. They may not be aware of it, but they have trouble staying on the subject of conversation and flit from one topic to another. They cannot answer a simple question simply.

The mental state that most closely reassembles this is mania. Indeed, grandiosity, unrealistic feelings of well-being, and paranoid ideas along with hallucinations, mostly visual, can accompany periods of dyskinesia, but so can a pervasive sense of anxiety, the sense that things are not right, and the sense of endangerment. It is very difficult for caregivers to deal with this, as they often are the targets of delusional suspiciousness. Fairly straightforward methods are available to deal with this. A slight reduction in the dose of L-dopa is often all that is needed.

Reducing the dose effectively controls all the symptoms of overdosage, but, rarely, it is not possible to control the motor symptoms of parkinsonism at a dosage of L-dopa that is low enough not to cause symptoms of overdosage. In other words, it is possible that no "happy median" may be found between underdosage and overdosage. In such instances, which are rare, it may be necessary to use clozapine to control psychotic thinking while using doses of L-dopa that are adequate to maintain mobility.

All the drugs used for the treatment of PD can produce nightmares, agitation, delirium, loose associations, visual and auditory hallucinations, delusions, and inappropriate affect. Toxic psychosis is most likely to develop in patients who have underlying brain disease outside of the dopaminergic system. Visual hallucinations early in the course of PD, with or without medication, are a feature of LBD. Patients with mixed disorders, such as Parkinson's plus, and older patients are also more prone to be demented as well as to develop toxic psychosis with visual hallucinations. For this reason, it is wise to start any antiparkinsonian drugs at relatively small doses to be sure that the patient can tolerate them. It is also incumbent on the professional to use the least amount of medication consistent with the control needed to maintain function.

Weakness

When a parkinsonian patient complains of an overwhelming sense of weakness, the inexperienced clinician may incorrectly assume that the PD symptoms are worse and that they require more antiparkinsonian medication. Weakness is the word that PD patients most often use to describe the feelings that postural hypotension imposes. Because all the antiparkinsonian medications can cause or aggravate postural hypotension, this assumption can be a dangerous medical error. The falls that occur when patients faint can break hips and other bones, and this can be life threatening and painful.

While patients are sitting or reclining and trying to avoid the sense of weakness imposed by postural hypotension, they may nap excessively during daylight hours. Then they are unable to sleep at night. Frequently, patients who are awake at night go to the toilet for want of anything else to do and report to the doctor that they are awake all night, going to the bathroom. The common medical response is to prescribe sleeping pills or anticholinergic drugs, or both, to help the patient sleep and to lessen the sense of bladder fullness. These classes of medication cause or aggravate confusion, however, and both should be avoided in parkinsonian patients.

The only way to diagnose this condition is to be aware that patients who complain of weakness may really mean lightheadedness. If this is the case, the weakness is most intense when the patient stands and is alleviated if he or she sits or reclines. Certain diagnosis is easy if the blood pressure is measured while the patient is standing. The diagnosis may be missed if the blood pressure is taken while the patient sits or reclines. When the blood pressure thus obtained is normal and increasing doses of antiparkinsonian drugs do not help, or even aggravate the sense of weakness, frustrated physicians and caretakers may seek a psychiatric explanation of the symptom.

Postural hypotension is a primary manifestation of autonomic failure in multisystem atrophy, the Shy-Drager syndrome. It is also encountered in ordinary parkinsonian patients and is aggravated by L-dopa and all the other antiparkinsonian drugs. The medication that is most helpful in overcoming postural hypotension is the salt-retaining steroid fludrocortisone (Florinef). Up to six tablets a day (0.1 mg each) may be necessary to control postural hypotension. A new pressor agent, midodrine, is now available to treat postural hypotension.

Nature of the Disabilities

Disability refers to the functional (behavioral) consequences of the pathology or the impairments, or both. The WHO definition of disability is "any restriction or lack (resulting from an impairment) of ability to perform an activity within the range considered normal for a human being."[4] This can include difficulty in getting around, communicating, dressing, and so forth. The effect of the disease and its subsequent impairments on patient function is an essential factor in consideration of treatment initiation. Later, if one cannot prevent or overcome the impairments such as the motor symptoms with dopamine replacement, one must address the functional problems that now remain. The aim must be to reduce the degree of disability by training the actions that remain so as to compensate for those that are affected and to learn to use technical aids as necessary.

The disabilities refer to the effect(s) that the impairments have on the life of the person. Not all impairments are disabling. Although various motor impairments such as tremor and masklike facies are pathognomonic, they may not actually interfere with the function of the patient. They may not be identified as disabling by the persons involved. Certain impairments of the motor system such as postural instability are more likely to be identified as causing problems in the life of the patient. Falls can occur, and the "freezing of movement" can be significant to some.

The identification of the functional limitations that are truly troublesome to the specific patient or caregiver, or both, is a result of the interaction between the type and severity of the impairments and the person who is experiencing them. As such, they cannot be deduced merely from the neurologic examination. Input from the person or the caregiver, or both, is necessary for their proper identification. The specific disabilities to be ameliorated vary with the goals and the character of the person and the environment in which he or she needs to function. For example, if the patient is working, is his or her employment threatened? It may be the unpredictability of his or her functional status that is the most disabling.

Although the motor impairments are most evident to the examiner, they may not be the ones that are most disturbing to the patient. An example is a 63-year-old retired man with stage II disease. He stated that he was not particularly concerned about his trouble in getting around. He was able to travel extensively, although he would stumble on uneven ground. With attention to his dosage regimen and scheduling of his activities, he had been able to compensate for his problems in getting around. In answer to the question as to concerns, he stated that his speech was most troublesome to him. He found himself having to repeat what he was saying because his words became slurred and could not be understood by others. He had particular trouble when he ran out of breath at the end of a sentence. He found several strategies offered by a speech therapist useful by which he could make his speech better understood. These included taking a deep breath to increase the volume of air available and making his sentences shorter, enabling him to take more frequent breaths.

In general, the treatment must be appropriate to the condition. Patients with disordered gait must be given practice in walking and transferring to and from a chair. They must practice what to do if they become frozen and shown how to arise if they fall. Gait freezing and other motor blocks can be helped by techniques that involve the use of imagery. Other methods incorporate techniques by which one learns to substitute a conscious motor program instead of the malfunctioning automatic motor program.[6]

Poor equilibrium can be ameliorated with visual cues in some cases. Other methods require the patient to be trained to consciously center the feet under the body when first arising and, when turning, to make a relatively wide arc rather than a narrow-based, sharp pivot. Wearing a small bicycle helmet is sometimes necessary to prevent serious injuries in falls. In general, treadmills and strengthening exercises do not help people with PD-like symptoms. Stretching exercises can be useful in maintaining range of motion and flexibility.

Equipment, such as canes, walkers, and wheelchairs, can be helpful. Special tools such as eating utensils with thick handles are more easily grasped by patients who have limited finger and hand dexterity. A lazy Susan on the front seat of the car can greatly assist an impaired driver in entering the vehicle and swinging the feet around from the sidewalk to the accelerator.

Many intervening variables can affect the connection between the ongoing impairments and the reduction of the disabilities, that is, the functional consequences in the life of the person. One is the ability to learn compensatory strategies, dependent as such learning might be on concomitant cognitive and emotional issues. Cognitive issues can affect learning, but emotional issues are particularly significant in affecting the willingness or ability to commit one's energy as well as ideas to the development of compensatory methods.

Some of the best ideas about physical methods of lessening the burdens of PD and its related disorders can come from other patients or caregivers. Support groups provide a venue for the exchange of ideas. The National Parkinson Foundation (telephone number: 1-305-547-6666 or 1-800-327-4545) provides information about the location of such groups across the country and the world.

The fear of telling friends and employers about the disease can be particularly disabling. One wife describes her experience and that of her husband: "People with PD may want to conceal the things they are not able to do. And because their symptoms are not there all the time, they can be pretty successful. The hard part is that, as a result, they don't get the support and understanding they need. I felt very isolated during the 4 years I didn't tell my friends and coworkers, and it must have been even worse for him."

Eventually, this couple found that it is better to open up, dispel doubt, and allow people to adjust their image of what one can do. This woman's husband, a lawyer, described himself in this way: "I have a couple of really good clients who don't mind waiting the extra time it takes me to prepare the documents they need. I've been honest with them, and they have been really grateful. When people understand what is going on, they are really wonderful." It is the fear of discovery that must be dealt with so the person can deal with the depression that can ensue.

Another man vividly describes his relationship to his disease as having "a cat by the tail."[7] He makes the analogy to the growth in severity of the disease over the 14 years to the changes from a "small kitten . . . to a large, angry cat." The progressive nature of his disease process had the effect of "slowing my step and stooping my back. He has slurred my speech and caused me to shake. He has stolen my balance and disturbed my sleep. The damage he does is both progressive and irreversible." The emotional impact has perhaps been the most significant. "I have finally learned to ask for help when I need it. . . . Each time I ask for or accept help, I feel little bits and pieces of my independence slipping away. . . . A friend told me that she thought I should get a wheelchair for those times when I needed one. I said that I didn't want to be wheelchair-bound. 'How about housebound? Is that what you want?' End of argument."

Treatment of the person with the disability frequently includes training and ongoing support for caregivers. The availability of caregivers is crucial to living in a community setting. Problems in interpersonal relations and the need for ongoing emotional support for caregivers become particularly important in the management of persons with PD. The wife and the children—the entire family—have the disease, not merely the patient. This same patient goes on to describe the effect on his wife: "My wife has my PD; she worst of all. . . . Her responsibilities increase as my abilities decline. We who carry the cane get the attention. They who walk beside us with tired steps, weary faces, and sad eyes, they who care for us, get none. Yet they bear a heavy burden, and they need support and encouragement."

Most moving is the statement by this same man about what has enabled him to deal with his disease over the years. "My cat has taught me that I have within me reserves of strength and patience and courage that I would not have thought possible. I have learned that stubbornness and contrariness are virtues. . . . My success in remaining useful . . . has come at least 50% from my stubbornness. . . . My cat's gift to me has been the gift of unwelcome truth. He holds before me the mirror of self-revelation and forces me to stare at it, unblinking. Until I see myself as I am."

The person with PD has the experience of dealing with his or her disabilities on a daily basis. The role of physicians must be to relieve suffering. Such relief partially comes from the effective use of regimens to reduce impairment. Any interaction between the professional must also contribute to the enhancement of the ability of these persons and their families to continue to maintain their courage in dealing with the sometimes inexorable course. The next section of this chapter describes some of the characteristics of such a relationship.

Character of the Solution

The management of the person with PD is an example of the management of a person with chronic neurologic illness. Care of the person with chronic illness is considered to be an ongoing planning process. Problems are identified, goals set, activities (including medication regimens) designed, and time established for review and revision of the initial plan. At the time of review, status is assessed, and the regimen by which those results have come about is reviewed before a new plan is made once again. A basic set of planning questions are addressed. Particularly important is awareness of the degree to which the patient, the caregiver, or both are enabled by the health professional to participate in answering these planning questions. The goal is for these "primary participants" to learn their self-management in the ongoing interaction with the professional staff. This reiterative process is described in detail in Chapter 2.

The person with PD has a progressive disease that can vary in its rate of progression. The impairments can change over time not only in terms of severity but also in kind. Although motor impairments are the most dramatic, others, including cognitive and emotional aspects, may become paramount. Both the impairments and the resultant disabilities can vary, as changes occur not only in the disease process but in the situation in which the person finds him- or herself. Priorities can change as conditions change. One principle of proper care would be to provide continuity of care over time to deal with such changes.

The professional components of the treatment team vary depending on the phase and therefore the range and severity of the problems. Coordination of a comprehensive range of interdisciplinary services may become necessary, particularly in the later stages of the disease process. The intensity and duration of overall services and thus the costs also vary with the phase. Given the side effects, one must optimize the effects of the medication and emphasize other nonpharmacologic treatments. The need for use of ancillary therapies as well as dietary changes along with the more complex medical regimen in the later stages requires a greater degree of participation on the part of the patient or caregiver, or both, in collaboration with the professional staff.

Continuity of Care

The life of the person with PD is divided into three phases of unequal duration wherein the frequency and intensity of the planning and treatment process vary. The initial stage can last for the longest time, in the range of 5–10 years, wherein the intensity and frequency of treatment are least. Stage II requires somewhat more attention to management and can also last in the range of years. Stage III is the shortest in duration but requires the greatest intensity and frequency of intervention. The value of ongoing care is reflected in the following cases that illustrate the early stages, when relatively little intervention can lead to major benefits in the maintenance of function.

The making of the diagnosis of PD and the initiation of treatment in itself require a commitment to ongoing review: A 74-year-old woman, very youthful in appearance, complained of a tremor in the right hand that had started approximately 6 months earlier. It embarrassed her when she played bridge but did not affect her tennis game. She had a typical resting tremor that was present intermittently and was dampened by movement. No other symptoms of PD were found.

Some physicians would not treat this patient's relatively nondisabling symptom with L-dopa for fear of accelerating the degenerative process or losing the good years of L-dopa responsiveness. The author finds no convincing evidence that L-dopa treatment accelerates the course of PD or that the period of L-dopa responsiveness is limited in most cases that start with the typical tremor. As an initial symptom of PD, the tremor is usually a very good

sign. The tremor is very responsive to carbidopa–L-dopa, and the prognosis for a course of progression that is confined to the dopamine system is good; that is, it is likely that all the PD symptoms that develop in the future will be reversible with dopamine replacement therapy. Even if the patient is destined to develop symptoms from degeneration of neurons outside the dopamine system, one cannot choose the years of dopa responsiveness, saving them for a future time when the patient "will really need" L-dopa. The patient is complaining of the tremor; it is disturbing to her. The means of treating it are available, and treatment can be started with the most effective, least toxic, and cheapest drug available: L-dopa.

A 64-year-old man with similar findings did not find his resting tremor at all disturbing. Although he was concerned about the diagnosis, he felt that he could easily deal with the tremor in his role of museum docent. He was able to unobtrusively place his hand in his jacket pocket while speaking and preferred not to use any medication at this time. It would be important for this man to seek help when his symptoms become disabling to him.

The value of such continuity of care is further illustrated by the case of an 83-year-old woman who manifested the symptoms of PD for 7 years with an excellent smooth response to carbidopa–L-dopa 25/100, one tablet three times a day. Over the past several months, however, her response to therapy had become irregular. Her complaint was that "the medication does not work at all anymore." A more thorough history and referral to a diary she kept for several days revealed a different story. With a more precise analysis of her response, it became clear that her PD symptoms diminished after 30 minutes of her first dose, and she became normal in terms of her motor system. The beneficial effect of each dose lasted approximately 3 hours. After taking her first dose at 8:00 AM, she was in relatively good shape for most of the morning. After 3:30 PM, however, when the noon dose wore off, her PD symptoms returned. Until her 6:00 PM dose became effective, she was quite uncomfortable, experiencing cramps in the calves and being unable to walk or to rise from a chair without assistance. She was very unstable when undermedicated and almost fell on several occasions. Her daughter, with whom she lived, had to work and was afraid her mother might sustain serious injury by falling at home in the afternoon. The patient was concerned about her inability to carry out afternoon activities in preparation for dinner so that she would not be a burden to her daughter when she returned home after work.

On examination in the afternoon, the patient had postural instability and the short-stepped, narrow-based gait that is typical of dopamine deficiency. Festination and pulsion, but not tremor, were present. Her hands reflected none of the symptoms of PD, even at times when she was unable to walk. No dementia was present.

The variation in effectiveness of L-dopa that is linked to the time of dosing is the wearing-off effect. When fully medicated, the patient was totally normal. By changing her dosing schedule, it was possible to re-establish a smooth response during her waking hours. She started to take one tablet of carbidopa–L-dopa every 3 hours, from the time of awakening at 7:00 AM until her bedtime at 11:30 PM, a total of six doses in 24 hours. If she awakened after 1:00 AM with cramps, she took another dose at that time. If she was late in taking her pill, she experienced bradykinesia and cramps that lasted until the next dose became effective. A pill-box with a timer was a great aid in reminding her that the next dose was due.

The painful cramps in the patient's legs that had been especially troublesome in the afternoon and that recurred at night represented dystonia. Dystonic cramps in PD reflect low brain dopamine levels. The cramps disappeared when the L-dopa was administered on schedule. The absence of tremor and the sparing of the upper extremities are two of the many variations in the distribution and kind of symptoms that parkinsonian patients manifest. The absence of a tremor has some prognostic significance, as symptoms that result from degeneration of neurons outside the dopamine system were more likely to develop in this patient. Dementia is one such symptom that she had not begun to display.

What appeared to the patient at first to be a complete failure of the medication was easily remedied with return to full functional status. What seemed to be an overwhelming sense of deterioration and loss of control over her body was resolved. Continuity of care was an essential ingredient along with an adequate diary describing the symptoms in relation to the dosing schedule. Her own participation in keeping a diary helped her to regain the sense

that what was happening to her was in some way a result of her own actions in taking her medication. Knowledge of the relationship between the two increased her acceptance of the more frequent medication regimen. She contributed in part to the solution of the problem by remembering when to take the medication.

Comprehensive and Coordinated Care

The various phases in the life of the person with PD require different sets of skills. Coordination of a comprehensive range of interdisciplinary services, including physical and occupational therapy and speech therapy for treatment of swallowing as well as speech, may become necessary in the later stages of the disease. Attention to the psychosocial issues also becomes more necessary with support of the caregiver relationship. The need for nonpharmacologic approaches in stage III can include modification of the diet.

A case illustrating the need for a comprehensive approach is that of a 48-year-old man who worked as a judge. He had an early onset and was now in the fifteenth year of PD. The illness had begun with the typical tremor. His symptoms in the unmedicated state had developed into total immobility except for a resting, wide-amplitude tremor of both arms and legs. During periods of undermedication he was so immobilized that he was literally unable to scratch his nose. He would perspire profusely and was helpless. When carbidopa–L-dopa "kicked in" he was transformed into a normal person. He was able to carry on his work as a judge and his personal care. For several years, however, he had not been able to predict when such periods of good function would occur. He had been treated with dopamine agonists, selegiline, long-acting carbidopa–L-dopa (Sinemet), trihexyphenidyl, and drug holidays, none of which had helped to maintain his function satisfactorily.

The unpredictable variability in the patient's response to L-dopa was remarkable, and the shifts from mobility (on) to immobility (off) were startlingly rapid, occurring within seconds. At times he was normal, walking, talking, and using his hands without any sign of impairment. Such periods were brief but occurred daily. More often he was completely incapacitated: immobile, totally unable to initiate any movement of the arms or legs. His voice at such times was weak, and he was barely able to swallow his medication.

When the patient was immobilized with bradykinesia and tremor, he had severe cramps in the calves and had a tremendous desire to move but feared that he could not do so (akathisia). He begged his wife to move and massage his legs at such times. She had many other responsibilities, such as shopping, cooking, caring for their child, and augmenting the family income by pursuing her career as a lawyer. She deeply resented the burden she was experiencing and felt that he was behaving in an unreasonable manner.

The patient hated the immobility and much preferred the hypermobility of dyskinesia. Therefore, when he felt himself becoming immobile, he would take several tablets of carbidopa–L-dopa at once. Shortly thereafter, he would become wildly dyskinetic. At such times, he had to lie on a mat on the living room floor to avoid hurting himself as his arms and legs would otherwise fling wildly into the furniture. He had many bruises. He lost weight and was in danger of malnutrition. His mother suspected that his wife was abusing him and called adult protective services. They investigated but found no evidence of abuse. This did not improve harmony within the family.

The patient's wife was mortified by his wild gyrations when they occurred in public. Because neither could predict when he was going to turn on or off, he could not leave the house to go to a restaurant or movie. His wife felt herself to be a prisoner, as she had to be with him at all times at home, without respite, except to go to her office. It was clear that the couple had a serious marital problem along with the other issues. A comprehensive and coordinated approach was necessary.

The first step was to maintain mobility without creating the severe dyskinesia. Three obvious therapeutic problems needed to be assessed: How much L-dopa should be administered at each dose? How often should these doses be given? How could it be ensured that the L-dopa in the patient's bloodstream entered the brain at a constant rate?

It was necessary to establish the level of mobility that was to be sought. Because the problem was shared between the patient and his wife, the planning reflected them both. They agreed that some

tradeoff might be needed between his concern about his immobility and her concern about the dyskinesia. However, they also both agreed on the need to establish a more predictable smoothing out as their highest priority. Such predictability would enable them to regain a greater degree of freedom in their lives and enable them to go out once again in public. Given these objectives, it was possible to monitor the results by a diary and establish the dosage of $1^1/_2$ tablets carbidopa–L-dopa every 90 minutes. At this dose, the patient was fully mobile all day long but still moderately dyskinetic at peak, approximately an hour after dosing. Yet episodes of bradykinesia still occurred at irregular intervals. Something more would need to be done to achieve the predictability of function that was their joint goal.

Protein Redistribution Diet

Reasoning that plasma LNAAs are derived mainly from dietary protein and that such alimentary-derived LNAAs may antagonize the clinical effectiveness of oral L-dopa, Pincus and Barry[8] offered a low-protein diet for breakfast and lunch to patients who were experiencing daily on-off fluctuations. Patients with fluctuations were studied on a research unit for several days. Doses of L-dopa were held constant during the study. The patients received a low-protein diet totaling 1,600 calories that included 7 g protein divided into two meals (breakfast and lunch). On the next hospital day, the patients received a high-protein diet totaling 1,600 calories that included 160 g protein administered in equal aliquots hourly between 8:00 AM and 4:00 PM. On the next day, patients received a regular hospital diet consisting of a 250 caloric breakfast with 25 g protein and a 755-calorie lunch with 40 g protein. On each day of the study, all patients received a regular evening supper that more than made up the minimum daily protein requirement (0.75 g/kg body weight). Hourly samples of plasma were obtained for the determination of serial concentrations of L-dopa and LNAAs, and video documentation of the patients' clinical status was performed hourly and assessed.

All patients receiving the high-protein diet or the regular hospital diet became bradykinetic. Some demonstrated no response to L-dopa. All patients receiving the low-protein diet became mobile, even dyskinetic, within 2 hours of the first dose of L-dopa and remained so throughout the day. The LNAA plasma concentration bore an inverse relationship to the clinical status of each patient. The level began to rise within 1 hour after the first high-protein meal. When the LNAA plasma level increased to 2.5 times fasting levels, all patients became immobile. When the level dropped, bradykinesia lessened or patients became dyskinetic.

The diet remains effective in patients for long periods as a means of maximizing the efficacy of L-dopa. The redistribution of dietary protein is inexpensive, safe, and effective. A response can be achieved in hours. Because the diet requires no prescription, it lacks corporate sponsors. The diet benefits all patients with on-off fluctuations who have not obtained satisfactory relief from manipulations of their L-dopa dosage and the addition of adjunctive therapies.

The diet carries one major drawback. Protein is an essential nutrient, and even end-stage parkinsonian patients must consume the minimum daily requirement to maintain their health. The diet usually requires one high-protein meal each day. This meal is virtually always followed by 1–3 hours of unavoidable bradykinesia. The patient can choose which hours are least inconvenient by altering the timing of the daily high-protein meal, but at least one period of bradykinesia occurs each day, after the ingestion of protein. Dopamine agonists (pramipexole, ropinerol, pergolide, bromocriptine) can reduce slightly the disability imposed by dietary protein, and this, in our opinion, is the chief indication for their use.

The protein redistribution diet is effective only in stage III. Patients accept and follow through with dietary protein redistribution for the on-off state. The benefit is immediate, and the consequences of not following the regimen are obvious to the patient. Once the patient realizes that he or she can benefit from daytime protein restriction, liberalization of the diet can provide a more palatable and varied menu. Trial and error determine how much protein each patient can tolerate. In general, fruits and vegetables, including potatoes, yams, and rice, as well as butter, bacon, condiments, preserves, and certain breads are low in protein content; meat, fish, eggs, beans, nuts, pasta, most breads, and dairy products are high.

In the case of the judge described earlier, the episodic bradykinesia of the on-off state reflected the inability of circulating L-dopa to enter his dopamine-depleted brain. He no longer had any dopamine stored in his brain. If dopa from his plasma was delayed in entering his brain, no other source was available that could mitigate the deficiency. Without any dopamine stores, he was exquisitely sensitive to exogenous dopamine. The intermittent rises in large amino acids in his circulating plasma kept L-dopa from reaching the transporting mechanism that brings both L-dopa and LNAAs into the brain. The large amino acids were largely derived from his diet. By placing him on a protein redistribution diet that virtually eliminated protein from breakfast and lunch and gave him his needed protein supply just before bedtime, one could eliminate almost all the periods of immobility. Moreover, this ended the crippling unpredictability of episodes of being off that had prevented him from leaving home.

Only one persistent period of immobility remained that predictably occurred regularly every day. This was the period after his single, high-protein evening meal. For approximately 2 hours after dinner, all his symptoms of PD returned: bradykinesia, cramping, tremor, inability to stand or move, and overwhelming anxiety centered on a desire to move. To modify the severity of this now predictable off period, the dose of L-dopa was doubled at dinnertime, and a dopamine agonist was added to the regimen. By eating shortly before going to bed and taking a sedative, he was often able to sleep through periods of bradykinesia and avoid the cramping and the distress of these episodes.

He is now able to go to the movies and to a restaurant with his wife, although what he can eat at a restaurant is quite limited. He recently described his protein sensitivity when he said, "I never eat at a McDonald's when unaccompanied. Otherwise it gives new meaning to the term 'carry out service.'" Moreover, the process by which predictability returned to his life was important. It served to strengthen the crucial relationship between him and his wife. The setting of objectives enabled them to reach agreement as to their priorities. They then shared the responsibility of monitoring the outcomes in relation to their objectives. In addition, the need for significant modification in his diet required the cooperation of both. Their marital problems abated not only because they had achieved an important goal but by virtue of their sharing the process of solving their joint problems.

Cost-Effective Care

The intensity and duration of overall services and, thus, costs, also vary with the phase and LOS in each stage of disease. Coupled with concern about costs must be concomitant measurement of outcomes to optimize cost effectiveness. Given the side effects and difficulties of drug management, it is essential to take an approach to overall management that maximizes the effects sought while minimizing those that are unwanted. One must have clear objectives as a basis for monitoring the impact so as to assure maximal effect. In designing the more complex treatment regimens, it becomes increasingly important for the person with PD or the caregiver, or both, to participate in the tradeoffs that may need to be made. The objective that is common to all is optimization of treatment.

The limitations of dopamine replacement must be recognized. A case illustrating this issue is that of a 78-year-old priest in whom a disorder of gait had developed. He had to try several times to rise from a sitting position before he succeeded. When he walked, he took tiny steps rapidly. Turns were especially difficult; a 180-degree turn required eight steps. He was very unstable. When one pulled on his shoulder while standing behind him, he would fall if not protected. He was cheerful. His personality, memory, and ability to speak were unchanged. Although he appeared to be suffering from PD, he had no response to carbidopa–L-dopa even when the dose was raised to levels that caused agitation and vivid nightmares that persisted into the waking state.

This patient's disorder can perhaps only be distinguished from PD through microscopic examination of the brain. One must increase the dose to toxicity and ensure that the L-dopa is ineffective. Uncertainty might deny a dopamine-depleted patient the most effective and least toxic of the available drugs. However, it is pointless to administer useless medications. If L-dopa does not help, none of the other drugs can help either. Physical and occupational therapies are available to develop strategies to prevent falls and prolong independent functioning.

The case of the judge described earlier illustrates the ongoing problems in dealing with progression of the disease. Over the next several years, other problems developed in this patient that required modification of his original regimen. Visual hallucinations began to appear at the doses that were required for mobility. To control hallucinations, he was started on clozapine (Clozaril), 25 mg at bedtime and 12.5 mg in the morning. This eliminated the hallucinations without worsening his PD symptoms. The use of Clozaril was followed by spells of weakness, which he experienced when standing. His blood pressure when standing was 85/45; sitting, it was 110/75. This discrepancy confirmed the diagnosis of orthostatic hypotension, which in turn responded to Florinef, 0.1 mg twice a day. After these issues were resolved, the patient became increasingly depressed and irritable. These symptoms responded to fluoxetine (Prozac), 20 mg daily. Depression in PD is common and cannot usually be explained as a psychological response to the illness but rather as the result of the chemical disturbance of the brain.

The only remaining problem has been immobility when the patient awakens at night and wishes to go to the toilet. Long-acting Sinemet was not effective in dealing with this problem. However, it has been somewhat helpful to take the carbidopa–L-dopa during the night along with a dopamine agonist before bed. Despite all these problems, he has kept his sense of humor, as evidenced by his statement about the likely consequences of indulging in his love of hamburgers. The participation of the patient and his wife in decisions about the objectives of each of these changes adding to the complexity of their regimen helped maintain their sense of control in the midst of the progression of the disease.

Optimizing Medical Treatment

The opportunities for maximizing the effectiveness of any drug regimen depend on knowledge of the characteristics of the drugs available and their indications. (See Olanow and Koller[6] for a review of the criteria for various alternative treatments.)

One common problem lies in adjusting the dosage of dopamine to reduce the degree of impairment without causing side effects, particularly in stage III. The manner in which L-dopa is formatted can make a slight reduction in dose difficult to accomplish, especially if a patient must take the L-dopa dose every 2 or 3 hours. The smallest dose of L-dopa contained in a pill is 100 mg. This can be broken in half accurately, but the pill cannot be further divided. Some patients require a dose of L-dopa that is more than 50 mg and less than 100 mg.

For such patients, the best answer is for them or their caretaker to make a solution of L-dopa by dissolving 1,000 mg (10 pills) in 1,000 ml water along with 1,000 mg ascorbic acid (vitamin C). The resulting mixture contains 1 mg L-dopa in each milliliter of water, and in the ascorbic acid it is stable for 2 days. By trial and error, adjusting each dose, the patients can find the dose of L-dopa that is exactly correct for them. If they need 60 mg, they can swallow 60 ml at each dosing interval. Because of the frequency with which the solution must be freshly mixed—every 2 days—the patient, not a pharmacist, must prepare it.

Clozapine. In some patients with PD, it is not possible to adjust the dose of L-dopa to provide relief of the motor symptoms without inducing a toxic psychosis. In such patients, it is necessary to use L-dopa in combination with an antipsychotic drug. Because the antipsychotic drugs, even most of the newer "unconventional" neuroleptics, block dopamine receptors, none can be used safely in patients with PD without causing regression of their motor symptoms. Clozapine alone reliably provides antipsychotic effects without aggravating PD.

Clozapine is sedating, causes or aggravates postural hypotension, and, in 2% of cases, causes severe leukopenia that necessitates discontinuance. Weekly blood counts add to the expense of the use of this medication, but it is an extremely effective drug. It is rarely necessary to use more than 50 mg per day to control toxic psychosis in PD, a fraction of the effective doses necessary to control other psychoses.

Amantadine. Amantadine inhibits the dopamine uptake mechanism and is mildly effective in relieving bradykinesia and tremor in mild PD because it prolongs the duration of action of released dopamine. It is relatively ineffective in relieving the symptoms of severe PD when no dopaminergic cell is left on which it can act and, therefore, no uptake mechanism exists to inactivate.

Amantadine also effectively reduces L-dopa–induced dyskinesia and is useful in late-stage PD for this purpose. This effect is counterintuitive and was first reported 34 years after the introduction of amantadine for the treatment of PD. This is an example of how physicians can often not see what they do not expect to see. No convincing theory for amantadine's efficacy in treating dyskinesia has yet been offered.

Belladonna Compounds. Anticholinergic compounds (trihexyphenidyl, benztropine) may be mildly effective in stage I PD. Belladonnas reduce tremor and some of the other symptoms of stage I parkinsonism, yet they are very effective in reversing the neuroleptic drug–induced parkinsonism that results from dopamine receptor blockade. Belladonnas are relatively ineffective in relieving the PD symptoms of patients with stage II and stage III PD.

Belladonnas, like amantadine, inhibit dopamine reuptake. This can lead to a significant increase in dopamine concentration at the dopamine receptors when some intact dopaminergic neurons remain on which the belladonnas can act. By blocking the inactivation of released dopamine, the belladonna compounds can overcome the action of neuroleptics and some symptoms in patients with mild, stage I PD.

Dopamine reuptake inhibition is not an effective mechanism for relieving the symptoms of advanced PD. In stages II and III, virtually no dopaminergic neurons are left on which the belladonnas can act.

The belladonna drugs are anticholinergic, and most neurologists mistakenly attribute their antiparkinsonian activity to the anticholinergic action. Anticholinergic compounds are supposed to restore a balance between acetylcholine and dopamine. This theory envisions the normal state of the brain as being one in which the transmitters acetylcholine and dopamine are in balance. In PD, an imbalance exists between them because dopamine is insufficient and acetylcholine is normal. By reducing the normal levels of acetylcholine, a new balance can be achieved between acetylcholine and the degraded state of the dopamine system, and, thus, normal motor activity can result.

The balance theory is quaint but woefully mistaken. This model fails to explain the mechanisms by which drugs that have anticholinergic effects impact PD. Every drug has at least two effects, the one that is well known and the other(s) that are not so well known. Anticholinergic drugs affect PD only through their ability to affect dopamine.

A brief review of the pharmacology of three classes of anticholinergic drugs indicates that their anticholinergic activity is completely irrelevant to their PD-relieving capacity. These drugs include neuroleptics, belladonnas, and tricyclic antidepressants (TCAs).

Neuroleptics, such as chlorpromazine, are strongly anticholinergic but cause PD symptoms.

Belladonna compounds, such as trihexyphenidyl, are strongly anticholinergic but relieve parkinsonian symptoms. TCAs, such as amitryptyline, are strongly anticholinergic but do not affect PD symptoms at all. The interaction of each of these anticholinergic classes of drugs with dopaminergic systems provides the only explanation for their differential effects on PD. Neuroleptics block dopamine receptors and, therefore, induce parkinsonism or worsen its symptoms. Belladonna compounds block dopamine reuptake and, therefore, improve symptoms of parkinsonism. TCAs have no effect on dopaminergic mechanisms. They block serotonin and norepinephrine uptake. They are antidepressants with no effect on the motor symptoms of PD.

Dopamine Agonists. Dopamine agonists, including the oldest such agent, bromocriptine, and three newer ones, pergolide, ropinerole, and pramipexole, directly activate dopamine receptors. They are not taken up by presynaptic cells, need not be released at a particular time, and require no inactivation mechanism. Theoretically, they should be very effective, but they do not work very well. Bromocriptine is inferior to the others. No study has been done that compares the three newer agonists. All are prone to causing unacceptable cognitive side effects, and all are expensive compared with generic L-dopa.

Monamine Oxidase Inhibitor. The monoamine oxidase inhibitor selegiline (Deprenyl, Eldepryl) inhibits beta monoamine oxidase inhibitor, the enzyme that breaks down dopamine. By inhibiting the catabolizing enzyme, the monoamine oxidase inhibitor provides a minimal symptomatic benefit because the intracellular dopamine concentration is slightly increased within the dopaminergic neurons. Of course, this minor benefit is limited to those PD patients with disease that is mild enough that some dopaminergic neurons remain. It is, therefore, more helpful in mild than in severe PD. This drug is now being used clinically in an attempt to slow or to prevent the advance of PD symptoms. Research that was said to indicate that selegiline slows the course of PD has been severely criticized. The best that can be said for this drug is that it is relatively safe. It is expensive and ineffective.

Catechol *O*-Methyltransferase Inhibitors (Tolcapone). Catechol *O*-methyltransferase inhibitor inhibits the enzyme catechol *O*-methyltransferase, an enzyme that is responsible for the degradation of L-dopa. By reducing L-dopa breakdown, tolcapone elevates blood levels of L-dopa and prolongs their elevation. The use of tolcapone with L-dopa has allowed patients with fluctuating responses to L-dopa to take it less frequently. The deaths from severe liver failure of several patients who were taking tolcapone has dampened enthusiasm for this expensive drug, despite the marginal advantages it provides.

Surgical Treatments

Transplants. Adrenal transplants do not work. Fetal cell transplants also do not work despite isolated reports of success for each. The choice of patients for this kind of "curative" surgery has posed a serious problem. Many conditions of the brain cause PD-like symptoms that do not respond to dopamine replacement therapy. Presumably, such symptoms result from disease outside the dopaminergic system. Motor problems that do not result from dopamine deficiency are not reversed when dopamine is replaced. The transplant, if it worked, would function as a biologic dopamine pump. It can only be efficacious in someone who has simple dopamine deficiency. If a person has motor symptoms that do not result from dopamine deficiency, a dopamine pump cannot relieve those symptoms.

How would a physician know whether a patient had dopamine deficiency? The patient's symptoms would respond to dopamine replacement. If the patient's response to dopamine replacement is only intermittent, then by definition he or she has on-off symptoms or stage III PD. The patient should be given frequent doses of L-dopa and placed on the protein redistribution diet. This simple, safe, and uniformly effective approach has not always been attempted before patients have been declared medically intractable and referred for surgery.

Pallidotomy. Pallidotomy has been said to relieve both bradykinesia and dopa-induced dyskinesia. The operation is claimed to permit both the use of less L-dopa and the use of more L-dopa. Dyskinesia in PD usually results from L-dopa overdosage and responds to the use of less L-dopa. Nonetheless, pallidotomy is now being used primarily to reduce the dyskinesia that results from L-dopa overdosage. It costs approximately $30,000 for a unilateral pallidotomy.

Complications of the procedure include hemorrhage, infection, paralysis, aphasia, blindness, and cognitive changes. Very few patients have had complete psychological testing before surgery and then after operation. Most reports have emphasized the advantages conferred by the operation but have minimized the cognitive declines that follow surgery. Few surgeons are willing to perform bilateral pallidotomies because of the high prevalence of adverse cognitive changes that follow bilateral surgery. The literature fails to support this justified reticence to perform bilateral pallidotomies because poor results are often unreported. Fragmentary evidence indicates that the incidence of cognitive decline after unilateral pallidotomies that is attributable to the operation is approximately 25%.

Brain Stimulation. A permanently indwelling electrode placed into the subthalamic nucleus bilaterally and stimulated can reduce the tremor of PD and other diseases. Some of the other, more disabling, symptoms of PD can also be favorably affected, but the greatest efficacy of this procedure is in treating tremor. It is advertised as a reversible procedure and, therefore, safer than pallidotomy. The stimulator can be turned off and the electrodes removed without the extent of harm or risk associated with pallidotomy. Operation on each side costs approximately $40,000. Bilateral operations can be "safely" performed.

Neither pallidotomy nor stimulation is without risk. In the author's opinion, the risks of the surgery have been underestimated, the expense of operation has been understated, and the efficacy of the procedures and the duration of the symptomatic relief they provide are unknown. All the patients subjected to such operations were considered medically intractable but in very few had the protein redistribution diet been tried.

Collaborative Care

Underlying the overall management plan is the development of the capability for self-management by the primary participants, namely, the patient and family. The planning and treatment process must be a collaborative one that leads to conjoint contribution of both energy and ideas. The identification of the significant functional issues in the life of the person and the caregiver provides the context for the design of the treatment and its evaluation. No treatment can necessarily deal with all aspects in their entirety. Tradeoffs must be made in terms of results versus the cost and complexity of the regimens recommended. The process of involving the patient and the caregiver in the decision making does not aid only in making the evaluation of the regimen more meaningful. The very process of involvement can enhance the sense of control that serves to mitigate the helplessness that the management of a progressive disease engenders.

The case of a 63-year-old physician illustrates the problems in designing a regimen in the context of a mixed syndrome owing to Parkinson's plus. It also demonstrates the value achieved in an imperfect result by attention to the involvement of the family in the decision-making process. The patient had been diagnosed as having PD 3 years before. He was being treated with a complex regimen of selegiline, 5 mg twice a day; pramipexole, 0.25 mg three times a day; and Sinemet CR, 50/200 three times a day. His symptoms were bradykinesia, postural instability, and a marked tendency to tilt to the left as he sat in a chair. He had fallen at home, injuring himself on several occasions. His wife had to call 911 on two occasions to obtain assistance in helping him up off the floor. His wife reported that he was having visual hallucinations and delusions. He had once been a very active person, involved with other people and with his work, but he was now content to sit in his living room, watching television and dozing.

On examination, he had restricted upward gaze. He held his head erect but tilted to the left. He had difficulty standing and initiating gait: He would take a few stuttering steps at first. Once he got started, he was better able to continue. Often he walked too quickly and came dangerously close to bumping into furniture that might have tripped him. He was mildly demented and had physical signs of frontal lobe disease.

The combination of the patient's motor problems, personality change, and restriction of upward gaze pointed to the diagnosis of PSP, a degenerative disorder that involves the upper midbrain region. PSP can be associated with some degree of dopamine deficiency. Despite the limitations of the treatment with dopamine replacement in this situation, a treatment regimen could be designed to maximize function. Although the patient had multiple problems, the highest priority according to the wife was to deal with the issue of his safety, to protect him from falls, and to develop some training by which she could help him to get up without having to call 911.

The first question to be answered was that of medication toxicity. Was dementia partially or wholly the result of the medication? The next question was whether dopamine replacement therapy was helpful.

Discontinuation of the drugs other than Sinemet CR led to diminution of the hallucinations without adverse effect on the motor problems. The Sinemet CR was then discontinued, with substitution of the generic carbidopa–L-dopa 25/100 on a milligram-per-milligram basis. His condition remained unchanged. The dopamine was then tapered by half a pill each day. When the dosage reached three times a day, his motor capacities had improved to the extent that he walked less dangerously. He seemed a bit more interactive socially, and his hallucinations and delusions had also been reduced. However, when his dosage was reduced further, he became unable to rise out of a chair or to initiate gait. It became clear that he had been toxic on the medication that he had been receiving at first, but he needed some L-dopa for optimal function.

Titrating the dose was helpful, but major functional difficulties remained, particularly in dealing with the patient's postural instability and resultant falls. In designing the treatment for his falls, it was important to identify the specific conditions under which he had fallen. The combination of the difficulty in initiation and the ongoing rapidity of his gait led to several recommendations. Physical and occupational therapists provided training in the use of assistive devices. A walker was recommended along with a lazy Susan for the car and chairs at the table that made it easier for the patient's feet to swing around. The wife was taught techniques by which she could raise him more easily without injury. In addition to the modification in the medication regimen and the training in the use of assistive devices, a more comprehensive approach included membership of the wife in a support group that provided her with ideas for overcoming practical problems and also offered her the comfort of shared difficulties.

Although not all the problems could be solved, and the problems that were alleviated could not meet the full need of returning the patient to his previous status, the situation had been improved. To the extent that improvement lay in the areas that the husband and wife had identified as important, it served to strengthen their ability to continue. The role of the physician in dealing with the management of persons with chronic, ultimately progressive, neurologic disease must recognize the limitations of medical management of the disease. One must focus as well on giving validity to the knowledge that the persons involved have acquired to enable them to carry on their lives. The very process of interaction by the physician and the patient and caregiver can serve to support such a sense of hope and self-efficacy that is so necessary.

Measuring Effectiveness

The distinction made by such classification schemes as that of the WHO between impairments, disabilities, and handicaps (QOL) is an important one in measuring the effectiveness of treatment. As was pointed out earlier, the management of persons with PD provides an extraordinary opportunity in that one can alleviate many of the motor impairments by dopamine replacement. However, those are not the only symptoms of the disease particularly as it progresses. In addition, the effects of medication can lead to further impairments. In the proper pursuit of reducing impairment, one must not lose sight of the person(s) in whom these impairments continue to exist and the impact of the long-term and progressive nature of the disease on their functional status and QOL.

Measurement of Impairment

Hoehn and Yahr Scales

The Hoehn and Yahr scale was the first scale used to describe the progression of disease.[9] A modified version has been incorporated as a component of the unified PD rating scale.[10] It consists of descriptions of various stages in evolution of the disease. For example, stage 2 is described as "unilateral disease." Stage 3 reflects both measures of degree of impairment and some measure of disability: "mild to moderate bilateral disease; some postural instability; physically independent." Stage 5 is "wheel-chair bound or bedridden unless aided." The scale mixes presumed pathology (unilateral-bilateral) with impairments and disabilities.

Parkinson's Disease Impairment Index

The Parkinson's Disease Impairment Index[11] is a prototype of a number of scales developed for use in measuring the effects of dopamine replacement therapy.[6] This scale lists the common impairments with varying weights for each, ranging from "akinesia" (6) and "dementia" (8) through "tremor" (5) and "depression" (5) to "postural abnormality" (3) and "mask facies" (1). Each finding would then be multiplied by a severity score ranging from 0 to 2 to provide a total score in which 0 is normal. One may note that the lower score reflects better function. This scale is interesting in that it measures not only the degree of severity but also some value to be attached to one or the other impairment. Major drawbacks include a lack of clarity as to the basis for the weights that are to be applied. Nevertheless, it is described as one of the potential measures if one could establish an appropriate basis for the weights to be assigned.

Unified Parkinson's Disease Rating Scale

The Unified Parkinson's Disease Rating Scale has been the most widely used scale in research studies.[10] It consists of six separate parts. Section I relates to secondary features of the disease, such as mentation, behavior, and mood. Section II, entitled "Activities of Daily Living," is described later in this chapter (Measurement of Disabilities). Section III concentrates on motor impairments but also includes some aspects of disability such as gait problems. Section IV, entitled "Complications of Therapy (in the past week)," contains an assessment of the presence of dyskinesia, another dealing with clinical fluctuation, and a third dealing with other complications. Section V is a modification of the Hoehn-Yahr staging as described previously. Section VI, entitled "Schwab and England Activities of Daily Living," is a numeric scale that ranges from 100% ("completely independent, able to do all chores without slowness or difficulty") through 60% ("some dependency, can do most chores but exceedingly

slowly and with considerable effort and errors") to 20% ("does nothing alone; can be a slight help with some chores; severe invalid").

This scale has been used in most research projects but is cumbersome for clinical use. Reliability has been assessed. Section I (mentation, behavior, and mood) contains four separate measures, such as intellectual impairment, thought disorder (owing to dementia or drug intoxication), depression, and motivation-initiative, with a scale ranging from 0 (normal) to 4. Section III (motor examination) is similarly a semiquantitative, relatively complete measure that consists of 14 separate items with each scored from 0 to 4 when 0 = "normal."

The variation in patient performance to dose and time of day makes any scale per se difficult to apply as a basis of guiding therapy. Described here is a briefer adaptation of the impairment measures to the clinical setting as a means of measuring the effects of treatment. When the patient enters the door, he or she is asked to walk to the opposite wall, turn around, and come back. One can time this with a stopwatch and count the number of steps. One can also determine the number of steps that are necessary to turn 180 degrees. Standing behind the patient and gently pulling on the shoulders three times, one can see if he or she can maintain postural stablility. Blood pressure can be taken while the patient is still standing. Once sitting, the individual can be asked to open and close the hands, and the time (seconds) taken to carry out 10 such motions in either hand is determined. All these activities provide a numerical score that can be used to assess the progress of therapy.

In general, gait disturbance may or may not be helped by increasing L-dopa. In most instances, broad-based gait cannot be assisted and results from conditions other than dopamine deficiency. Narrow-based, small-stepped gaits are typical results of dopamine deficiency and are more likely to respond to therapy.

Time since the last dose should be recorded. If the medication is at its peak (between 1 and $2^{1}/_{2}$ hours since the last dose), one can assume that this is the best response that can be produced by that dose. If dyskinesia is present, one can lower the dose. If bradykinesia or other signs of PD are found, one can raise the dose. One can determine, by history or patient diary, how long the therapeutic effect of the dose of L-dopa lasts. That determines the frequency of dosing. The patient diary should list the timing and content of meals, the timing of doses, and the effects of the medications.

The need for more frequent dosing and changes in diet can be assessed by asking whether the effect of the medication is smooth throughout the day or whether it has a tendency to wear off and, if so, how long it takes the medication to start to work; one should also ask how long the medication remains effective before wearing off. Furthermore, it is important to ask whether the medication ever seems not to work. If the answer to this is yes, a protein distribution diet may be effective. Patients should be weighed as a measure of their nutritional status. Weight loss can be prevented by a special drink of whole milk, ice cream, and "instant breakfast" mixed just before bed. The immobility that such a high-protein drink might induce in late parkinsonism can be rendered benign if it occurs during sleep.

It is important in assessing the effectiveness of any regimen to evaluate the impact on the patient's actual functioning during the course of the day. Assessment of the disabilities is ultimately the measures that can aid in maintaining QOL and can determine the priorities to be measured.

Measurement of Disabilities

Activities of Daily Living Scale of Unified Parkinson's Disease Rating Scale

Section II of the Unified Parkinson's Disease Rating Scale[10,11] continues to be recommended for use[12] to assess functional disabilities. Reliability is sought with good results in the hands of nurses as well as trained physicians.[13] Like the other components of the Unified Parkinson's Disease Rating Scale, this section consists of a number of separate items, each with a scale that ranges from 0 to 4, in which 0 is normal. Most of the items do reflect functional status, such as "speech, swallowing, and handwriting" in the area of communication. "Cutting food and handling utensils, dressing, and hygiene" addresses some of the more usual ADL activities. Mobility issues are addressed in "turning in bed, falling, freezing when walking, and walk-

ing." Additional items that do not reflect functional issues are such impairments as "salivation," "tremor," and "sensory complaints."

Self-Assessment Parkinson's Disease Disability Scale

The Self-Assessment Parkinson's Disease Disability Scale serves as a prototype of a number of others that can be helpful in clinical settings to aid in design of the objectives of treatment plans.[13] A five-point scale is used to assess performance, ranging from 1, able to do without difficulty, to 5, unable to do at all. Intermediate is 2, able to do alone with a little effort; 3, able to do alone with a lot of effort or a little help; and 4, able to do only with a lot of help. Twenty-five items are listed that explore a broader range of activities, including items such as "travel by public transport," "dial a telephone," and "hold and read a newspaper." The items that reflect those on the Unified Parkinson's Disease Rating Scale are more finely grained. For example, items related to hygiene include "get into a bath," "get out of a bath," and so forth.

Although a number of scales have been devised, identification of the functional disabilities needs to reflect the specific experience of the person with the impairments and the family. In setting goals that are meaningful to these persons and that can truly measure the value of treatment, one must help them to identify the problems that they face in their lives. One way to do this easily and effectively is by going through the process of a day. One must ask: Can you turn in bed unassisted? Can you arise from bed? Can you walk to the bathroom and get up off the toilet? Can you brush your teeth, comb your hair, zip or tie or button clothes, put on a jacket or sweater, drive safely, get in and out of a car, and so forth? Do you do these activities slowly? Can they be done with assistance or not at all?

It is not only the listing of the problems but their relative importance that only the patient and the caregiver can adequately assess. In helping them to do so, one can increase the effectiveness of any treatment. One must enhance the ability of these persons to then participate in the setting of goals and the subsequent monitoring of the degree to which they are accomplished. This is important in maintaining hope and a sense of accomplishment.

Such information in the experience of the patient and caregiver can provide the basis for their further understanding of the relationship between the results achieved and the actions taken by them. These actions can include carrying out the medication regimen or whatever other efforts are being taken. In the course of optimizing their participation in such ongoing planning and assessment lies the maintenance of the sense of hope and satisfaction that are necessary to alleviate the suffering that results from the chronic progressive disease.

References

1. Goedert M, Sillantini MG, Davies SW. Filamentous nerve cell inclusions in neurodegenerative diseases. Curr Opin Neurobiol 1998;8:619.
2. Sillantini MG, Crowther RA, Jakes R, et al. Filamentous alpha-synuclein inclusions link multisystem atrophy with Parkinson's disease and dementia with Lewy bodies. Neurosci Lett 1998;31:251.
3. Lippa CF, Fujiwara H, Mann DM, et al. Lewy bodies contain altered alpha-synuclein in brains of many familial Alzheimer disease patients. Am J Pathol 1998;153:1365.
4. World Health Organization. The International Classification of Impairments, Disabilities and Handicaps. Geneva: World Health Organization, 1980.
5. Tandberg E, Larsen JP, Aarsland D, et al. Risk factors for depression in Parkinson's disease. Arch Neurol 1997;54:625.
6. Olanow CW, Koller WC. An algorithm (decision tree) for the management of Parkinson's disease: treatment guidelines. Neurology 1998;50(suppl 3):S26.
7. Andes GM. Mark Twain's cat. Ann Intern Med 1998; 128:1043.
8. Pincus JH, Barry K. Influence of dietary protein on motor fluctuations in Parkinson's disease. Arch Neurol 1987; 44:270.
9. Hoehn MM, Yahr MD. Parkinsonism: onset, progression and mortality. Neurology 1967;17:427.
10. Lang AET, Fahn S. Assessment of Parkinson's Disease. In TL Munsat (ed), Quantification of Neurologic Deficit. Stoneham, MA: Butterworth, 1989;49–67.
11. Wade DT. Measurement in Neurological Rehabilitation. New York: Oxford University Press, 1992;328–335.
12. Bennett DA, Shannon KM, Beckett LA, et al. Metric properties of nurses' ratings of parkinsonian signs with a modified united Parkinson's disease rating scale. Neurology 1997;49:1580.
13. Brown RG, MacCarthey B, Jahanshahi M, et al. Accuracy of self-reported disability in patients with parkinsonism. Arch Neurol 1989;46:955.

Chapter 10

Management of Persons
with Seizure Disorders*

Robert J. Gumnit

Nature of the Problem

Extent of the Problem

The term epilepsy defines a condition in which a patient has recurrent seizures, that is, more than one seizure on more than one occasion. Three seizures during a bout of meningitis would not qualify the person as having epilepsy; two unprovoked seizures 6 months apart certainly would.

Incidence and Prevalence

It is difficult to produce reliable demographic information in the absence of clear-cut definitions that can be reproducibly applied. In the case of paroxysmal events such as epilepsy, this is particularly difficult. The physician is dependent for the most part on the observations of excited and alarmed lay people. Furthermore, the studies that have been carried out throughout the world use a variety of definitions. Despite this lack of uniformity, reasonably good estimates can be made of the incidence and prevalence of epilepsy.

In a study carried out in Olmstead County, Minnesota (where the medical records of every inhabitant can be reviewed), Hauser and Hesdorffer[1] concluded that close to 9% of the population will have one seizure sometime in their life. Just over 2.5% are simple febrile seizures that do not develop into epilepsy and that appear only during early childhood. Approximately 3% of the population had one seizure in their life and no more. Another 3% had more than one seizure on more than one occasion and went on to develop epilepsy.

When one considers that Olmstead County, Minnesota, has more neurologists per capita than the United States has physicians per capita, the 3% of individuals who have only one seizure must include a number of people in whom a diagnosis was promptly made and treatment quickly initiated. It is remarkable, given the high level of expertise immediately available, that these authors also found that only one-half of the patients were diagnosed within 5 months of their first seizure and that, after 5 years, only 80% of the patients had been diagnosed as having epilepsy. This comes about because of the ephemeral nature of the symptoms and the reluctance of many midwestern Americans to seek medical attention until the problem can no longer be denied.

In the last quarter of the twentieth century, the incidence of new-onset seizure disorders in the United States population was approximately 30 to 57 per 100,000. This translates to approximately 120,000 new cases of epilepsy each year, or about

---

*Portions of this chapter, including some sections that are the length of a full paragraph, are adapted or reproduced from other works by the author. The author holds the copyright to these works and has granted the publisher of this book the use of this material in its present form for the purposes of this edition only.

3 per day in a metropolitan area of 2.5 million. When one divides that number by the number of primary care physicians in a metropolitan area, the average primary care physician will see one new case of epilepsy every 2 or 3 years. The incidence is higher in people younger than 20 years and older than 60 years. It is particularly high in the group younger than 1 year and in those between the ages of 60 and 80 years.

Hauser and Hesdorffer[1] defined active epilepsy as taking antiepileptic medication or having had a seizure within the past 5 years. The rate was 6 per 1,000 in Olmstead County. Applying this estimate to the United States with a 7% inflation of the figure for those who do not seek medical care (an underestimate in the author's opinion), the prevalence is approximately 1.5–2.0 million cases of active epilepsy in the United States.

A slight preponderance of men over women is found in the incidence figures, but the prevalence is uniformly higher among men. The incidence figures approach one-tenth of 1% in individuals younger than 9 years and two-tenths of 1% younger than 1 year. The prevalence rate again increases in patients older than 60 years, and unpublished figures from a survey of a large national nursing home corporation indicate that 6–10% of the patients in nursing homes are taking antiepileptic medications.

Mortality

Nearly all patients with epilepsy recover completely after an epileptic seizure. Nonetheless, age-adjusted overall mortality is increased two- to threefold in patients with epilepsy when compared with the general population. Much of the mortality associated with epilepsy is related to the diseases that cause the seizures such as cerebral infarctions or neoplasms. Mortality is also increased with status epilepticus or seizure-associated accidents, both of which are potentially preventable. However, between one-fourth and one-third of deaths in epilepsy are sudden and unexpected without preceding illness or other obvious causes. This sudden unexpected death in epilepsy (SUDEP) is alarming to physicians and devastating to families. The patient was usually getting along quite well and then suddenly is dead. Family members wonder what caused the death, whether the death might have been prevented, and why they were not told that sudden death can occur in epilepsy.

The contemporary definition of SUDEP requires that patients have a documented history of epilepsy, that the death must have occurred unexpectedly while the patient was in a reasonable state of health, that the death must have occurred suddenly while the patient was engaged in normal activities, and that the death must have no obvious cause. It is now clear that this is a genuine entity. Several hundred cases of SUDEP have been published, and the individual situations are remarkably similar. Most of the reported patients abused alcohol or street drugs, and noncompliance appears to be common. Virtually all reported patients suffer from generalized tonic-clonic seizures. Many also experience other seizure types. The seizures tend to be poorly controlled. Most of the time, the patients are found dead in bed after an uneventful day. The great majority of the time, the sudden death occurs at home.

How often does SUDEP occur? In population-based studies, which include a high proportion of people with infrequently occurring seizures, the annual incidence ranges from 3 to 15 per 10,000 people a year. In general epilepsy clinics, frequencies range from 20 to 30 per 10,000 people a year. In studies of patients with seizures that occur frequently enough to warrant treatment with experimental drugs, 30–60 sudden deaths per 10,000 patients a year are reported. Highest frequency occurs in patients whose seizures are severe enough to warrant evaluation for epilepsy surgery or in whom epilepsy surgery has failed. Between 90 and 150 per 10,000 patients a year experience SUDEP in these circumstances. Thus, approximately 1 in every 100 patients with severe epilepsy experiences SUDEP in any given year. These data predict that a patient has an approximately 30% chance of experiencing SUDEP during 30 years of severe intractable epilepsy. The risk of SUDEP in severe epilepsy is 40–70 times risk in the nonepileptic population—2 per 10,000 patients per year. Therefore, it is not clear that risk is elevated in patients with well-controlled epilepsy, but it appears to be substantially elevated in poorly controlled epilepsy. These findings strongly support aggressive treatment of epileptic seizures and referral to comprehensive centers when seizures are not easily controlled locally. Frequent, persistent seizures not only have an indelible psychosocial impact but also increase the risk of death.

Nature of the Disease

Seizures can be divided into two broad categories: epileptic and nonepileptic. An epileptic seizure is an episode of disturbed brain activity that results in abnormal behavior. The main problem lies within the functioning of the neurons of the brain. A nonepileptic seizure is an episode of abnormal behavior that is not primarily caused by a disturbance of neurons. Nonepileptic seizures may be physiologic or psychogenic in origin. For example, an abrupt drop in blood pressure produced by Stokes-Adams disease, or severe hyponatremia, may cause a physiologic nonepileptic seizure. Certain psychological problems are manifested by the patient behaving in an abnormal manner that may resemble an epileptic seizure. This event would be diagnosed as a psychogenic nonepileptic event.

Epileptic Events

The appearance of seizures has both general and specific risk factors. Anyone is capable of having a seizure; it is within the repertoire of response of the normal brain. The threshold at which a seizure appears, however, is polygenetically determined. If an airplane should suddenly depressurize and stay at high altitude, eventually everyone on the airplane would have a seizure from hypoxia. The distribution of time of onset would tend to follow a bell-shaped curve. In addition to polygenetic determinations, recessive and dominant genetic diseases have seizures as a prominent symptom. However, the brain reacts with seizures from all kinds of mechanical and metabolic insults. Head trauma; CNS infections; hypoxic changes from vascular problems of the sort that cause cerebral palsy, mental retardation, and stroke; degenerative diseases such as AD; toxins such as alcohol; and repetitive bouts of metabolic strain and hypoxia associated with prolonged complex febrile seizures are all risk factors for the development of epilepsy later in life.

The idea that people "grow out" of epilepsy is a myth. Technically speaking, we are discussing the risk of recurrence after a first seizure or the probability of remission once an individual has been diagnosed with epilepsy. Subsets of this include the risk of relapse after withdrawal of antiepileptic drugs in a patient who has been well controlled for a long time and the likelihood of remission (or success) after epilepsy surgery. In general, of patients who have an initial unprovoked seizure, recurrence is likely in close to 50% of them. High recurrence rates are associated with patients who have a remote symptomatic etiology (e.g., an old serious head injury), seizures that are partial in onset, or an abnormal EEG. Recurrence is less likely if the seizures were primarily generalized, occurred during sleep, and were associated with sleep deprivation.

Once patients are diagnosed as having epilepsy, the likelihood of their never experiencing another seizure is, again, approximately 50%. People are less likely to have future seizures if the seizures began when the patient was young and they were generalized in nature, the neurologic examination was normal, and no proximate etiology could be identified.

Patients who are well controlled on antiepileptic drugs (AEDs) follow a similar remission pattern except that it is likely that recurrence will occur sooner if they have had frequent seizures, clusters of seizures, and an abnormal EEG. A permanent neurologic deficit (including mental retardation) and a symptomatic etiology also increase the risk of relapse. A full discussion of the remission and recurrence rates after surgery for the treatment of epilepsy is found later in the chapter. Of course, if the patient has a progressive neurologic disorder, such as AD, Down syndrome, postirradiation encephalopathy, or certain inborn errors of metabolism, or if the individual has what is loosely called Lennox-Gastaut or mixed-seizure disorders, the likelihood for recurrence approaches 100%, and the prognosis is for gradually increasing difficulty.

Nonepileptic Events

Nonepileptic events include a broad range of conditions that are lumped together under a variety of names: hysterical seizures, pseudoseizures, nonepileptic seizures, nonepileptic events, and psychogenic seizures. These problems are fairly common, yet they are very difficult to diagnose and treat. Nonepileptic seizures represent 20% of the referrals to our specialized epilepsy center. Patients with nonepileptic events are frequently inadequately diagnosed

Table 10-1. Physiologic Nonepileptic Events

Problems in perfusion
    Rhythm disturbances, e.g., Stokes-Adams disease
    Transient ischemic attacks
    Emboli from carotid plaques
Decreased oxygen tension from poor saturation
    Acute respiratory disease, e.g., pneumonia leading to confusion
    Internal lung shunts leading to transient hypoxia
    Pulmonary emboli
Metabolic causes
    Decreased blood glucose levels from excessive insulin and other causes of hypoglycemia
    Electrolyte shifts, hyperosmolality, calcium ion shifts, low serum sodium
    Toxic reactions, e.g., excessive concentrations of antiepileptic drugs, especially from erratic absorption
    Street drugs, e.g., lysergic acid diethylamide, amphetamines
    Prescription drugs, e.g., sedatives or cimetidine
    Alcohol
    Foodstuffs: "wooziness" associated with some herbal teas and ingestion of garlic, onion

and treated. They use an inappropriately large amount of medical resources, not only in visits to physicians' offices but also in visits to emergency rooms and admissions to hospitals.

It is all too easy to accept the patient's history as reality. Misdiagnosis by a physician, nurse, parent, or other caregiver is most common in severely mentally retarded individuals with motor mannerisms who are described as having many seizures per day. If a misdiagnosis is made by the physician or nurse on the basis of the history, the family will report frequent seizures. The physician will be tempted to use ever-increasing doses of AEDs for what may simply be a misinterpretation of a mannerism, a normal physiologic sensation, or some benign psychological issue. Until video-EEG is performed, the diagnosis is obscure, and disabusing the informant of a mistaken belief is futile.

Nonepileptic events that at first appear to be seizures can be divided into physiologic events, psychogenic events, and malingering. They do not have any single presentation. The diagnosis cannot be made with certainty on the basis of any one characteristic or even on the basis of a single EEG recorded during the ictus. The physician must always be aware that the first impression is likely to be wrong. Technical problems add to the difficulty. A scalp recording does not always reveal ictal activity deep in the brain, and ictal events that are potentially visible with scalp EEG recording may be obscured by muscle and movement artifact. Depth-electrode studies of complex partial seizures have revealed that behavior manifestations may occur minutes or even hours before the surface EEG changes can be seen.

Although most of the cardiac and respiratory causes of physiologic nonepileptic events occur later in life, a few can be seen in younger patients. Disturbances of consciousness produced by decreased oxygen tension to the brain can cause behavior that mimics psychogenic or true seizures (Table 10-1).

Some clinical characteristics are fairly common in certain nonepileptic events, especially psychogenic seizures and malingering episodes that mimic generalized tonic-clonic seizures. Malingerers rarely present at specialized epilepsy centers but may be quite a problem in the primary care setting, especially if the patient is forced to seek treatment by the courts, a spouse, or an employer. Prisoners and those in military service are particularly likely to be malingerers. Malingerers have, on occasion, mimicked generalized tonic-clonic seizures so well that even experienced epileptologists have been confused. Video-EEG recording of the events during the ictus is mandatory for the diagnosis. The absence of postictal slowing during the recovery phase is often helpful. A careful search for primary gain often helps make the diagnosis. On occasion, it is only when the patient confesses or boasts to another about fooling the doctor that the diagnosis is made.

Psychogenic seizures are particularly difficult to diagnose and treat. They rarely begin in children younger than age 6 and rarely start in middle or old age. Classic psychogenic seizures may occur in children as young as 8 or 10 years. Younger children with nonepileptic paroxysmal behaviors more often have mannerisms that are misinterpreted—parasomnias, hyperventilation attacks, breath-holding spells, syncope, or movement disorders—but frank episodes of psychogenic unresponsiveness or "convulsion" may be seen toward the end of the first decade of life. This possible diagnosis should not be forgotten in pediatric patients with persistent episodes and repeatedly normal EEGs.

The diagnosis can be made only with the help of video-EEG recordings during the ictus. At the same time, testing of consciousness and reaction to startle response should be carried out. The diagnosis cannot be made on a single event; often the first impression is wrong. Patients with true epileptic seizures may occasionally experience a psychogenic seizure during video-EEG monitoring out of a desire to be helpful. Unless the witnessed psychogenic seizure is identical to the seizures that occur at home, a false diagnosis will be made. Secondary gain nearly always plays a role in psychogenic seizures but tends to serve as a reinforcer rather than as an etiologic agent per se (Table 10-2).

Our experience is that physical and sexual abuse play an etiologic role in many patients with psychogenic seizures, especially females. Female patients are three times more likely than male patients to have psychogenic seizures. One can often provoke a psychogenic seizure by suggesting that the patient will have a seizure. However, simply because a psychogenic seizure occurred, one cannot conclude that this is the event that prompted the patient to seek medical care. The witnessed event must be compared carefully with the presenting complaint. Physicians strongly disagree about whether to use an injection of placebo to provoke seizures. In our experience, it gives too many false-positive results.

Mixed cases present a similar problem. Many patients have frequent psychogenic seizures in addition to occasional epileptic seizures that can be well controlled with AEDs. Treating each entity properly (but differently) is difficult and time consuming. Psychogenic seizures may mimic any type of epileptic attack: partial motor, partial sensory, drop attacks, complex partial, myoclonic, generalized tonic-clonic, and, rarely, absence seizures. In none of these is a description of the clinical behavior alone particularly helpful. The physician should look for "la belle indifférence" or clear secondary gain.

Certain serum hormone and enzyme determinations can be used to help separate psychogenic seizures from true epilepsy. However, they are useful only in severe, full-blown seizures that appear to be generalized tonic-clonic. From a practical point of view, obtaining the specimen in a timely manner and interpreting it may be difficult. Because all of these hormones have circadian fluctuations, control values must be based on samples drawn from the

Table 10-2. Classification of Psychogenic Seizures

Misdiagnosis/misinterpretation by
  Patient
  Caregiver/parent
  Physician
Elaboration (simple sensory or motor seizure followed
    by a more elaborate psychogenic seizure)
  Fear
  Attention seeking
  Reinforcement of dependent role
  Conditioned response
Inappropriate coping strategy
  In a patient with limited intellectual resources
  Psychological conflict or personality issues

patient at the same time of day when no event has taken place. The concentrations go up and down so rapidly that the measurement has to be made during the peak. A serum prolactin level drawn 5–15 minutes after a generalized tonic-clonic seizure can be compared to one drawn 90–120 minutes later. A rise of $2^{1}/_{2}$ times the control provides approximately 90% reliability in determining a true generalized tonic-clonic seizure. A negative result has no value in distinguishing psychogenic from complex partial seizures (40% false-negative rate).

Because nonepileptic seizures have diverse causes, treatment must be tailored individually. Misdiagnosis is fairly easy to treat if the patient has confidence in the new diagnosis. Anxious patients who misinterpret normal sensations may need a comprehensive approach based on reassurance. Misinterpretation of the diagnosis by caregivers is best avoided by educating and reassuring them. However, if the caregiver has psychological needs that are met by the misdiagnosis, prolonged counseling and family therapy may be necessary.

Simply informing the patient that the seizures are nonepileptic is not treatment. Denial and doubt are routine reactions to be expected from the patient. They are often healthy responses that are necessary for individuals who require more time to process the diagnosis. Patients whose nonepileptic seizures represent a significant psychological defense mechanism cannot simply be told the diagnosis. Leaving such patients defenseless without providing alternative coping mechanisms can be and has been catastrophic. Suicide attempts occur and are occasionally successful.

Treatment of psychogenic seizures is complex and time consuming. If treatment is to be successful, the diagnosis must be accurate, or at least the physician must be willing to risk being wrong and to act with great confidence. Any ambivalence provides an opportunity for denial or further manipulation by the patient. The diagnosis should be delayed until one is certain; a too facile or a premature incorrect diagnosis creates a loss of confidence that may never be overcome.

Psychogenic seizures are learned behavior. Proper treatment focuses on the patient's ability to learn new coping skills. The patient with limited intellectual resources often resorts to psychogenic seizures as a way of avoiding conflict or of influencing a highly structured and restricted environment. In that case, treatment is directed at the family and the caregiver. Patients whose psychogenic seizures arise from psychological conflict or personality or character disorders are the most difficult to treat. They require a team of professionals skilled in the techniques of modern psychology and psychiatry. Our experience is that ad hoc task forces created from general hospital support staff do not achieve rates of success comparable to those of a dedicated team in an epilepsy center. The treatment of psychogenic seizures requires extensive resources, an experienced team, and a lot of time. It is usually better not to tell the patient of one's suspicions. The patient should be referred to a specialized epilepsy center, which should make the diagnosis and provide the necessary psychological and psychiatric care at the time that the diagnosis is made.

If the precise diagnosis is not known, the physician does not know what he or she is trying to treat. The choice of treatment then becomes a guessing game, and the likelihood of success is markedly decreased. Given the possible toxicity of antiepileptic medication, it is particularly important to differentiate epileptic from nonepileptic seizures. In general, it is very difficult for ordinary physicians to know what they are treating in most cases of epilepsy. The historical information is unreliable, the laboratory determinations are complex and time consuming, and the possible etiologies of seizure disorders mount into the hundreds.

Nature of the Impairments

Seizures are an episodic disorder. Therefore, one must be very cognizant of the differences between the impairment created by the seizure disorder (the problems associated with the seizure itself), any impairments created by the underlying etiology, and the impairments, including the side effects, of treatment.

Primary Impairment

With rare exception, seizures last only a minute or two, and the postictal confusion and somnolence rarely persist for more than a few minutes or a few hours. This is the duration of the actual impairment. If seizures occur infrequently and do not involve profound hypoxia, measurable damage is minimal. Frequent seizures over many years clearly cause brain damage and can develop into a progressive encephalopathy.

Patients injure themselves in seizures. They fall, break bones, get burnt, and drown. If they are operating a motor vehicle or machine tools, they can hurt themselves or others. Nevertheless, although the risk of these injuries creates a disability, it is relatively small compared with the substantial degrees of secondary disability that face the patient with epilepsy.

Nonmedication Impairments

Persons with certain types of epilepsy have impairment of cognition independent of that which is attributable to medication. One of the most commonly reported of these impairments is memory impairment. This is not often measurable in the routine office visit because of the limitations of the "bedside" mental examination. Also, it may be very specific. An example is a patient who appeared to function normally but reported memory loss. Although the full-scale IQ of this individual was 109, memory was severely impaired, with 0 of 15 objects presented in a formal neuropsychological examination recalled after 60 minutes.

A number of epilepsy syndromes have memory loss or intellectual impairment as part of the syndrome. For example, persons with head injury have a number of difficulties. These may include poor impulse control, memory deficits, difficulties with foresight and planning, and loss of previously learned skills. AEDs could make these problems more severe. However, one must carefully evaluate the contribution to these issues from AEDs. Lowering medications too much and precipitating seizures can also cause problems. Often, memory functioning and other cognitive functions are impaired for several days after a tonic-clonic seizure. (See Chapter 6 for a more detailed discussion of persons with head injury.)

One of the more common causes of epilepsy in adults and children is mesial temporal sclerosis (MTS). The hippocampal structures, one of the main groups of anatomic structures that serve memory, are damaged and are a source of the seizures. With carefully performed MRIs, small losses of tissue may be detected. Although these patients have normal intellectual functioning, they have significant loss of memory. For example, persons with dominant speech hemisphere MTS may have profound difficulties with verbal memory but not visual memory, and vice versa. The seizures of MTS are complex partial (formerly called psychomotor or temporal lobe seizures) and are particularly refractory to treatment with AEDs. On the other hand, these patients can be candidates for surgery with a rate of elimination of seizures as high as 75%.[2,3] This can have a dramatic effect on the life of the patients, permitting them to drive and find employment and perhaps freeing them from the need to remain on AEDs with their consequent side effects.

Medication Impairments

Many patients with epilepsy complain that the side effects of AEDs are a greater problem than the seizures themselves. Difficulty with thinking, focusing thoughts, remembering, sleepiness, a sense of depression, and the loss of sexual desire and performance are serious impairments that need to be addressed by the physician.

All AEDs cause some degree of cognitive impairment even at "therapeutic" concentrations. Patients often describe this, but because very few studies have been reported in the medical literature, this issue is often not fully appreciated by physicians. Also, most of the tests of neuropsychological functioning are not sensitive enough to detect subtle cognitive impairment. In one study, volunteers who do not have seizures were given phenytoin and carbamazepine in doses similar to those used in patients with epilepsy. Both of these AEDs caused a statistically significant decrease in performance in some of the tests, but no difference was found between carbamazepine and phenytoin.[4] Our experience has been that some persons with epilepsy are not aware of cognitive side effects, but often, when admitted to our diagnostic unit and withdrawn from medications to record seizures, they report feeling much more awake and often are reluctant to resume medications. We have observed this with all of the standard AEDs, (valproate, phenytoin, carbamazepine, and phenobarbital), with phenobarbital causing the most impairment.

Particularly important can be the effects on learning and memory in schoolchildren placed on AEDs. One woman recalls how difficult she found it to read or to organize her thoughts to take tests when she was in high school. For example, she was unable to select answers when given multiple choices let alone take essay-type tests. Her grades in school were uniformly poor despite the fact that she worked very hard. She has, in adulthood, been able to take a graduate-level degree and glean information from reading material of even a very complex nature now that she is no longer on medication.

The goal of treating epilepsy is to achieve complete control with the least amount of drug. Many patients may have achieved complete control at a price that is too high in terms of side effects. Seizures may occur only a few times a year, but toxicity is present every day. In those patients whose seizures cannot be completely controlled anyway, it may be better to have a small increase in seizures with much less toxicity. Also, the type of seizure must be considered. Simple partial seizures—those with no loss of consciousness—often cannot be controlled completely. Attempts to do so usually result in toxicity. However, because patients often report these seizures as troublesome, attempts are made to suppress them with doses of medication that lead to toxicity. The patient should be educated as to the relative severity of seizures. Simple partial seizures do not, in many states, impair the ability to obtain a driver's license. For example, in Minnesota, the law specifies "loss of consciousness or loss of control" as the factors that restrict eligibility for a license. Thus, persons who are having only simple partial seizures may drive.

Nature of the Disabilities

People with seizures that cause a loss of consciousness cannot operate a car. This leads to severe handicaps in obtaining and retaining work, dating, and participating in community life. The social and psychological secondary disabilities of epilepsy are severe. In many ways, they are an artifact of modern civilization. In any case, most patients with epilepsy complain more about the secondary disability than the seizures themselves. People with epilepsy are discriminated against, both consciously and unconsciously. This makes employment and recreation more problematic. These individuals have difficulty in obtaining life insurance and health insurance as well.

Even though good seizure control has been reached, other problems may arise that affect the patient's QOL. Epilepsy is a complicated disorder. Patients who have their seizures controlled may have problems in functioning to their fullest capacity. These problems arise for a number of reasons. First, because the medicines used to treat epilepsy act in the CNS, they can cause neurotoxicity, which may not be easily recognized by others or even the patient. Also, many of the antiepileptic medications have metabolites that are not usually measured but may be present in toxic concentrations due to drug interactions or individual patterns of metabolism. Second, epilepsy may be caused by conditions that damage the brain. One example is damage to the hippocampal structures associated with MTS, which leads to significant difficulties with memory. Finally, because of the social stigma of epilepsy, many patients have internalized the negative feelings of society and lack self-esteem and the ability to function in a competitive job environment. Although important, control of seizures is not the only hurdle that must be overcome.

One should avoid severe and unnecessary restrictions for the patient. The risks should be graded on the degree of seizure control and the level of common sense that the patient displays. A patient is more likely to die from drowning in a bathtub than from an accident at work. Most patients with seizures require few limitations. One

girl recalls being removed from playing the flute in her school orchestra on the grounds that it might be too stressful. As a result, she was deprived of the only area in which she could excel and of the opportunity to feel part of one of the important social organizations in her school.

For many years, physicians talked about the so-called epileptic personality. Abnormal behavior may result from the same disturbance in brain function that produces seizures, but the personality problems of the patient with seizures usually result from a downward social spiral. Patients with seizures develop fears and anxiety, which can lead them to withdraw socially. Social withdrawal leads to social isolation, which in turn leads to frustration, anger, and alienation. A frustrated, angry patient is a difficult patient. Often, these factors also lead to personality disorders, neuroses, and psychoses. Avoiding social stigma must be part of any total management of persons with epilepsy.

It is important not to speak of the patient with seizures as "an epileptic." This tends to make the fact that the patient has seizures more central to individual identity than gender or name. Many patients with intractable seizures have become so isolated from society that they truly think of themselves as "epileptics." Although it takes more words, it is much better to speak of someone who "has epilepsy" or has "recurrent seizures." When the cause of the seizures has been identified, it is better to speak of a patient as having a brain scar that causes recurrent seizures.

In summary, seizures are relatively common in the population (9%); epilepsy, or recurrent seizures, is somewhat less so (approximately 3%). Despite this, seizure disorders are among the least well-understood medical conditions by general physicians and the population at large. The diagnosis is loaded with a broad variety of negative connotations, creating substantial psychological and social difficulties. Compared with the management of other chronic disorders such as diabetes or asthma, the U.S. health care system in general does a poor job. The reasons for the failure of the health care system reflect the relatively small amount of attention that has been given to organized systems of care and the development of appropriate centers of excellence.

The causes of the psychological and social problems with which the diagnosis of a seizure disorder becomes enmeshed are the result of the cultural environment in which we live. That culture abhors loss of control. By its very nature, a seizure disorder means that the individual has "lost control." If this is coupled with incontinence of bowel and bladder, attracting attention by falling to the ground or wandering around making funny noises, and the historical association of seizures with such diseases as tertiary syphilis and chemical dependency, the reason why major social problems exist becomes evident. In a bizarre manner, epilepsy is the last of the pornographic diseases. Our presidents talk openly of their cancers and of AD, sexually transmitted diseases are discussed at dinner or in church, and a major campaign is under way to talk about the various forms of mental illness, particularly depression. Yet almost no public figure has talked openly about seizures and epilepsy, even though this problem has touched the families of some of our most prominent leaders.

The physician who would do well by his or her patient with a seizure disorder must take on a broader job than simply making a proper diagnosis and writing a prescription. The physician should not only encompass the modern concepts of the treatment of persons with chronic disease (to which this book is dedicated) but also should recognize an advocate's role, removing the myths that surround the disorder and assisting the patient in dealing with the injustices that persons with seizures face in society.

Character of the Solution

Overall Plan

It is instructive to think of epilepsy as an example of a chronic disease. By definition, a chronic disease is a condition for which no quick cure is known. That means the patient must accept the fact that the aim of treatment is to live successfully with the problem, that it is not going to go away, and that compromises must be made. Perhaps the trickiest task is to get the patient to accept that this is a long-term process, which means that the patient must abandon the idea that he or she can be a passive recipient of treatment and walk out cured in a brief time. Once the patient understands this, it is possible to begin the steps that are necessary for successful treatment.

In treating chronic illness, it is important that the following needs are kept clearly in mind: (1) the need for clear therapeutic aims, (2) the need for a careful treatment plan, and (3) the need for the patient's cooperation and understanding. The structure of an ongoing treatment and planning process is described in detail in Chapter 2. The character of such an ongoing relationship for the management of persons with seizures must meet the criteria described in that chapter for continuity of care, comprehensive care, cost-effective care, and collaborative care. The goals of the ongoing interaction of the professional staff and the patient with epilepsy must be to lead to self-management. The professional staff should strive to maximize the patient's participation in the planning and treatment process. This involves the ability to participate in setting the objectives of treatment and monitoring the outcomes. It also involves the patient's recognizing the relationship between the outcomes and the actions taken as a basis for participation in the design of the treatment regimens. To the extent that the professional staff enables this participation, one creates in the person a sense of control. The very character of the disease is to have loss of the sense of control over one's body and one's life. Thus, the process of interaction as described in detail in Chapter 2 and as applied in this chapter to the problem of epilepsy specifically addresses the issue that the disease presents.

The goals of treating patients with epilepsy are straightforward: (1) freedom from seizures, (2) freedom from the disabling side effects of treatment, and (3) a full opportunity to enjoy all that life has to offer with minimal disease-related limitations (probably the most important measure of QOL). Successfully treating seizures while ignoring the chronic impact of the disease usually does not improve QOL. On the other hand, aggressively addressing the impact of seizures may significantly improve QOL even if medical treatment is not entirely successful. The comprehensive approach recognizes that both the seizures and their impact on the patient, in the patient's particular situation, must be addressed.

Aiming for complete freedom from seizures may seem excessive, but careful consideration reveals that this is not the case. Patients generally cannot drive unless seizures with impairment are completely controlled. Loss of driving privileges is a major handicap in most regions of the United States. The anxiety experienced by most patients with epilepsy derives from the inability to predict when the next seizure and the ensuing disruption of life are going to occur. This anxiety persists even if seizures occur relatively infrequently. Finally, most studies agree that employment prospects do not improve significantly unless seizure control is more or less complete.

What are the consequences of continuing seizures? Many caregivers and even some patients feel that one or more complex partial seizures per month are acceptable and do not require further aggressive attempts at seizure control. However, most evidence suggests that the risks of continued epilepsy are high. Longer duration of epilepsy has been consistently associated with decreased vocational status and increased emotional and psychiatric disability. Some evidence has been found that longer duration of epilepsy is associated with worsening memory. Other studies have suggested that the longer seizures are allowed to continue, the harder they are to control. Chronic treatment with some AEDs may cause neuropathy or dysmorphic effects or worsen the tendency for osteoporosis in women. Mortality in epilepsy is two to four times that in the general population. This is owing in part to the diseases associated with epilepsy. However, a substantial portion of increased mortality is due to accidents associated with seizures or the seizures themselves. Some of these, such as drowning or seizure-related motor vehicle accidents, can be prevented with appropriate education, but many cannot. Patients with epilepsy die suddenly and unexpectedly far more often than the general population. SUDEP occurs once every 300–1,000 patient-years and appears to be especially common in young patients with frequent seizures. One study has suggested that sudden death occurs more often in patients with continuing seizures than in individuals who have been successfully treated by epilepsy surgery.

In contrast, the risk of death associated with epilepsy surgery is almost nonexistent. The rate of significant complications with standard anterior temporal lobectomy is 1–2%. Clinically significant memory loss is rare, and patients with nondominant resections may actually experience some improvement in memory. The risks associated with epilepsy surgery in other regions of the brain may be somewhat higher but are generally acceptable.

Overall, studies indicate that the risks and disabilities associated with continuing seizures are higher than had been anticipated, while advances in surgical techniques continue to lower the risks of surgical treatment. It is therefore important to consider surgical intervention early, before the social and vocational disability associated with the longer duration of epilepsy has taken hold.

Fewer than 5% of patients treated with the newer AEDs or with vagal nerve stimulation have prolonged cessation of seizures. This is an important point because QOL improves significantly only when seizures are completely controlled for long periods of time. Furthermore, reduction of seizure frequency with the newer AEDs is generally not striking. Standard temporal lobectomy stops seizures in more than two-thirds of patients and in more than 80% of patients with MTS.[4] Studies in our patients have revealed that these benefits persist over the long term. Epilepsy associated with discrete cerebral lesions has a similar rate of success. Seizures outside the temporal lobe that are not associated with lesions generally respond somewhat less favorably, and the risk for complications is somewhat higher.

A thorough evaluation is necessary to determine the likelihood of surgical cure and the risk of complications. This is best performed at a comprehensive epilepsy center with extensive surgical experience. The risks and benefits of the various treatment options can be determined and discussed with the patient and the best possible treatment initiated. Epilepsy surgery is indicated when (1) seizures are disabling and medically refractory, (2) seizures emerge from a single discrete region, and (3) that region is not critical for normal function. How many medications should be tried before a patient's condition is considered refractory? The best evidence indicates that only approximately 20% of patients who do not respond to aggressive treatment with a single appropriate antiepileptic medication will respond to treatment with another antiepileptic medication. Only approximately 10% of the patients in whom two trials of monotherapy fail will respond to a third AED or two AEDs used together. Further manipulations are even less likely to help. Thus, epilepsy surgery should be seriously considered in patients in whom two trials of monotherapy and a trial of duotherapy fail. These trials can usually be completed in less than 2 years. A comprehensive re-evaluation should not be put off further to minimize the social and psychological disability associated with longer epilepsy.

The only definite contraindications to epilepsy surgery are a progressive neurologic disease or a medical illness associated with poor prognosis. Seizure foci in the dominant hemisphere, EEG evidence of bilateral abnormalities, moderate developmental delay, or psychiatric illness are not contraindications in the modern era. Similarly, practitioners should not be put off if seizures appear to emerge from a critical brain region. A comprehensive evaluation often enables one to make the distinction between areas of seizure onset and eloquent cortex, allowing surgical treatment.

Establishing an Individual Treatment Plan

In treating epilepsy, our aim is no seizures, no side effects, and a healthy outlook on life. It is important to try to get the patient completely seizure free. Despite being impaired by seizures for only a few minutes a year, the patient may be totally disabled. The patient with even one or two seizures a year is unable to drive, finds it much harder to obtain employment and educational opportunities, is discriminated against for both health and life insurance, and lives with constant fear and anxiety.

To achieve these aims, it is necessary for the patient to learn the following:

What is wrong (that he or she has seizures)
Why it is wrong (the cause of the seizures)
What the possibilities are for complete seizure control
What the prognosis is for a normal life

The treatment planning process must include the following:

Coming to an accurate diagnosis and sharing this with the patient
Establishing a goal for treatment together with the patient
Choosing an appropriate AED(s) as part of an overall regimen
Taking necessary steps to assure the patient's cooperation, understanding, and active participation in setting goals, monitoring outcomes, and helping to define the appropriate strategies, including the use of medications

This planning process necessitates no high-tech facility but does require time and thought. First, patients must be taught the general facts about epilepsy. They want to know about the types of epilepsy, the general types of causes, what tests and treatments are carried out, and information about AEDs—their use, side effects, and costs.

Using this as a base, patients should be taught the specific facts about their problem. They should know about the type of epilepsy, the etiology (if known), the results of the diagnostic tests, what drug is being prescribed, why the drug is being prescribed, when blood level tests are indicated, and the pharmacokinetics of their specific drug regimen. The choice of an AED(s) should be made according to seizure type, syndromic diagnosis, cost, the potential relative risk of side effects in the particular patient, and other factors.

The patient should also be taught about keeping a calendar of when seizures occur and when medicines are taken. The patient becomes a monitor of the degree to which he or she meets the goal and the effectiveness of the regimen. This permits reconstruction of events to see whether a deviation from the treatment plan has occurred or if the patient is simply not responding to what the physician thought was an appropriate AED. A general discussion of nonspecific precipitating factors, such as menstruation, loss of sleep, too much caffeine, stress, and so forth, and how they raise and lower the seizure threshold, is important. The patient must also be made aware of the possible interaction of AEDs with other drugs, including prescription, over-the-counter drugs (e.g., antihistamines), or illegal drugs. Finally, and hardly the least important, one must be sure that the patient and the family understand first aid for the specific seizures that the patient has, how to recognize the seizures, and what to do in the case of status epilepticus. No physician can make a patient accept the diagnosis, but every doctor can provide a confident assessment, empathy, and sympathy for the challenges that the patient faces, as well as support while the diagnosis and its implications are assimilated.

The value of such basic self-knowledge is illustrated in the following case. Joan T. felt hopeless and helpless. Her experience, she said, was that seizures seemed to occur no matter what she did. Over the years, she had seen several different physicians and had reached the conclusion that nothing could be done to help her. At the initial consultation, it was clear that Joan T. had no idea when her seizures occurred, whether she was taking her medication, and when she might be missing her medicines. Her sense of helplessness and hopelessness seemed to be all-pervading. The concept of maintaining an adequate blood level was explained to her, and she agreed to keep a careful diary to see whether the seizures were occurring because the choice of medicine was wrong or because not enough medicine was present in her body. Because it was obvious that she was not taking her medicine regularly, a nurse clinician set up regular weekly appointments with her to supervise the loading of her pillboxes and to review the calendar that she was keeping.

At the end of the month, it was clear that, now that she was taking her medicine regularly, seizures were under better control, but serum anticonvulsant determinations indicated that, for some reason, this patient was a rapid metabolizer and would benefit from higher than normal doses. The dose of her AED was increased to an appropriate point, and she became seizure free. Not only did her seizures come under control, but her pervasive sense of suffering, of feeling helpless, improved as she began to see that it was her actions in taking her medication that largely contributed to her control.

One cannot conclude that an AED is ineffective unless the patient keeps an accurate diary so that the physician together with the patient can determine seizure frequency in relation to adherence to the drug regimen. In association with blood levels and good adherence, one can make an initial evaluation of the rate of metabolism as well. The sense of control that the patient achieves by keeping an accurate diary and recognizing the association between adherence to the regimen and effectiveness of treatment is crucial to ongoing adherence.

Continuity of Care

Continuity and follow-up are essential. Once patients understand the basic facts about their condition, the physician can help them take charge of their life, teaching better coping skills and providing support during times of situational stress. Patients will become receptive to the importance of taking AEDs on schedule, especially when the use of a cal-

endar can show a direct relationship between not doing this and the occurrence of seizures.

The value of continuity of care is illustrated by the following case. Michael F. is a young man with juvenile myoclonic epilepsy whose seizures had been brought under complete control with valproic acid. Although it was difficult, he adhered to his regimen and took his medicines regularly four times a day. However, when he left home to go to college, seizure control was lost. At first, Michael and his family attributed the change to the stress of adjustment to college. However, when his seizures continued, they returned to the epilepsy clinic to review what could be done. With his agreement to the careful use of a calendar, it became clear to Michael as well as his physician that in the excitement and busyness of his college day, he was frequently missing one of his doses, usually the noontime one. In discussion with Michael, he selected from the choices offered the pattern that would be most reliable for him. The decision was to take his medication in conjunction with his usual pattern of brushing his teeth in the morning and again in the evening before going to bed. Although the dosage times would not be exactly every 12 hours, they appeared to be acceptable. By switching to divalproex sodium (Depakote), which can be taken twice a day, adherence improved, and seizures once again came under control.

With the initial choice of AEDs, and again with each change, the medication prescription, the half-life of the particular drugs, the dosing interval being used and why, and what to do in the case of missed doses should be reviewed with the patient. Patients tend not to take their medicines regularly. Those who are doing very well often forget their medicines and need to be reminded. Those who are doing poorly think the medicines are useless and do not take the regimen seriously. Both kinds of patients are best handled by random checks of blood levels. Variations of more than 20% suggest noncompliance and the need for renewed patient education.

One of the most valuable tools is a clinic run by a nurse clinician. Patients can come in as frequently as weekly, load their pillboxes under the supervision of the nurse clinician, ask questions, receive reassurance, and learn to participate in a social ritual that encourages long-term adherence to the treatment regimen. The patient should be allowed to help design the dosage regimen for his or her convenience. Complex dosing regimens are hard to follow, especially if the patient is leading a busy life. Many patients find it difficult to take a midday dose. Therefore, a twice-a-day dosage (breakfast and dinner or "every time you brush your teeth") should be used whenever possible. It is simple to remember and avoids losing an entire day's dose if pills are taken only once a day. Once-a-day dosage can be risky because missing one dose puts the patient at very high risk for a seizure.

Pillboxes with seven compartments are helpful. Patients should use two: one for AM and one for PM. In this way, they can tell at a glance whether they remembered to take their medications and can take a catch-up dose sooner, resulting in less risk of seizures or toxicity.

One should address common concerns and misunderstandings even if the patient does not voluntarily voice them. Many people have questions that they do not ask, such as

> If I have seizures, does it mean that I am going to go crazy?
> What about taking all these drugs? Am I going to get hooked on them?
> Will I die from a seizure?
> If I have children, will they get epilepsy?
> What about feelings of embarrassment after a seizure?
> Did I get epilepsy from my parents?

It is important to help the patient overcome the sense of hopelessness and helplessness. It is also important that the patient who is newly diagnosed with seizures be returned to employment as quickly as possible. After 4–6 months of unemployment, the likelihood of the patient becoming chronically unemployed or permanently disabled increases substantially.

Optimal Use of Antiepileptic Drugs

Crucial to the accomplishment of the goals of seizure control has been the appropriate use of medications. This requires ongoing follow-up to establish an optimal regimen. Except for circumstances that require management at specialized centers, a simplified classification is adequate to help select AEDs. Table 10-3 provides a description of seizure

Table 10-3. Classification of Seizure Types

Generalized seizures
Primary
   Absence
   Juvenile myoclonic
   Major motor (i.e., hereditary generalized tonic-clonic)
Secondary
   Lennox-Gastaut
   Mixed seizure disorder
   Secondary generalized
   Localization-related seizures:
Simple partial (no disturbance of consciousness)
Complex partial (with a disturbance of loss of consciousness)
Secondarily generalized
   Generalized tonic-clonic, secondarily generalizing from a partial seizure

types. Table 10-4 lists preferred antiepileptic medications in relation to type of seizure.

In general, the efficacy of a given drug is optimal within the therapeutic serum concentration range. However, this is a population statistic. Patients require individualized dosing, which may be higher or lower than the average, and, at a given dose, blood concentrations may be higher or lower than usual. This is particularly important for drugs with a narrow therapeutic window, such as AEDs. Some patients have seizure control with greater than or less than the so-called therapeutic serum drug concentration range without side effects. One of the most important tasks for the physician is to assure optimal treatment with medications. This requires the physician to be familiar with usual drug dosing and the therapeutic drug concentrations as well as to recognize the exceptions to those rules.

Optimization of an AED is the process by which the dose of an AED is slowly increased until seizure control is achieved or intolerable side effects occur. Ideally, seizure control is reached before side effects occur. Underlying this process is the awareness that the physician cannot be confined to the recommended dosing regimen or so-called therapeutic range.

All of the major AEDs are generally used on a milligram-per-kilogram-per-day dosage with more or less defined therapeutic serum concentrations. For example, if a phenytoin (Dilantin) trial is initiated, the package insert recommends starting the

Table 10-4. Preferred Antiepileptic Medicines*

Seizure Type	First Line	Second Line	Contraindicated
Simple partial	Dilantin	Felbatol	
	Tegretol	Mysoline	
	Neurontin	Topamax	
	Lamictal	Gabitril	
	Phenobarbital	Sabril	
		Klonopin	
Complex partial	Dilantin	Depakote	
	Tegretol	Gabitril	
	Lamictal	Topamax	
	Neurontin	Klonopin	
	Sabril	Mysoline	
	(West syndrome)	Phenobarbital	
		Felbatol	
Secondary	Dilantin	Topamax	
	Klonopin		
	(Lennox-Gastaut)		
Generalized absence	Zarontin	Lamictal	Phenobarbital
	Depakote		Mysoline
Generalized tonic-clonic	Dilantin	Lamictal	
	Tegretol	Topamax	
	Depakote	Phenobarbital	
		Mysoline	
Tonic/drop	Depakote	Klonopin	Phenobarbital
	Felbatol	Topamax	Mysoline
	Lamictal		
Myoclonic	Depakote		
	Klonopin		
	Lamictal		
	Zonisamide		

*Except for phenobarbital, all are registered trademarks.

patient on 300 mg per day. Studies show that fewer than 50% of the patients are in the therapeutic range (between 10 and 20 mg/liter) after that recommendation. A better approach is to calculate the initial maintenance dose as 4–7 mg/kg per day and to consider patient-specific criteria. For example, the elderly population of seizure patients needs lower milligram-per-kilogram-per-day dosing, whereas children need higher dosing. Questions to consider are

Is the patient on mono- or polytherapy?
How severe is the patient's seizure disorder?
Is the patient a hypo- or hypermetabolizer?

How sensitive is the patient to medication side effects?
What other drugs is the patient taking concomitantly?

The newer AEDs, such as gabapentin (Neurontin), lamotrigine (Lamictal), and topiramate (Topamax) may need slower or faster titration schedules based on a milligram-per-day dosing. Lamictal and Topamax must be titrated to maximum dose very slowly over 8–12 weeks to minimize the incidence of side effects. For example, clinical trials have shown that if Lamictal is added to a Depakote regimen too fast, the incidence of rash is increased. To guide use of those medications, titration guidelines and the maximum doses used in clinical trials are cited in the package insert.

Doses chosen for the clinical trials often are the best guess at the doses that can lead to seizure reduction and minimal side effects. Therefore, when optimization of the newer AEDs is attempted, a daily dose that may be higher than the package insert recommendation may be used. Patients whose doses are higher must have closely supervised care, including frequent complete blood counts, chemistry profiles, and AED levels. Frequent clinic and phone follow-up visits are used to evaluate treatment by monitoring seizure frequency and side effects.

The use of drug levels in seizure control is important primarily because the relationship between the serum concentration of the active drug and therapeutic effect is ordinarily closer than that between dose and effect. The same is true for minimizing side effects. In general, for each AED, a desired therapeutic effect is achieved within a specific range of serum levels. For the newer AEDs (Neurontin, Lamictal, Topamax), this relationship has not yet been established. It is thus particularly important to monitor drug levels despite some manufacturers' package insert claims to the contrary. Every patient has his or her own therapeutic level at which seizure control occurs or side effects appear. The data from the clinical trails were analyzed comparing plasma levels from all patients with reduction in seizures. The individual patient response versus individual plasma was not evaluated.

In cases of breakthrough seizures, measuring AED levels determines whether seizure increase might have been the result of lower AED levels, thereby guiding decisions in drug therapy (e.g., increasing the dose, assessing adherence, and so forth). Treatment with more than one drug at the same time often results in drug interactions from changes in absorption, protein binding, or elimination, thereby changing the therapeutic outcome in the patient. Serum levels reveal noncompliance in patients and can be used to help ensure that they take their medication as prescribed. The growing number of AEDs on the market continues to complicate therapy management for monitoring seizure frequency and side effects. Keeping pace with the usual dosing guidelines for all of the AEDs is a task in itself, and current literature advises the reader to do so.

Although problems may be present in persons being treated with a single AED, they are compounded in those who receive more than one drug for the treatment of epilepsy. This is often overlooked in persons receiving two or more antiepileptic medications who have blood levels in the low therapeutic range. For example, a patient with a carbamazepine level of 4.5 mg/liter (therapeutic range = 4.0–12.0 mg/liter) and a phenytoin level of 12 mg/liter (therapeutic range = 10–20 mg/liter) may have symptoms of toxicity that are overlooked or not considered to be from drugs because levels are low. However, the CNS of these patients is exposed to the total amount of drugs, which is quite high. Furthermore, the 10,11 epoxide of carbamazepine should be measured, as it also causes toxicity.

Blood levels can be misleading. Phenytoin and valproate are highly protein bound, but the usual methods for measuring these drugs determine only the total level. However, it is the unbound or "free" level that is in equilibrium with the receptor site and thus pharmacologically active. In some circumstances, the total level may appear to be low or in the therapeutic range, but the patient is experiencing toxicity. Because the levels are not elevated, one may not attribute the symptoms to the medicine. For example, phenytoin is 90% bound and 10% free. Thus, under normal circumstances, a total phenytoin level of 15 mg/liter is associated with an unbound concentration of 1.5 mg/liter, and the usual therapeutic range of 10–20 mg/liter based on the total is the equivalent of 1.0–2.0 mg/liter. Valproate is 90–95% protein bound, and the unbound fraction is larger at higher doses. Protein binding is abnormal in many situations. The most dramatic of these is in renal failure, in which protein binding is markedly abnormal and the free fraction may be as high as 20%. This translates into a total level of 15 mg/liter being associated with a free level of 3.0 mg/liter, well in the range of toxicity.

One common situation occurs in patients treated with both phenytoin and valproate, two drugs that compete for the same binding site. Almost always, when they are used together, the total levels may appear to be low, and still the patient experiences toxicity. Thus, it is not unusual to see a patient receiving both of these drugs whose total phenytoin is 15 mg/liter and total valproate is 60 mg/liter (therapeutic range = 40–100 mg/liter total or 4–10 mg/liter free) experience toxicity; however, the free phenytoin is 2.5 mg/liter and the free valproate is 20 mg/liter. Whenever a patient is experiencing symptoms of toxicity and the levels are in the normal range, one should suspect a problem with binding and order a free level.

Another pitfall arises from the fact that carbamazepine has an active metabolite, the 10,11 epoxide. Although it is relatively easy to measure this compound, it is not measured routinely. This metabolite is usually present as 20–40% of the parent drug. Thus, if the carbamazepine level is 8 mg/liter, the epoxide level may be 1.6–3.2 mg/liter. The epoxide is metabolized by an enzyme, epoxide hydrolase, which is inhibited by valproate or may be deficient genetically in some individuals. It is not unusual to see a patient who is receiving valproate and carbamazepine appearing toxic, but with a carbamazepine level of 8 mg/liter. However, this person may have an epoxide level of 5 or 6 mg/liter. Because the parent and epoxide are similar in potency, this is the equivalent of a carbamazepine level of 13–14 mg/liter.

Occasionally a person who is genetically deficient in the epoxide hydrolase enzyme is encountered. This may occur in up to 5% of the population. An example is a patient who had ataxia and nystagmus that were not considered to be related to her carbamazepine, the levels of which had been measured to be between 4 and 7 mg/liter. Her 10,11 epoxide level, however, was higher than that of the parent drug, in the 6–9 mg/liter range. Symptoms resolved when carbamazepine was discontinued.

The value of continuity of care in relation to the optimal use of AEDs is illustrated by the story of John F. His was an apparent success story. He experienced his first complex partial seizure as a teenager. He was treated with Dilantin successfully and was seizure free for more than 30 years. He married, raised a family, and considered himself under complete control. His QOL began to deteriorate as he approached the age of 50 years. He felt depressed and had difficulty maintaining an erection. After consulting with his family physician and psychiatrist, he sought a consultation at the epilepsy clinic to see if something in his AED regimen could be adjusted. An evaluation revealed that the Dilantin in his blood had gradually crept up to toxic levels, manifested in part by end-point nystagmus and slight ataxia. His Dilantin dosage was adjusted, and he felt more energetic but still had difficulty in maintaining an erection. Rather than attribute this problem to his age alone, he was started on carbamazepine (Tegretol), and the Dilantin was discontinued. He continued to be seizure free but no longer had erectile dysfunction. This particular problem cannot be attributed consistently to any one drug. Some patients do better on Dilantin than Tegretol. However, any inquiry into the QOL of persons with epilepsy should include sexual function.

Comprehensive Care

Physicians soon realize that drug management alone does not ensure that patients with epilepsy will be able to learn, work, and live normally. Children with seizures can have physical and cognitive problems that require coordinated interdisciplinary care. Many youths and young adults face difficult life decisions that are further complicated by their epilepsy. If physicians limit their role to manipulating medications, they fall short of ensuring the patient's well-being.

The value of a broader approach to the management of seizures is illustrated by the following case. Phillip W. had a difficult time achieving complete seizure control. However, on a combination of Tegretol and Lamictal, his complex partial seizures with rapid secondary generalization had been brought under complete control. Phillip went off to college and soon recognized that lack of sleep, excessive caffeine intake, and beer drinking were particular problems for him. After a stormy first semester, he took control of his life and, despite the intense nature of his college experience, he again achieved seizure control. After he graduated from college, however, to his dismay, seizures recurred. He was adhering to his drug regimen and getting adequate sleep and did not use caffeine or alcohol. Nonetheless, seizures occasionally recurred. He returned to the epilepsy clinic for advice. We knew Phillip to be a very intense, high-strung young man. His new job thrust him into constant contact with the public, and he had to be "on." He was taught the basics of meditation and encouraged to use simple sitting-at-your desk meditation techniques, particularly controlled breathing. Phillip learned to recognize when he was getting overly excited and to use meditation to center himself. He has subsequently been seizure free and has been promoted to sales manager of his company.

The physician cannot and should not feel responsible for directing all aspects of life for the individual with epilepsy. The physician should, however, take a leadership role within the broader human services system. A large part of disability suffered by most patients with seizures lies in the area of self-esteem and coping. If patients believe that they are of little worth and if they have no mechanisms with which to cope, they almost certainly become passive and aimless. Early intervention is necessary to avoid the development of this defeatist attitude. The use of counselors, psychologists, social workers, and group therapy to deal with the problem once it has developed is essential if these individuals are to be helped. Patients with seizures are physically impaired only a few minutes to a few hours each year when the seizures are actually occurring, but a great many are totally disabled because of the related social and psychological problems.

The diagnosis of epilepsy can have far-reaching psychological effects in the life of the person. One cannot overestimate the importance of the changes that have occurred over the past years with the development of more openness in dealing with the stigma of the disease. This is illustrated in the story of Kathy H., who is now in her 40s. As a 5-year-old child, she had the first of two grand mal seizures. She recalls being placed "in a cage" when she was put in a crib to have an EEG. She did not understand what had happened and why she was told that she was someone special who had to take medication in school by going to the nurse's office each day. Her family did not discuss what had happened to her to justify their concern, expressed as anger, when she did not take her medication. Her family also discouraged her from being physically active. She felt not only that she was different but also that she must have done something very bad to justify being deprived of what other children were permitted to do. As a high school student, she became more informed about having had a seizure on the occasion of her second grand mal, yet her knowledge remained limited. She recalls only that she found herself back in bed that morning after having gotten out of bed at her normal time. Only after this episode was the word fits used. She remained on Dilantin and later became pregnant without being informed of any contraindications to doing so. She eventually ceased taking medication because of its continued effects on her memory when she entered a college program after the birth of her son. She has remained free of seizures associated with loss of consciousness while off medication for the past 25 years. However, she still recalls the sense of social isolation as a teenager that affected her entire life.

Schools, vocational agencies, public health programs, and other community agencies often call on the physician for consultation. Providing medical information about epilepsy may help more than in any other way to eliminate unnecessary concerns and restrictions imposed by authorities who may not fully understand seizure disorders. Individuals and families rely on the physician's recommendation and endorsement of programs and services. The issues may range from eligibility to attend summer camp to fitness for an occupation. In these cases, the physician's knowledge of which specialized programs are available can make an important difference.

It is difficult to change programs, residential opportunities, and vocational opportunities. A physician's position of leadership in the community gives him or her a special opportunity to bring about favorable change. Accurate medical knowledge and support are needed if community officials are to be helped to increase the options that are available to individuals with epilepsy.

In addition to controlling seizures, the physician may need to address certain other problem areas:

Personal feelings of the patient about seizures, especially poor self-image and social withdrawal

How the patient deals with these feelings

How the patient copes with the real problems created by the seizures

How family members deal with their feelings and with those of the patient

Changes in lifestyle, such as revised safety precautions at home and at work, failure to receive a driver's license

Discrimination in employment

Women of Childbearing Potential

Women of childbearing age who also have seizures have special needs and encounter unique risks. Their management is an example of a comprehensive approach to persons with epilepsy. One must help them make wise choices, especially about pregnancy and childbirth. Most women with epilepsy can have a healthy baby. Like all women, they can avoid pregnancy if they choose. Because of the special risks that epilepsy and antiepileptic medicines create for women who can have children, however, all women with epilepsy should plan their pregnancy carefully.

All women who can possibly become pregnant should take vitamins, even if they are not sexually active. Many authorities recommend that they take two multivitamins per day, providing 0.8 mg folic acid. Women who are not using birth control and who are taking valproic acid (Depakene), Depakote, or Tegretol need more, at least 3 mg folic acid per day. Taking 3–4 mg folic acid a day has been shown to reduce spina bifida in the babies of women who are taking Depakote or Tegretol.

Overall, the birth control pill provides the highest degree of reliability for contraception. Women who are taking antiepileptic medicines require special attention from their doctors in choosing the proper pill. The AEDs speed up the metabolism of the liver, and the minipill is rarely strong enough to provide adequate protection. One should use a pill with a higher dose of estrogen and progesterone. Breakthrough bleeding between menses is a marker that may identify a woman who requires a larger dose. Another concern is the effect of hormones on seizures. Some women notice increased seizure activity at the time of ovulation or menses, or both, referred to as catamenial epilepsy. Treatments for catamenial epilepsy have included intermittent acetazolamide therapy and hormonal supplementation with varied results. Hormonal therapy has been reported to have an effect on seizures in animal models of epilepsy: High doses of estrogen are epileptogenic, whereas progestins decrease epileptogenic activity. Few women with seizures have changes in seizure activity when using hormonal contraception. Hormonal supplementation in menopause has not been well studied but, as far as we know, is well tolerated.

For most women, the biggest risk surrounding pregnancy is to have a baby that is not formed perfectly. Many women try to avoid taking any medicines while they try to get pregnant and while carrying the baby for fear of potential harm. Stopping antiepileptic medicines, however, is very dangerous. Especially if they are stopped abruptly, frequent and serious seizures can result.

The issues that face a woman who takes medicines to control seizures are complex. Both seizures, especially generalized tonic-clonic seizures, and AEDs can present a risk to the unborn baby. Seizure control may change during pregnancy. Approximately one-third of the women who get pregnant find that their seizures get worse. About one-third get better, and about one-third report no change. In many cases, the seizures get worse because the pregnancy speeds up liver metabolism, and the blood level of the antiepileptic medicine drops. This tends to be particularly true during the last 3 months of pregnancy. For this reason, all pregnant women who are taking AEDs should consult closely with their neurologist and obstetrician. They need to be closely and regularly followed and their antiepileptic medicine blood levels closely monitored.

Particularly important is the prevention of birth defects by taking folic acid. Most birth defects are mild, correctable, and impossible to detect before birth. Spina bifida (and similar neural tube defects), however, is detectable. At appropriate times during her pregnancy, a woman who is taking AEDs should have a serum α-fetoprotein level drawn. This is usually done at 15–16 weeks of gestation. Whether this is positive or negative, a high-definition ultrasound examination by an experienced examiner should be performed at 19 weeks. Women with babies with proven neural tube defects can elect to have a therapeutic abortion. Amniocentesis should only be performed if the α-fetoprotein level is elevated and the high-definition ultrasound fails to positively exclude a neural tube defect.

Any woman with epilepsy is considered to have a potentially high-risk pregnancy. Nonetheless, nearly all of these women go through their pregnancies without trouble. Certain complications of pregnancy are increased to a small degree in women with epilepsy. These include preeclampsia, abruptio placentae, polyhydramnios, and intrauterine growth retardation. A more frequent problem may be an increased tendency for the baby to bleed. It seems that the liver metabolizes vitamin K more quickly when a woman is taking antiepileptic medicines. Just before delivery, many obstetricians give a vitamin K supplement to a pregnant woman who is taking these drugs.

Cost-Effective Care

Ordinary cases of epilepsy respond to ordinary doses of ordinary medicine. If the primary care physician is confident of the diagnosis of seizure type and the syndromic diagnosis, it is relatively straightforward to choose among current AEDs. If two AEDs have been tried in monotherapy and the patient is still not responding to care, a referral is indicated. The referral should be to a comprehensive epilepsy center if the primary care physician practices in a community where one is readily available. If not, or if one's usual neurologic consultant manages intractable epilepsy well, the neurologist should be consulted. A neurologist should be capable of coming to a reasonably precise diagnosis of seizure type and syndromic diagnosis. After the patient has been tried on three major antiepileptic medications either in monotherapy or in combination, he or she can be considered medically intractable, and a referral can be made. If the neurologist has not achieved complete seizure control within 1 year, the matter should be discussed between the primary care physician and the neurologist, and a referral to a high-quality comprehensive program should be considered. On the average, intractable epilepsy continues for 10–15 years before referral to a center such as MINCEP Epilepsy Care. Exposure to the risk of SUDEP can be decreased by earlier referral. The reality of SUDEP may prompt earlier consideration of epilepsy surgery, especially if the patient has one of the surgically remediable epilepsy syndromes.

A leading managed care text has reviewed the treatment of epilepsy.[5] This review proposes a plan centered on a specialized epilepsy center based on the criteria for referral as described previously. The model includes

> An accurate diagnosis of whether the patient has epilepsy, some other problem, a mixture, or both
> A precise, accurate diagnosis of seizure type and syndrome
> A treatment plan for long-term care, including whether pharmacologic, surgical, or other treatment options, or some combination, are appropriate
> An evaluation of the psychosocial and social factors that affect the disorder

Systematic consultation and follow-up to other treatment physicians, including assistance in the event of acute difficulties in particularly intractable cases
Education of the patient to offer additional control to the patient, provide tools for self-management, and minimize the sense of isolation and of being different
Treatment of a sufficient number of patients with a wide range of seizure disorders to enable the center to offer a full range of diagnosis and treatment modalities
Creation of a detailed treatment plan articulating the specialized center's role and the primary treating physician's role and identifying useful patient and community agencies
A care management team to carry out treatment plans for patients with intractable seizures or to collaborate with treating physicians as they carry out the treatment plan
Measurement of the success of individual treatment plans to enable their appropriate modification when necessary
Collection of cost information
Modification of plans when appropriate in consideration of cost data
Assistance to the patient to obtain approval for coverage from insurer or health maintenance organization for specialized epilepsy services

A specialized epilepsy center is staffed full-time with an interdisciplinary team that focuses on epilepsy diagnosis and treatment issues and includes

Clinical neurophysiologic diagnostic technologists and support staff
Clinical psychologist (with specialized experience)
Epileptologist (neurologist with additional fellowship in interpreting diagnostic tests for seizures and treating patients with a wide variety of seizure disorders)
Neuropsychologist (with specialized experience)
Nurse clinician
Pharm.D. (Doctor of Pharmacy)
Health care professionals from related practices, including neurosurgeon, radiologist, and social worker
Affiliation of the epilepsy team with appropriate hospitals and receiving appropriate univer-

sity credentials (some medical schools have little or no knowledge base about the modern treatment of epilepsy)

Administrative leadership with advanced degrees in finance, accounting, and law who are responsible for understanding the purpose, goals, and procedures of the specialized epilepsy center

Nothing can substitute for clear communication with the treating physician, especially if the treating physician is a generalist and the patient cannot return regularly to the specialized center. A precise diagnosis, a clearly described treatment plan, outcome measures, and ready telephone consultation help ensure a good outcome. The Centers for Disease Control and Prevention of the U.S. Public Health Service has accepted the definition of seizure control as "no seizures and no side effects." A few patients have such severe brain damage that this goal cannot be reached. However, the great majority of patients who today continue to have seizures or have unacceptable side effects can reach that goal with expert help.

Consideration for Surgical Treatment

Any patient whose seizures have not responded to antiepileptic medications should be referred for an evaluation to determine proper treatment. QOL is an important consideration in determining when a patient should be referred to a seizure specialist. AEDs may not be the appropriate treatment, and it may be necessary for the patient to undergo surgery for epilepsy. This is best determined by an experienced group of epileptologists at a comprehensive epilepsy center. A good working definition is that patients have uncontrolled epilepsy or refractory seizures when one or more major AEDs have failed at levels pushed to the point of toxicity. When the diagnosis has been correctly made and is precisely known, the likelihood of a patient responding with complete seizure control to a second AED (when the first has failed) is approximately 30%. After the first two AEDs are tried, the likelihood of response to a third drops to less than 10%. The percentage decreases with each increasing drug trial. On the other hand, if the diagnosis has been improperly made (e.g., diagnosing complex partial seizures instead of juvenile myoclonic

epilepsy), a simple outpatient visit may result in complete seizure control.

Physicians who are unfamiliar with the major advances and the safety and efficacy of all brain surgery, and especially of elective procedures, are often unduly concerned about subjecting their patients to neurosurgery. Why should a patient take the risk of surgery for the treatment of seizures? The logic is really based on weighing relative risk. Someone who is completely controlled without any side effects obviously should not consider surgery. However, someone who is having frequent seizures and is at risk for injury or death, or is totally disabled (not able to work or drive), would certainly want to consider taking the risk. Weighing the factors of those patients who are in between requires a thorough understanding of the type of seizures the patient has, the prognosis of that particular type of epilepsy, the relative likelihood of successful outcome from surgery, and the likelihood of complications. The goal of the treatment of epilepsy is no seizures and no side effects. A patient may be completely disabled by side effects but may be impaired for only 3 minutes a month with seizures.

Evaluation first aims at confirming the diagnosis of epilepsy and epilepsy syndrome. Of patients who present for comprehensive evaluation, 20–30% actually have nonepileptic events that mimic epileptic seizures. This distinction may be impossible until habitual attacks are observed. Similarly, comprehensive evaluation allows secure diagnosis of epilepsy syndrome. This assures that appropriate AED therapy has been given and that simply using another class of AEDs will not result in substantial improvement.

Video-EEG monitoring conclusively addresses these two issues and is critical in the evaluation for epilepsy surgery. Clinical features of the seizures and examination during the seizure yield further useful clues regarding side and location of seizure onset. Longer samples of interictal activity including computerized spike and seizure detection reveal areas with higher likelihood for seizure onset. MRI detects cerebral lesions and MTS. Routine MRI is not sensitive enough; special sequences and thin serial sections parallel to the long axis of the hippocampus are necessary. Neuropsychometric testing establishes a baseline and helps detect areas of cerebral dysfunction. Intracarotid amobarbital (Amytal) testing establishes the hemisphere of language dominance and indicates whether learning can occur with resection of either temporal lobe. Functional MRI readily identifies cerebral regions that are necessary for simple motor function. Functional MRI investigations of the cerebral networks used in learning and other cognitive tasks have yielded complicated results that do not have clinical utility at present. A thorough psychological evaluation is critical to determine patient expectations and readiness for invasive procedures or surgery.

More than two-thirds of the time, location and side of seizure onset can be determined with this noninvasive information alone. Furthermore, intracranial recording is not necessary in seizures that start in the dominant temporal lobe if MTS is present. On the other hand, intracranial recording generally is necessary if side of seizure onset is unclear, if an epileptogenic lesion or MTS is absent, if noninvasive evaluation is contradictory, or if seizures appear to emerge from areas of functional cortex. With intracranial recording the precise area of seizure onset can usually be determined. Cortical stimulation studies can be used to define functional areas of cortex. The surgical approach is then tailored to remove areas involved in seizure onset while sparing areas that are vital for normal function.

The various surgical procedures have been detailed.[4] Anterior temporal lobectomy removes 3–5 cm of anterior temporal neocortex and virtually the entire hippocampus. This is the most common form of epilepsy surgery and is indicated for seizures that emerge from the temporal lobe. Lesionectomy removes epileptogenic lesions and a small area of surrounding cortex; it is indicated when seizures are associated with a discrete epileptogenic lesion. Nonlesional neocorticectomy removes areas of brain that are involved in seizure onset; because no lesion is present to guide the neurosurgeon, extensive intracranial recording is necessary. Hemispherectomy removes an entire cerebral hemisphere; this is indicated when seizures emerge from one hemisphere and that hemisphere is severely damaged by a congenital lesion. Although this may seem a dramatic and radical intervention, congenital lesions usually result in transference of function to the healthy hemisphere. Complete resection of the diseased hemisphere generally results in cure without loss of function. Corpus callosotomy sections the white matter pathways that connect the two hemispheres; this procedure is very effective with atonic seizures but does not help with other seizure types. Multiple

subpial transection consists of multiple superficial incisions in cortical gray matter perpendicular to the cortical surface. In theory, this procedure interrupts lateral spread of seizures while allowing normal function. This may be a helpful adjunct when the seizure onset zone includes vital cortex, and thus, cannot be entirely removed. At present, little indication has been found that multiple subpial transections by themselves are helpful, and neurologic function after these procedures has not been carefully evaluated.

Patients with MTS or discrete epileptogenic cerebral lesions, such as low-grade tumors, cavernous hemangiomas, or hamartomas, should be considered for epilepsy surgery after two or three AED trials have failed. These patients generally have good outcome after surgery, with 70–90% achieving complete control of seizures. It is important not to delay longer so that the social, psychological, and vocational consequences of chronic epilepsy can be prevented. We have had good success in most other circumstances as well, although the likelihood of cure may be somewhat lower. Overall, surgery is substantially more likely to result in cure than further AED manipulations in these situations. Therefore, even "less than ideal" patients deserve an aggressive evaluation and an informed discussion of the various treatment options available so that they can help decide whether to proceed with intracranial evaluation or further anticonvulsant treatments.

It has long been clear that seizure surgery usually stops seizures or significantly decreases their frequency. Several studies confirm that this surgery also improves employment and mood. Studies in our patients have further confirmed that patients use fewer medical resources and feel more confident socially after epilepsy surgery. However, thorough education before surgery and further support after operation are important to maximize benefit. It is important to set realistic goals before surgery.

The NeuroCybernetic prosthesis (vagus nerve stimulator) has been approved, offering yet another treatment option. Once in place, the stimulator delivers a mild electrical current at intervals of approximately every 5 minutes for a duration of approximately 1 minute. This causes hoarseness so that the patient and others know the device is on. The stimulator parameters can be altered externally, and a software program is available to adjust the device for the optional settings for each patient. In addition, the prosthesis can be activated by patients when they experience an aura. This is done by placing a magnetic device on the stimulator. Overall, a few patients have been rendered completely seizure free, approximately 30% have had greater than 50% reduction in seizure frequency, and the remaining patients have had some or no improvement.

People with seizures need access to early, accurate diagnosis of the disorder. The following case studies clearly illustrate how early intervention and a well-defined, long-term management plan could have had a positive impact on QOL issues for these patients, often many years earlier.

At the age of 6 months, J.S. had a severe head injury and experienced a 12-hour seizure. A second seizure occurred when he was 10 months old, and he was treated with phenobarbital. This did not control his seizures, which continued at the rate of two or three per month until he was 13 years old. He was completely seizure free on other AEDs for 4 years. Medicine was discontinued, and he remained seizure free for 2 years. When he was 20 years old, however, seizures recurred with increased frequency and severity. They were primarily complex partial, although he did have two generalized tonic-clonic seizures. After 3 years, his neurologist concluded that this patient qualified as having intractable epilepsy. After an appropriate workup, a right temporal lobectomy was performed, and he has been seizure free for the last 4 years without medication.

M.D. is a young woman who was 13 years old when she experienced her first seizure, initially diagnosed as absence in type. However, a few years later, this diagnosis was recognized as being incorrect, and a diagnosis of complex partial seizures was made. An MRI suggested a lesion in the mesial temporal portion of the temporal lobe. Despite the presence of a lesion and clearly focal seizures that were intractable to several antiepileptic medications, her physicians continued to try varying combinations of medications. She was referred to an epilepsy center when she was 21 years old. Presurgical workup indicated the onset of seizures from the right temporal area. The final pathologic diagnosis was that of a well-differentiated astrocytoma. The lesion was completely excised, and the patient has been seizure free without medications for 4 years.

B.G. is a 48-year-old woman who lives in a rural town in a very rural state. She has a 31-year history of intractable epilepsy. Symptoms began when she was 17 with a complex partial seizure in which she suddenly began speaking gibberish. Over the past 31 years, the seizures have tended to cluster. B.G. may go 3 weeks without a seizure but then have five or six in 1 day. She had her only generalized tonic-clonic seizure when medicines were withdrawn for abdominal surgery. Initially seen by a family physician in a rural town, she consulted with neurologists beginning approximately 10 years before she was seen at an epilepsy center. Past medical records indicate that the seizures were identified as being focal in nature more than 20 years ago and that they probably involved the left side of the brain.

By the time B.G. was evaluated, the focal nature of her seizures was clear, as was the left hippocampal atrophy, but she had already kindled and she had involvement in both temporal lobes. Under the circumstances, she could not be offered surgery.

One could proceed with a careful pharmacotherapeutic analysis addressed at how best to manage B.G.'s medications. One trial of Tegretol had previously failed, but before that was thoroughly tried, she was switched to Neurontin. She had been on phenobarbital all of her life, so we have no idea whether it is effective. She had been on Dilantin for 30 years. This medicine had good efficacy but had never been used in monotherapy. A detailed treatment plan was worked out, emphasizing Dilantin monotherapy, subsequent to retrial of Tegretol or, if that fails, trial on Lamictal.

S.S. is a 29-year-old woman whose seizure onset occurred at the age of 5 years while she was in kindergarten. She has never gone longer than 3 months without seizures since then. The seizures are stereotyped and are complex partial. The focal nature of her seizures was noted by the first of three neurologists whom she consulted over the years since puberty. At no point was the possibility of a surgical intervention suggested despite the fact that she had been on all the major antiepileptic medications. Evaluation revealed a left MTS with onset of seizures from the left temporal lobe without any indication of right temporal involvement. Neurospsychological studies revealed that, although she is left hemisphere–dominant for speech and language, verbal and visual memory are both mediated by the right hemisphere, with the left hemisphere having limited memory capacity. Despite the fact that she had uncontrolled seizures for 27 years, she had not yet involved the right temporal lobe in an epileptiform process. She is thus a candidate for a left temporal lobectomy.

Millions of dollars are wasted every year on AEDs that are ineffective, CT scans that are useless, MRIs that are technically inadequate or provide data that are not properly used, and EEGs that are meaningless. If we are to provide cost-effective care, we must overcome the habit of performing unnecessary diagnostic tests and providing ineffective treatment. The most cost-effective strategy is for the initial evaluation to be performed by the most qualified expert and for the day-to-day treatment to be carried out according to a careful, expert treatment plan by the family doctor. Any patient who is not completely seizure free without side effects should be evaluated in an expert center.

Collaborative Care

Most patients with uncomplicated seizures can be brought under complete control and will have no further seizures within 90 days from the start of treatment. Using the principle of starting with one drug and increasing the dose to just short of toxicity solves the seizure problem for the great majority of patients. This assumes, of course, that the type of seizure has been properly identified and the appropriate drug has been selected. The difficult patient, therefore, is one who continues to have seizures despite standard treatment.

If the patient continues to have seizures, one of three situations must apply. Either the diagnosis is wrong, the treatment is wrong, or the treatment is theoretically correct but the patient is not carrying out the regimen. This seemingly simple statement provides a clear guide to the orderly thinking that is necessary to come to grips with the patient who is not doing well. Physicians faced with a patient who continues to have seizures need to re-evaluate the diagnosis, treatment, and patient adherence to the treatment plan. At the same time, physicians should do some self-examination. Are they the right physician for this patient at this time? Do they have a good relationship, does the patient trust them, does the patient require the attention of a specialist?

Is the Diagnosis Correct?

Does the patient have epilepsy or something else? The differential diagnosis with epilepsy includes both physiologic and psychological nonepileptic events, migraine headaches, breath-holding attacks, and so forth. The diagnosis of epilepsy can rarely be made with certainty in the absence of capturing one of the seizures with combined video and EEG recording. Nonetheless, most patients can be treated on the basis of a presumptive diagnosis, and if they respond to treatment this is good enough. However, when the seizures do not stop, one must re-examine the diagnosis and go back to fundamentals.

If the patient does indeed have epilepsy, does he or she have one or more than one kind of seizure? Perhaps the AED chosen is working for one kind of seizure but does not control a second type. Often the patient and the family are unable to make a distinction until the physician has witnessed all the types of seizures on video-EEG and can help them make that distinction.

Is the Treatment Correct?

It must be remembered that the patient, not the blood level, should be treated. One cannot be sure that the patient has been tried on adequate dosages of the drug until that drug has been pushed to toxicity. It should not be assumed that the drug is ineffective until the pharmacokinetics of that drug are reconsidered in the context of this particular patient. If the dosing intervals are too long, the drug may be effective for only a portion of the day. It should be remembered that half-lives decrease with polypharmacy and may be decreased by self-induction of certain drugs such as Tegretol. One should try checking both fasting levels and the level just before a subsequent dose—it may answer this question.

It should be kept in mind that Dilantin and Tegretol occasionally paradoxically produce seizures if the serum level is too high. The increased levels may occur without signs of clinical toxicity. This problem should be considered if the Dilantin level is more than 40g/ml or the Tegretol level exceeds 10 g/ml.

Is the Patient Carrying Out the Regimen?

If the diagnosis and the choice of anticonvulsant are right and the patient is still having seizures, one should ask oneself whether the patient is following the treatment plan. If he or she is not, it is necessary to undertake a different series of maneuvers. In general, a simple way to determine whether the patient is taking the medicine is to measure serum

Table 10-5. Managing Nonadherence

When the problem is lack of information:
  Use patient education materials
  Use staff members as a resource for education
  Check to see if the patient understood the explanation given at the previous visit
When the problem is psychological:
  Remove rewards for inappropriate behavior that seeks secondary gain
  Give rewards for appropriate behavior
When the patient uses denial:
  Confront the patient in a nonthreatening manner
  Use a gradual and gentle approach
  Provide emotional support but also provide reality
When the problem is cognitive:
  Identify the problem and work with those who care for the patient so that they are able to help him or her comply
If the patient is drug dependent or an alcoholic:
  Seizure control cannot be approached while the patient is drug dependent and metabolism is fluctuating rapidly
  Consider recommending social intervention or sheltered living

drug levels on three different occasions. Preferably, the blood samples should be taken at the same time of day, and the patient should not be aware that noncompliance is suspected. If the three serum drug levels, measured at the same time in relation to the dose, show variation of greater than 20% among them, the question of poor adherence to the dosage schedule should be raised.

Particularly important for effective care is enlisting the patient to the maximal extent possible in managing the regimen. Use of the term compliance or noncompliance implies a relationship in which the patient is to follow orders in the form of prescriptions. More appropriate to the management of chronic problems that require long-term and frequently far-reaching commitment is a higher degree of patient participation in the design and ongoing review of treatment regimens. The use of terms such as adherence can reflect a higher level of collaboration in the design of plans, with subsequent greater commitment to follow through. Measurement of the level of participation achieved can enhance the likelihood of higher levels of participation. A scale is described in Chapter 2. It deals with the varying levels of verbal participation in the planning process—definition of goals, monitoring of progress in relation to the goals, and design of regimens.

If the patient is not adhering to the treatment plan (Table 10-5), one should consider whether the patient

Understands the need to do so
Understands what is necessary to do
Wants to adhere
Is permitted to follow the physician's treatment plan

The patient who does not understand the need to follow instructions may not have understood the initial explanation. Most people need to hear instructions several times. Some patients may be of very low intelligence. Particularly troublesome is the patient with a short memory span. The impaired memory may be the result of the organic brain damage that initially led to seizures, can be an effect of brain damage and senility in older age, or can be related to toxic effects of the prescribed AEDs. These persons are usually dependent on other people: parents, spouse, or counselors. It is necessary to train these other individuals to help the patient. Simple overlearning techniques to help the patient are often effective. A week's supply of pills can be laid out in an egg carton or a pillbox. The patient is instructed not to go to bed at night without taking all the pills that are left from that day's section.

The patient may have understood exactly what the physician wanted but did not understand why it is so important. Such a patient needs to be re-educated. One should explain again to the patient what needs to be done and why. It may be worthwhile to have the patient visit the office nurse on several occasions for reinforcement. One helpful maneuver is to have the patient keep a log of the drug that he or she takes, the time it is taken, and when the seizures occur. This reinforces the importance of taking medicines regularly and helps the patient to draw his or her own conclusions.

The patient may not be able to comply because of psychological incapacity: Many patients use denial. They become so anxious at the thought of having seizures and of having to take medicines indefinitely that, psychologically, the problem becomes too difficult to face. The patient should be confronted, but in a nonthreatening manner. A gradual and gentle approach is required. On the other hand, it is important to help the patient face reality. Alternatively, the patient may become so frustrated and unhappy over the thought of having to take medicines and over the implications of having seizures that he or she becomes angry. The same phenomenon is seen in patients with juvenile diabetes. If the physician can avoid getting angry in return, the problem usually can be worked out.

Much more troublesome are the patients who have a substantial amount of secondary gain as a result of having seizures. They get a great deal of attention, and their dependency needs are met. For example, perhaps the only way to get financial help from parents or the welfare system is to be disabled. It is necessary to remove the reward and give the patient some other type of gratification. This is easier said than done, especially with the patient whose dependency needs are seemingly limitless.

If the patient is alcoholic or drug dependent, seizure control can rarely be successfully approached. Rapid changes in metabolism and erratic behavior are to be expected. Social intervention, and possibly sheltered living, may be necessary before seizures can be brought under control.

In general, one of the most effective techniques for helping patients take their medicine regularly is close attention. If patients are seen frequently, as often as once a week, by a nurse, adherence rapidly improves. The nurses emphasize the importance of taking the medicine regularly. They help the patients count their pills for each day and, if necessary, assist them in putting the tablets into a pillbox or egg carton. Patient can readily check before going to bed whether they took the day's dosage. Patients appear to respond to having someone care about them. It may not be practical for the physician to see the patient this often, but someone in the physician's office can. The cost of these regular visits is small compared with the cost of hospitalization when seizures go out of control.

Increased individual attention by a nurse, physician, or other health professional seems to be crucial. The several strategies all depend on monitoring by the treating team so that the patient is given objective facts about his or her behavior. Instructions are given on each visit about taking the medicines and when to take them. To the extent possible, the patient needs to be the one to eventually monitor his or her status in terms of seizure control in relation to the goals that were established. Furthermore, the connection can be made by the patient between the results achieved and the actions that he or she takes.

Thus, the use of calendars, individualized medication programs, and pillboxes is helpful. The patient must understand at the outset that the behavior eventually expected is complete self-medication. Many patients, especially those of limited intelligence, have to be helped to develop appropriate responses through a series of successive steps. For example, one can help them pack their pillboxes on weekly visits to the office. Then, they can be told to do them at home and bring them in to show how well they have done. Eventually, they can do it on their own. Each step must be reinforced and no further steps taken until the previous one is mastered. In general, only positive reinforcement should be used. Minimizing approach-avoidance conflict makes the patient's visit to the physician or nurse a positive experience. Reinforcement must be given as soon as good behavior is observed, in small and frequent amounts. One should encourage positive reinforcement from the family and peers as well.

The more the patients understand their illness and have a role in the design and ongoing review of their treatment plan—the goals, the outcomes achieved, and the actions taken—the more initiative they can take. Thus, they can begin to play an active role in tailoring dosage intervals to suit their own individual lifestyle and make changes in their activities to maximize seizure control.

Measuring Effectiveness

Measurement of outcomes must be intrinsic to the management of persons with seizures. The effectiveness of the treatment of epilepsy can be evaluated by measuring improvement in three major areas. It has been helpful to consider the effects in terms of the WHO classification of impairment, disability, and handicap or QOL.[6]

The measure of impairment can reflect the frequency and severity of seizures. Other measures could include such issues as injuries that occur in the context of seizures. The disabilities are the functional effects of the impairments on the life of the person. These can include the problems with memory and psychosocial difficulties as well as hospitalization for treatment of emergencies or other illness associated with the seizures and their treatment. The third level of outcome is that of handicap or QOL. Measures include outcomes in terms of social roles and community integration along such parameters as schooling, employment, and general QOL. The overall goal of treatment is control—no seizures and no side effects.

Measurement of Impairments

A useful and generally accepted classification for seizure frequency was developed by Engel.[7] For example, outcomes from epilepsy surgery are scored as follows:

Class I: Seizure free
Class II: Rare seizures that do not interfere with life
Class III: Worthwhile improvement, but seizure frequency still interferes with daily living
Class IV: No worthwhile improvement

Control equals no seizures and no side effects.

Measurement of Disabilities

Patient satisfaction on a 1–5 scale has been a practical measurement device on a grid against such major life issues as seizure frequency, seizure severity, drug toxicity, housing employment, social life, sex life, and so forth. Measurement also can include number of hospital admissions and treatment in hospital emergency departments.

Measurement of Handicap–Quality of Life

In the early 1990s, a flurry of interest was shown in the revision and development of testing instruments to evaluate improvement or changes in the QOL of people with seizure disorders.[7] This is a highly technical subject that underwent a great deal of development but is currently in the doldrums. In the author's opinion, none of the instruments that are currently being tested are suitable for routine clinical practice. In general, they tend to be too long and too complex. Each of them has useful elements, and some of them are distinctly better than others.

A comprehensive review of the subject of the measurement of QOL and epilepsy can be found in Trimble and Dodson.[8] The chapter by Fallowfield provides an excellent overview of QOL measurements, and the reader is particularly directed to the instruments developed by Carl Dodrill (Washington Psychosocial Seizure Inventory, Chapter 8) and the QOL instruments developed under the leadership of Orrin Devinsky and Barbara Vickrey (Chapter 9).

All of this being said, the aspect that tends to be overlooked most often in day-to-day management is the necessity to have the patient set appropriate goals and to help the patient measure progress toward those goals. Although it may be salutary for a patient who, has, for example, a cord compression syndrome to set the goal of being able to walk freely without assistive devices, perhaps the more practical immediate goal is to be able to transfer in and out of a wheelchair and to maneuver that wheelchair around the home. In a similar manner, in dealing with a patient with epilepsy, breaking the long-range objective of no seizures and no side effects into shorter-range goals makes a great deal of sense. These shorter-term measurable goals include adhering to a medication regimen and maintaining blood levels between a certain range. Meeting such short-term goals can provide the basis to lead to the longer-term goal of seizure control. This in turn is a prerequisite for the improved QOL as measured by employment, schooling, and family life.

Thus, although the primary motivator for a young patient may be to get a driver's license, the practical issue is to have the patient adhere to the medical regimen well enough that the effectiveness of the medicine can be evaluated. The very process of evaluation carried out with the patient provides an opportunity for the person with seizures to develop a sense of control over a medical problem that by its very nature induces a sense of life being out of control.

References

1. Hauser WA, Hesdorffer DC. Epilepsy: Frequency, Causes and Consequences. New York: Demos, 1990.
2. Luders HD. Epilepsy Surgery. New York: Raven, 1992.
3. MINCEP Epilepsy Reports, vol I, no. 1. Minneapolis: MINCEP Epilepsy Care, 1993.
4. Graham FH. Comprehensive Management of Lower-Incidence Chronic Disease: the MINCEP Epilepsy Care Model in Disease Management Sourcebook. New York: Faulkner & Gray, 1998;144–155.
5. World Health Organization. The International Classification of Impairments, Disabilities, and Handicaps. Geneva: World Health Organization, 1980.
6. Engel J Jr, Pedley TA (eds). Epilepsy: A Comprehensive Textbook. Philadelphia: Lippincott–Raven, 1997.
7. Devinsky O, Cramer JA (eds). Assessing quality of life in epilepsy. Epilepsia 1993;34(suppl 4):1044.
8. Trimble MR, Dodson WE (eds). Epilepsy and Quality of Life. New York: Raven, 1994.

Suggested Readings

Aidardi J. Epilepsy in Children (2nd ed). International Review of Child Neurology Series. New York: Raven, 1994.
Commission for the Control of Epilepsy and Its Consequences. Plan for Nationwide Action on Epilepsy. DHEW Publication no. (NIH) 79-1115. Washington, DC: U.S. Department of Health, Education and Welfare, 1979.
Cramer JA, Spilker B (eds). Patient Compliance in Medical Practice and Clinical Trials. New York: Raven, 1991.
Dam M, Gram L (eds). Comprehensive Epileptology. New York: Raven, 1991.
Engel J Jr. Seizures and Epilepsy. Contemporary Neurology Series, no. 31. Philadelphia: Davis, 1989.
Epilepsy Foundation of America. Current Trends in Epilepsy: A Self-Study Course for Physicians. Landover, MD: Epilepsy Foundation of America, 1994.
Gumnit RJ. The Epilepsy Handbook. The Practical Management of Seizures (2nd ed). New York: Raven, 1994.
Gumnit RJ. Living Well with Epilepsy (2nd ed). New York: Demos, 1997.
Gumnit RJ. Your Child and Epilepsy. New York: Demos, 1995.
Gumnit RJ, Risinger M, Leppik IE, Maister B, Gil-Nagel A. The Epilepsies and Convulsive Disorders. In RJ Joynt, RC Griggs (eds), Clinical Neurology. New York: Lippincott–Raven, 1996;1–95.
Hopkins A, Shorvon S, Cascino G (eds). Epilepsy (2nd ed). London: Chapman & Hall, 1995.
Schmidt D, Leppik I. Compliance in Epilepsy. Epilepsy Research. Suppl 1. Amsterdam: Elsevier, 1998.
Temkin O. The Falling Sickness. A History of Epilepsy from the Greeks to the Beginnings of Modern Neurology (2nd ed). Baltimore: The Johns Hopkins University Press, 1971.
Wylie E (ed). The Treatment of Epilepsy: Principles and Practice (2nd ed). Baltimore: Williams & Wilkins, 1997.

Chapter 11
Management of Persons with Chronic Pain

Robert D. Gerwin

Nature of the Problem

The specialist, whether neurologist or physiatrist, is often asked to evaluate and manage problems associated with pain. Diagnosis is essential in the management of both acute and chronic pain. The management of acute pain encompasses pain relief and treatment of its cause. Most acute pain resolves within a short time and does not disrupt the social and economic life of the patient. The patient is often a passive participant in acute pain management, relying on the temporary use of analgesics until the condition resolves and pain abates.

Chronic nonmalignant pain (i.e., pain not associated with carcinoma), on the other hand, has a life of its own, notwithstanding the need to identify and treat the cause of the pain whenever possible. Pain itself is not a diagnosis, in that it is always caused by another medical or structural problem; however, pain can be considered as an impairment that can become the major disabling factor in a person's life. Pain can thereby become the illness.

Extent of the Problem

Chronic pain is a private problem that burdens an individual; a family problem that affects the relationships of parents, spouses, children, and siblings; and a social problem that affects the community at large. The costs of chronic pain to the person and to the community are staggering.

The problem is addressed herein through a review of some sources of chronic pain: musculoskeletal, myofascial, and neuropathic.

Chronic Low Back Pain

Chronic musculoskeletal pain of at least 1 month's duration has a prevalence of approximately 15%.[1] Back pain can be taken as an example of a chronic musculoskeletal pain that is common, is disruptive of family life and of work, and uses a disproportionate amount of medical care. It is one of the two most common pain complaints.[2] Back pain is the primary model of chronic pain that is discussed in detail to illustrate the principles set forth in this chapter.

The incidence of low back pain (LBP) in the United States is approximately 5% per year.[3] Lack of standardized diagnostic criteria has led to different estimates of the incidence and prevalence of LBP.[4] A survey of the literature by Linton[5] notes that 85% of the population has back pain at one time or another, but 6% of those with back pain use half of the total health care visits and consume the larger portion of sick leave and health care resources. The prevalence of chronic benign pain—that is, pain without a direct link to a specific cause—is approximately 15% of the adult population, with a range of 2–40% in different studies.[6] The relapse rate of LBP is high, estimated to be 70–80%, whereas approximately 5% is estimated to develop chronic back pain that persists for longer than 3 months.[4]

As an example of the burden of LBP, the cost of back pain in the Netherlands was equal to 1.7% of the gross national product, with only 7% of that cost going to health care. Indirect costs of absenteeism and disability equaled 93% of the total costs. Linton[5] further notes that, in Sweden, the health care costs for musculoskeletal pain tripled between 1975 and 1983, with 85% of the costs resulting from absenteeism and disability. The majority of the health care costs were devoted to advanced diagnostic testing, although most back pain is nonspecific and resolves within weeks. Only 6% of health care costs were related to primary care evaluation and treatment. Nevertheless, persons with chronic pain are among the most frequent users of the health care system.[7] Others have noted the high cost of back pain and the disproportionate expenditure of monies on a small proportion of patients.[8]

The cost to the individual with chronic back pain is likewise high; personal costs and out-of-pocket expenses consume almost one-half of the monies expended. Income decreases at a time when financial outlay for health-related needs rises. Musculoskeletal pain in general, including back pain and other spine and joint pains, increases the odds of having physical disability more than sixfold (and increases the likelihood of depression more than threefold).[9]

Linton[5] observes that the recurrent nature of chronic back pain is costly to the individual and to the community and that most of the costs are related to compensation. Nevertheless, compensation status and litigation by themselves do not affect the return-to-work outcome in LBP, and the high cost of compensation should not be seen as a bias predisposing to disability.[10,11] Instead, it reflects an emphasis on supporting the disabled, rather than diminishing disability through prevention and rehabilitation.[5]

Chronic Neuropathic Pain

The problems of chronic pain are very much the same for other conditions besides chronic LBP and other musculoskeletal sources of pain. Painful polyneuropathies are less common than musculoskeletal pain but can be equally disabling. The most common of these are diabetic neuropathy and nutritional neuropathies associated with excessive alcohol intake. Diabetic neuropathy is considered a model of chronic neuropathic pain because of its prevalence and severity. It is the most common acquired neuropathy in the United States and the most common painful neuropathy. Diabetic neuropathy occurs in more that 50% of patients with long-standing diabetes. Approximately 10% of persons with diabetic neuropathy have painful sensations, including burning pain. Other painful neuropathies are isoniazid neuropathy, pellagra, and amyloid neuropathy. Postherpetic neuropathy affects an increasing percentage of persons older than 60 years who contract shingles. The percentage of persons with postherpetic neuralgia after herpes zoster virus increases with age until it reaches 75% of those affected in their eighth decade, and it lasts for longer than a year for almost half of those who are affected.[12]

Other chronic pain syndromes include complex regional pain syndrome, previously called reflex sympathetic dystrophy, which complicates soft tissue or nerve injury. Burning pain and hypersensitivity in complex regional pain syndrome are so severe as to be almost uniformly disabling. Initial protective postures to protect the affected part of the body become harmful in themselves, leading to frozen joints, contractures, and disuse atrophy. Phantom limb and central neuropathic pain, such as post-stroke central thalamic pain, spinal pain in MS, and pain in dystonias and PD, are additional syndromes that are chronic and debilitating and can be challenging to treat. This listing is not meant to be comprehensive but serves to emphasize that the problem of chronic pain arising from the nervous system is widespread and can be extremely disruptive. These entities, as well as chronic headache, are discussed in other chapters in this book.

Myofascial Pain Syndrome and Fibromyalgia

Fibromyalgia and myofascial pain syndrome have been selected as other examples of disabling chronic disorders because they are so prevalent. These two soft tissue pain problems are perhaps the most common muscular pain syndromes that afflict humans. Fibromyalgia may involve 2–5% of all women aged 20–40 years. It is a chronic problem that can last for years and that alters the lives of those who have the disorder.

Myofascial pain often becomes chronic and can be so severe as to prevent sitting or standing to a degree that is disabling, interfering with work and with home life. The incidence of symptomatic myofascial pain syndrome is not known, but it is a cause of pain that accompanies or complicates a multitude of musculoskeletal conditions, including lumbar and cervical spondylosis, arthritis of the hip or knee, postlaminectomy pain syndromes, whiplash injury, and overuse syndromes. Myofascial pain syndrome can be regional, but it is often generalized, and in that way it is similar to fibromyalgia, which is a generalized chronic pain syndrome. It is frequently encountered in persons with LBP. Its successful management and treatment[13] require skills and approaches that are different from the usual simple analgesic approach to pain management and can be very effective.

In all these syndromes, patients can become prisoners of their pain. Pain and its avoidance become the focus of their lives. Chronic pain as dealt with in this chapter is by its nature unremitting and can be progressive. It takes great effort on both the physician's and patient's part for the person to take control of his or her life, to develop strategies to reduce pain to the extent possible, and to perform usual daily activities in the presence of pain. The chronicity of the problem leads to its high prevalence and burden. It is necessary to develop approaches to its management that can prevent the development of a pattern of chronicity and intervene to break the cycle of pain and resultant disability.

Nature of the Diseases

The structure of this section recapitulates the formulation developed by the WHO. The first aspect deals with the underlying changes at the cellular level and those of the pathophysiology. The level of the disease is the traditional focus of medical care leading to diagnosis. The natural history of the disease processes is the fundamental background on which the management of the patient must depend.

Low Back Pain

The publication in 1995 of the report Back Pain in the Workplace by the Task Force on Pain in the Workplace of the International Association for the Study of Pain[14] created a stir in the community of clinicians who treat chronic back pain. The general thesis of the task force is that nonspecific LBP

(NSLBP) is self-limiting and usually resolves within 6 weeks but that chronic NSLBP is a form of pain that has been "medicalized" when in reality it is "activity intolerance" and is not a medical problem. When NSLBP continues beyond 6 weeks, the individual must be re-examined for other (specific) causes of LBP. If none is found, it can be highly suspected that the problem is more than just a physical injury or impairment and that interaction with the environment (a worker-job "dissonance" or unhappiness) may be the crux of the problem.

Recognizing that persistent disability from LBP has become epidemic, the task force proposed that persons with unresolved NSLBP after 6 weeks of disability that has not been reclassified as specific LBP should be reclassified as unemployed and be given all of the resources available to the unemployed, such as vocational rehabilitation and training, but lose the benefits of workers' compensation, including ongoing medical care. In other words, NSLBP would cease to be a medical problem after 6 weeks, and the focus would be on marshaling those resources that facilitate return to work. The safety net for the individual is re-evaluation to identify specific causes of continued LBP that require a medical approach and warrant further disability status. However, it is acknowledged that only approximately 15% of persons with LBP have an identifiable pathoanatomic or pathophysiologic medical cause of their pain.

A serious limitation of the task force presentation is the small number of recognized conditions that are acceptable causes of specific LBP: disk herniation, spondylolisthesis, spinal stenosis, spinal instability, vertebral fractures, tumors, infections, and inflammatory diseases. Other persistent musculoskeletal causes of chronic pain, such as myofascial pain syndrome, fibromyalgia, and repetitive strain syndrome, conditions that are diagnosed based on clinical or physical criteria rather than radiologic or other laboratory criteria, are missing from this list.

Nonetheless, the task force focuses on NSLBP and contends that persons who experience it should be able to return to work. A rebuttal by Teasell and Merskey[15] argues that clinical conditions, such as chronic cervical whiplash, fibromyalgia, and regional pain, do not have the type of identifiable cause of pain that the task force specifies, although they have well-defined pain syndromes. Teasell and

Merskey also criticize the concept that associated psychological causes are considered causative of disability, whereas organic and physical causes are disregarded. They point out that the psychological manifestations of chronic disease are often the consequence of pain and are not the cause of it. This has been shown for chronic whiplash, in which psychological distress resolved when medical treatment eliminated the pain.[16]

Turk[17] notes, however, that rehabilitation efforts in chronic LBP have not been very effective. For example, many different regimens are in vogue for the treatment of LBP, but few have been found to be truly beneficial,[18–21] therefore diverting costs from rehabilitation toward compensation and disability payments.

Myofascial Pain Syndrome and Fibromyalgia

Muscle tenderness is found in both myofascial pain syndrome and fibromyalgia, but the presence of myofascial trigger points that reproduce the individual's pain distinguishes the two conditions. Myofascial pain syndrome can be an acute response to injury, but it can also be a chronic condition, usually perpetuated by uncorrected mechanical, postural, or underlying medical stresses. Thus, both conditions can be chronic and therefore a source of potential disability; family, social, and occupational dislocation; and despair.

Myofascial pain syndrome has as its central feature the myofascial trigger point that develops in response to acute or repetitive physical stress to the muscle. The pathophysiology of the trigger point is discussed in detail in Chapter 2 of Myofascial Pain and Dysfunction: the Trigger Point Manual.[22] The trigger point is always found on a taut band of muscle that is discrete within the muscle belly. Many of these taut bands may be found in a single distressed muscle. The trigger point is in reality a zone of hypersensitivity to mechanical stimulation. It has abnormal electrical activity. Myofascial trigger points show spontaneous needle EMG activity[23] that is composed of a low-amplitude (50–100 μV) discharge that looks like miniature end-plate potentials but occurs many times more frequently than spontaneous end-plate activity. Active trigger points show a superimposed irregular discharge of 500–1,000 μV. This background activity of the trigger point is reduced by 80% in response to the systemic infusion of the α-adrenergic blocking agent phentolamine.[24]

The characteristics of the persistent electrical activity at the trigger point are indicative of it being an abnormal motor end plate with a manyfold increase in the release of acetylcholine at the synaptic junction, modulated in some as yet unknown way by sympathetic activity. Hubbard and Berkoff[23] have proposed that the nature of the sympathetic control of trigger point activity is more in keeping with the muscle spindle and its sympathetically innervated intrafusal fibers being the central feature of the trigger point. This is the motor aspect of the trigger point. The sensory aspect has to do with the nature of trigger point pain. Substance P and other neuropeptides related to sensitization of peripheral nerve endings are thought to be released by the muscle at the trigger zone, resulting in peripheral sensitization and increased activity that in turn lead to sensitization of the dorsal horn neuron. The result of peripheral and central sensitization is the development of allodynia (the perception of pain in response to normally nonpainful stimulation) and hypersensitivity (the amplification of the pain response to noxious stimulation) and a spread of the receptive field seen by a particular dorsal horn neuron. Hence, two features of the trigger point are explained by this model that are supported by experimental studies: the unusual tenderness of the trigger point, which is a manifestation of hypersensitivity and allodynia; and referred pain or the perception of pain felt at a distance from the stimulus, which is a spinal cord phenomenon related to enlargement of the dorsal horn neuron receptive fields. The local twitch response of the taut band in response to mechanical stimulation depends on a spinal reflex but is not a tendon stretch reflex; rather, it is a contraction of the taut band alone.[25]

In clinical practice, the trigger zone is identified by physical examination. Identification of the features of the trigger point (tenderness in a taut band, twitch response, referred pain phenomena, and reproducibility of the usual pain syndrome) by manual palpation has been shown to have good inter-rater reliability.[26]

The pathophysiology of fibromyalgia, a condition in which there is chronic widespread muscle pain, is actively being investigated in a number of laboratories. Two outstanding features of the fibromyalgia syndrome are of particular interest and are probably related. One is the finding of hypersensitivity to a variety of stimuli, both mechanical and otherwise (e.g., thermal and aural).[27–30] The other is the observation that serotonin is decreased in plasma and substance P is increased in spinal fluid, suggesting that the neuropeptides that regulate pain transmission are abnormal in a way consistent with the development of widespread mechanical hypersensitivity and allodynia or widespread muscle, tendon, and bone tenderness.[31]

Chronic Neuropathy

Neuropathic pain in polyneuropathy is complex and has many different features that contribute to the clinical presentation. The peripheral nerve undergoes axonal degeneration and segmental demyelination, and a secondary dying of the related neuron occurs. These changes usually happen together, although systemic, metabolic, and toxic neuropathies are more likely to affect the axon, whereas immunologic disorders (such as Guillain-Barré syndrome) are more likely to affect the myelin sheath. The injury to the nerve may be metabolic, such as the accumulation of sorbitol or abnormalities in essential fatty acids in the nerves of diabetic patients. Injury can occur as a result of compression or of ischemia. Pain is not related to the fiber size of the affected nerves. The mechanisms that have been found to be responsible for neuropathic pain include sensitization of both peripheral afferent receptors and central dorsal horn neurons, ectopic discharges between afferent nerves, and ephaptic cross-talk. Peripheral sensitization that results in tenderness is induced by inflammatory mediators such as bradykinin. Sensory neurons become hyperexcitable and discharge at abnormal locations in the nerve fiber (ectopic discharges). Increased amplification of the response in the spinal cord and brain is known as central sensitization and is mediated by excitatory amino acids that activate NMDA receptors. Other spinal cord receptors that are activated and that amplify and spread the response to mechanical stimulation are the alpha-amino-3-hydroxy-5-methyl-isoxazole-4-proprionate and metabotropic glutamate receptors. These lead to calcium accumulation within the cell and subsequent activation of membrane-bound and cytosolic proteins that change the characteristics of NMDA receptors, leading to increased neuronal excitability and spread of pain impulses to adjacent neurons, thereby amplifying the response to afferent input.

Nature of the Impairments

Impairments are viewed as the direct consequences of the underlying pathology. They are the symptoms or signs such as one would assess in the course of the medical-neurologic examination. Normal medical practice uses impairments to deduce the underlying pathology or disease process. It is useful once again to use the WHO formulation and the distinction made between "impairment" and "disability." Impairment has been defined as "any loss or abnormality of psychological, physiological, or anatomic structure or function."[32] It thus can be considered to be at the "organ" level. A disability exists at the multiorgan level of function.

Impairment in chronic pain syndromes can be the result of the underlying disorder or of the pain itself. In the case of myofascial pain that causes LBP, shortening of the psoas and quadratus lumborum muscles, for example, as a result of the contracted bands that contain trigger points, leads to restricted range of motion. The loss of range of motion is the impairment, which is caused by the inability of the muscle to lengthen fully. Lack of normal lengthening of the muscle results in the inability to stand or sit fully erect, which is a disability. However, pain itself may prevent straightening of the back (as in pain from quadratus lumborum trigger points) and therefore an inability to stand upright. Pain in this case is itself an impairment that prevents a function (standing upright), which is a disability.

Whatever the disease process and wherever it manifests itself anatomically, the uniform problems discussed in this chapter are the effects of the existence of ongoing pain. One can specify the type and frequency of the pain as well as its duration and intensity. One objective of management is to reduce the degree of pain by appropriate treatment directed to its sources. In the course of doing this, one may find it useful to consider how one may seek to reduce the various components of pain. One may try to reduce intensity, duration, or frequency. For example, a man with central pain after SCI had as his goal carrying on his personal business during periods of reduced pain intensity that lasted the several hours during the day that were necessary for him to keep an appointment. Still another man sought a lower intensity of pain particularly at night to enable him to get adequate rest. The selection and dosage of medication or other treatment can be optimized to meet these specific objectives.

In the absence of abolition of pain or its extensive alleviation by direct treatment, and given its costs in terms of side effects of medication and so forth, the objective can also become reduction of the disabilities despite the continued existence of the impairment.

Suffering describes the impact of the pain on the person. According to Cassell,[33] it addresses the degree to which pain is perceived to be a threat to the person's integrity. Suffering can result from the inability to carry out one's roles. Pain and suffering are not the same, although they often are closely identified. Suffering can occur in the absence of pain. Conversely, pain can occur in the absence of a sense of suffering. It is important to recognize that one can alleviate suffering without necessarily doing away with the pain.

As Cassell[33] has emphasized, it is not necessarily true that the greater the pain, the greater the suffering. For example, some pain such as that in childbirth can be quite severe, but many women consider it uplifting. The amount of analgesia necessary to relieve labor pain varies with the woman's choice to exert control over the process of childbirth. The perceived meaning of the pain influences the amount of medication required to control it. The example is given of the person who achieved good control of her pain when it was attributed to sciatica but required much larger doses when it was attributable to the spread of cancer. Patients can writhe in pain from kidney stones yet not be suffering (by their report) because "they know what it is." In contrast, people may report considerable suffering from apparently little pain when they do not know its source.

People in pain may report suffering from pain when they feel out of control or when the pain is overwhelming. In the context of chronic pain such as is described in this chapter, suffering can be felt when the pain is apparently without end; this pain can be a source of suffering even if not overwhelming if it continues for a very long time so that it seems endless. Physicians tell patients that they "will get used to the pain," but that rarely happens. What patients learn is both how little tolerance other people have for their continued report of pain and how pain becomes less bearable the longer it continues. Still another aspect of pain that causes

suffering is lack of validation of the person's pain by the physician. If no disease is found, the physician may suggest that the patient is "imagining" the pain, that the pain is psychological in the sense that it is not real and that she or he is "faking."

Chronic pain arises out of physical illness but can also be caused by psychological stress associated with illness. Chronic pain syndromes do not develop in all persons with the same illness. Some persons with chronic illness see themselves as in chronic pain, and others do not. Some individuals with chronic pain think of themselves as victims. Others seem to master the causes of pain and, despite requiring medication or other treatment, do not see themselves as ill or as sufferers. The person with chronic pain develops a role in the family and in the community (at work, in the health care system, and in the social support system). The physician's role, as well as the role of those in society who interact with the chronic pain patient, can be supportive and enabling of successful coping with suffering or can be enabling in maintaining the role of chronic illness. Therapy is not only directed to the physical causes of illness and pain but to using specific reinforcements directed toward changing those aspects of life that perpetuate the role of the sufferer into actions that support control and mastery of life situations.[34]

Chronic pain has commonly been seen as either a physical or a psychological problem. In this construct, pain is either not validated as an integral part of a somatic illness in the physical illness model, or in the psychological model, the physical illness is not seen as relevant to the psychological problems that have produced and maintained the pain. The effects of this dichotomy are such that, if pain is considered to be caused by a physical problem, neither the patient nor the physician needs to be concerned with the pain as a source of suffering. According to the physical illness model, concentration is on treating the physical cause of the pain. This approach is not without validity when a definite physical cause of pain is present that can be effectively treated.[16] On the other hand, if pain is considered a manifestation of psychological distress, one can concentrate on the psychological meaning of the form that chronic pain and suffering take and not focus on physical causes.

The view expressed in this chapter is not a dualistic mind-body approach but rather attempts to understand the patient's suffering as a result of pain that is most often grounded in physical illness. The expression of pain and thence suffering is influenced by a person's life experience, and patients can use suffering as a form of communication with family or coworkers or as a means to avoid certain other conflicts or tensions in their lives.[35] Notwithstanding that, pain and its concomitant suffering, which result from physical illnesses such as chronic back pain or neuropathy, can be as much an impairment as are limited range of motion or loss of sensation in the legs. Physicians must recognize suffering as an aspect of illness that needs to be treated along with the underlying disorder. Indeed, when treatment of the underlying disorder is not completely effective, as is often the case in chronic back pain and in neuropathy, the issues of suffering can predominate. In these situations, the patient needs to find a way around the limitations presented by pain and alleviate the feeling of suffering. The physician needs to recognize the presence of suffering related to the continued existence of pain, assess its impact, and be able, with the patient, to minimize its role in his or her life.

Nature of the Disabilities and Handicaps

Each of the chronic pain conditions that are discussed in this chapter leads to a physical and mental impairment with the potential for very real disability and handicap that can be catastrophic for the individual and the family, disruptive of the workforce, and costly to the community. Disability refers to the functional (behavioral) consequences of the pathology or the impairments, or both. WHO has defined disability as "any restriction or lack (resulting from impairment) of the ability to perform an activity within the range considered normal for a human being."[32] Thus, the inability to stand on the floor because of the pain of diabetic neuropathy or the inability to sleep because of the fear of an attack of pain from trigeminal neuralgia is a disability that results from pain. Musculoskeletal pain (LBP, myofascial pain, and fibromyalgia included) has been shown to lead to physical disability in senior citizens in which they were three times more likely to have difficulty with three or more ADLs.[9] Both physical impairment and pain-induced suffering must be addressed to restore a normal life to the disabled individual.

Disabilities are the result of the interaction of the impairments with whom that person is. As such, they cannot be deduced entirely from the medical-neurologic examination. Input from the patient or family, or both, is necessary for their proper identification. The specific disabilities to be ameliorated vary with the goals and the characteristics of the person. Normal rehabilitation practice deals with this level of analysis. One of its aims is to reduce the degree of disability by training the actions that are unaffected so as to compensate for those that are affected.

Family relationships of the patient with chronic pain are disrupted: A provider becomes a receiver, a breadwinner becomes a disabled economic burden, and a patient manipulates family and friends to serve his or her needs. A person with chronic pain is depressed, physically impaired, and socially isolated.[36] A previously independent individual develops a dependent relationship with his or her family, doctors, and therapists. The continuous use of analgesics that may be needed determines the patient–physician relationship. The patient often has a loss of empowerment, a lowering of self-esteem, and the onset of depression with mourning for lost functions and abilities. No matter what the cause, whether it be LBP, complex regional pain syndrome, diabetic neuropathy, or fibromyalgia, pain becomes the impairment, and the source of disability and illness.

Disability status associated with chronic pain may have another unwanted consequence in that it provides an acceptable means for assuming the sick role and dependency.[37] Moreover, it often places the patient and the attorney who is seeking social security disability or compensation benefits in conflict with the physician, whose goal is to optimize function and well-being. Goal-directed rehabilitation has been shown to have a better outcome, at least in terms of return to work.[38]

A handicap is an inability to perform tasks or functions associated with the usual roles that are performed by persons of like age, gender, and background.[32] The loss of the ability to work at a job for which one is otherwise qualified, to attend school full-time, to eat dinner at a restaurant with friends, and to adequately care for one's family are all handicaps that can exist when one has a chronic pain syndrome. A handicap caused by chronic pain can be the result of a physical impairment that produces a disability, the effect of a psychological or emotional impairment and disability, or a combination of both of these factors. Impairment and disability, however, do not necessarily lead to handicap. A person may continue to function fully despite pain. For example, an individual may continue to work at a computer keyboard despite myofascial trigger points in the forearm muscles. On the other hand, pain can be so severe as to prevent normal sitting or standing, thereby impeding the performance of workday tasks (disability), and producing a partial or total inability to work (the handicap).

The disabilities caused by chronic pain vary not only with the quality and intensity of the pain but with the needs and resources of the person who experiences it. The effects of the various pain syndromes described vary with the demographics of each. Gender and age affect the roles and the handicaps. LBP mainly affects men of working age, the soft tissue syndromes mainly young women, and the neuropathic syndromes due to diabetes mainly elderly persons with long-standing disease.

The impact of injury and pain is idiosyncratic to the patient, as illustrated by the following case. A young foreman fell when a stairway under construction collapsed under him. He experienced a mild SCI that resulted in weakness of the proximal leg muscles and severe pelvic floor pain. Despite the persistence of his pain, he returned to work as soon as his leg recovered strength enough to permit him to walk about the construction site. However, questioning him about the effects of pain and his cord injury revealed that he had also lost the ability to sustain normal sexual function and was thereby having difficulty with his wife. Treatment of the pelvic floor myofascial pain and counseling both the patient and his wife resulted in an improvement in their marital relationship and in his sexual functioning, even though it had not returned to its preinjury state. In this case, the cord injury and the continued impairment from pain resulted in a functional problem in the life of the patient. The partial impotence is a disability that led to a handicap (loss of normal marital relationships) that had to be identified as a problem. A goal could be developed for the restoration of a more harmonious marital relationship during the recovery period. One end result of treatment was a desired pregnancy, even though the patient had not fully recovered from either the impairment or its functional consequences.

The physician must skillfully assess the individual's activities to see if he or she has an inapparent handicap in addition to those that are obvious. The definition of the disabilities and their effects on the person's role as husband and potential father cannot be determined merely on the basis of the impairment alone. The development of a treatment plan that allows the patient and the physician to be partners in the healing and rehabilitation process requires the contributions of the person who is experiencing the problem. In this case, both the patient and his spouse were involved in identifying the problems and participating in the solution.

The multifactorial nature of the disease process and the necessity for treating these several aspects are illustrated in the following case. A young woman in her 30s complained of recurrent pain in the shin muscles of one leg. The pain had started after she began to work in a job that required her to negotiate with persons who were senior to her in age and in position. She needed to dress up and therefore began to wear shoes with 2- to 3-in. heels. Pain in the muscle of the anterior lower leg began after approximately 20 minutes of walking. During a week when she was not working and did not wear high heels, she had no pain. The pain recurred when she resumed work. Her goal was to be able to wear high heels again, as she considered dress shoes an essential part of her work wardrobe.

Physical examination revealed myofascial trigger points in the anterior tibial muscle that reproduced her pain, confirming the diagnosis of myofascial pain syndrome, and trigger points in the gastrocnemius muscle that did not relate to her pain. She had already taken nonsteroidal anti-inflammatory drugs for this condition with little benefit. She could have simply been treated for the myofascial pain syndrome with trigger point injections or with physical therapy at this point. Instead, the evaluation proceeded to examine possible reasons for the myofascial pain syndrome to develop in the first place. She reported that she had fractured the ankle of the affected leg many years ago and that it had seemed to heal completely. Watching her walk revealed both a pronation of the affected foot and an impairment of dorsiflexion of the foot. Mobility of the tibial-talus junction was reduced. The hypothesis was that she had impaired dorsiflexion of the foot as a consequence of the old fracture but that it did not cause pain when she wore flats. However, the increased plantar flexion associated with high heels required more effort to bring the toes and forefoot into dorsiflexion to clear the floor when walking. The anterior tibialis muscle is the most important dorsiflexor of the foot, and it responded to the increased workload by developing myofascial trigger points.

Treatment was therefore not directed to the anterior tibialis muscle but rather to mobilizing the ankle and improving dorsiflexion. The cause of the myofascial pain syndrome had to be identified and treated to relieve the pain. The cause of her problem was identified through a mutual exploration of the patient's activities. She supplied the details needed to make a functional diagnosis. She had already begun to analyze her activities to understand what was happening to her and had identified the times when she was relatively free of the pain. The diagnosis was made on the basis of her story and a relevant physical examination, analyzing her foot placement when she walked and assessing the movement and flexibility of the foot itself. No local treatment was directed to the trigger points themselves. Our immediate goal was to mobilize the foot so that she could realize her long-term goal of wearing high heels. She understood the need to accomplish the short-term goal to achieve the long-term goal, and she participated readily in the office therapy and in the home exercise program.

The young woman in this vignette displays the characteristics of the patient who is a partner in therapy, setting goals and seeking effective means of treatment. In this regard, this patient provided the thrust to move her therapy along and facilitate her recovery. Far from needing motivation, she supplied it to the treatment staff. She did not, however, have the characteristics of a patient with chronic pain. Intervention occurred early in the course of her illness, and although impaired, she never reached the stage of disability and she never let her pain or limitations become the center of, and rule, her life. In contrast to the patient with chronic pain, this woman remained in control throughout the entire process of illness and pain, through rehabilitation to recovery.

Another case further illustrates important elements of myofascial pain treatment and management. A woman in her 50s complained of unilateral shoulder pain, especially when she abducted and extended her arm. Her work required that she fre-

quently reach up and pull an overhead machine down to eye level during the day. She was also a competitive long-distance swimmer. Her shoulder pain interfered with her ability to work and to swim. As a result, she became depressed and irritable, despite a very supportive family. Physical therapy before treatment consisted of ultrasound, electrical stimulation, some massage, and soft tissue mobilization to the shoulder muscles. In addition, strengthening exercises were prescribed, but they increased her pain. Her goals were well stated from the beginning: to work without impairment and resume competitive swimming. The initial evaluation showed that myofascial trigger points that reproduced her pain were present in virtually all of the muscles that controlled shoulder movement and that contributed to ipsilateral muscle control of neck movement. The involved muscles included the subscapularis, the levator scapula, the supraspinatus and infraspinatus, the pectoralis major and minor, and the scalene and sternocleidomastoid neck muscles, in addition to others. She explored different ways to bring the tool close to her to reduce aggravation of her shoulder pain and still allow her to work. To reach her other goal, she developed a routine of pool exercises even though swimming was not possible. Initial treatment was directed toward inactivation of the myofascial trigger points by both manual and invasive means (trigger point injection). She was given self-stretching techniques that eventually included all of the muscles that control neck and shoulder movement, which further actively involved her in the treatment program.

The result of an intensive treatment program was an increase in active range of motion that permitted all of her desired activity but did not maintain her in a pain-free condition. Moreover, her restriction in near-end range extension and abduction never improved. Radiographic examination of the shoulder showed degenerative arthritis that created a mechanical restriction. No surgical therapy was deemed appropriate by her orthopedic surgeon, but nonsteroidal anti-inflammatory drugs allowed her to do limited swimming and to work without restriction as long as she continued her exercises. She has coped with the inability to resume swimming at the same competitive level. Continued stretching exercises maintain the gains that she achieved.

The patient remains content with the level of persistent pain, which is less than before treatment, and with the level of her work and recreational activity. Her ongoing participation in identifying goals and carrying out treatment aided in establishing a result that she could accept and that was relatively effective in dealing with her disabilities, although she was not entirely free of pain.

Character of the Solution

Overall Plan

Treatment of chronic pain often entails risk taking for the practitioner, whether a physician or other kind of therapist. The patient has been treated previously, often with little success or unsustained relief, leading to a search for treatment that ends at the practitioner's doorstep. The "you are my last hope!" statement is an invitation to be entrapped in a situation in which neither patient nor physician emerges victorious. The patient may act passively, implicitly saying, "Treat me, but don't expect me to help, since nothing previously has worked." It often is a plea to prescribe whatever narcotic has been repeatedly denied. Most important, it establishes expectations that cannot be fulfilled and sets the stage for failure and blame. The physician who, in a moment of hubris, accepts the role of savior, is vulnerable to the ever-increasing demands of the desperate patient, whether or not effective treatment is available or whether or not the patient adheres to the recommended therapeutic regimen.

No practitioner is ever really the last hope, as someone else with a new approach can always be found. Treatment of the patient with chronic pain does require the practitioner to define the roles of the therapist and the recipient clearly, to define the limits of obligation and especially of responsibility on both of their parts, and to define, with the patient, goals that can be realistically attained and mutually agreed on. A fundamental step is to enlist the person with chronic pain in the process of solving his or her problem rather than assigning responsibility to another agent.

The physician or other therapist must have an understanding of both the biological and psychological aspects of the illness and know what therapies are available and how effective they are for the patient's problem. The principles of management of persons with chronic pain are those of continuity of care over time to deal with what is frequently a multifactorial problem as well as a focus on different aspects of the illness as care unfolds. The principle of comprehensive care also incorporates several different modalities as needed at any one time. Treatment of chronic pain embodies both specific treatments (e.g., sympathetic blocks for sympathetically mediated pain syndromes, trigger point injections for myofascial pain syndromes, and surgical diskectomy for herniated nucleus pulposus) and nonspecific or general treatments (e.g., cognitive rehabilitation, antidepressants, anticonvulsants, and physical therapy). A technical or procedural treatment or a pain pill is not a sufficient answer for a problem in which suffering has occurred, and the degree of suffering that is causing disability must also be understood and addressed by the physician.

Cognitive Therapy

Cognitive therapy is based on the concept that pain is the result of an interaction of the many events, including the effects of peripheral and CNS activation, modulation of such activation, and the cortical perception and responses to stimulation that are expressed behaviorally. Behavioral manifestations of the human response to pain are influenced by cultural and ethnic background and family and personal experience. The process of interpretation and the expression of suffering, avoidance of certain activities, and the reinforcement of pain behaviors are addressed by directing patients toward new cognitive and behavioral responses to their pain, so that they can forego the dysfunctional patterns that do not work for them but that reinforce the chronic pain suffering role. The process is meant to help patients resume healthy behaviors, improve their emotional state, enhance their ability to cope with the stresses of chronic pain, and return to productive activities, including work. A review and meta-analysis of randomized controlled studies of cognitive and behavioral therapy report good evidence for the effectiveness of active psychological treatment based on cognitive behavioral therapy.[39]

Pharmacologic Treatment

Pharmacologic treatment of chronic pain consists of the use of nonopiate analgesics as the first level of therapy. These drugs include the nonsteroidal anti-inflammatory drugs and acetaminophen. Adjuvant analgesics used to treat pain include the antidepressant drugs, the anticonvulsant drugs, the γ-aminobutyric acid inhibitors, and, for special purposes, the calcium channel blockers (for headache), the oral local anesthetics, the biphosphonates (for bone pain), the α$_2$-adrenergic agonist clonidine, and topical agents such as local anesthetics and capsaicin. Muscle relaxants are used for musculoskeletal pain. The opiate drugs are generally used when nonopioid drugs fail to give relief. The use of opiates in nonmalignant pain remains controversial but is becoming more acceptable in the medical community, especially with the awareness of the need to build in safeguards for the patient. An indication that the patient has been educated in their use and that the doctor is prepared to monitor the opiate medication appropriately is a narcotic informed consent or drug contract, which is becoming the standard of care when these drugs are used on a long-term basis.

Physical Therapy

Physical therapy is prescribed for chronic musculoskeletal pain almost universally, including most particularly the three conditions discussed in some detail in this chapter—LBP, myofascial pain, and fibromyalgia. The role of physical therapy in the treatment of chronic pain has changed over the years, and this change is described in detail in a publication of the International Association for the Study of Pain by Harding et al.[40] Chronic illness (and for that matter, acute medical conditions) is no longer treated by bed rest and passive modalities in which the therapist does the work and the patient is worked on. A biopsychological model of health is now recognized that emphasizes the positive role of activity in healing and concentrates on function rather than impairment. These authors point out that the new concepts of cognitive and behavioral principles of therapy and of goal-oriented rehabilitation have transformed physical therapy practice. "A patient-centered rehabilitative approach . . . emphasizes restoration of normal movement and function . . . as a vital component of the collaborative approach."[40]

This approach to physical therapy recognizes that elimination of pain may not always be achievable, but that physical function may nevertheless be improved and disability lessened. Deconditioning can lead to activity intolerance and what has been called the overactivity-rest cycle, in which patients persist in activity until they can do so no longer, either because of pain or exhaustion. The cycle is repeated over and over. This often leads to association of activity with pain and fatigue in the mind of the patient rather than recognition of the need to pace activities. As a result, the patient learns not to be active, reducing function that further reinforces negative psychological, physical, and social effects on the individual's behavior. In this situation, common in all of the syndromes discussed, pain has become the basis for illness and dictates the activities and limitations of the patient. Limitations in activity are no longer determined by neurologic impairment but by fear of producing pain.

Surgery

Surgery is reserved for conditions in which a clear-cut lesion is present that can benefit from such intervention. The indications for which surgery is unequivocal are those cases in which the patient has spinal cord or peripheral nerve compression. Destructive lesions have been used to interrupt pain pathways and include cordotomy, for example, for malignant lumbosacral plexus infiltration, and neurectomy and rhizotomy. These two latter procedures are nonselective in the neural deficits produced and are often too limited to address the widespread nature of pain. Radiofrequency lesions give better control over the extent of the lesion and have been particularly useful in treating vertebral facet joint syndromes in such injuries as whiplash with resultant chronic pain. Spinothalamic tractotomy, medial thalamotomy, and cingulotomy have all been used, but their roles need to be reinterpreted in light of their complications and the availability of newer drugs to treat pain, as well as the growing acceptance of the use of opiates in chronic nonmalignant pain. Spinal and other central stimulation (periventricular and periaqueductal gray matter or various brain sites) is used effectively for chronic pain, especially for extra-axial limb pain. Intrathecal or epidural administration of opioid by implanted pump avoids the higher doses and associated side effects of orally administered opiates and is useful when pain is intractable and chronic.

The mode within which any particular treatment is provided is crucial to its success. The importance of the interaction with the person who has chronic pain in the transaction has been increasingly recognized. The high cost of failure including loss of earning power requires attention to the prevention of establishing a pattern of chronicity with a sense of passivity. One must equip the patient and family with methods for dealing with their problems independently. In addition to the principles of continuity and comprehensiveness the pursuit of cost-effective care can lie in prevention of a sense of suffering by virtue of being overwhelmed. The ongoing interaction between the professional and the person with the problem should lead to a sense of self-efficacy in coping with the ongoing impairments. Details about the collaborative planning process that enable such growth are described in Chapter 2.

In the following sections, each of these principles is illustrated in the various pain syndromes. Case reports reflect the application of the principles.

Musculoskeletal (Low Back Pain)

Treatment of LBP of musculoskeletal origin, including persistent postoperative or postlaminectomy pain syndromes, has been controversial, particularly because many proposed treatments have been poorly supported by outcome studies or not studied at all. An often quoted example of a commonly prescribed treatment that turned out to be ineffective when examined critically, for acute LBP in this case, is bed rest. Neither short-term bed rest (2 days) nor extension and lateral bending exercises, which were also studied, were found to be better than ordinary activity.[19] The use of physical therapy modalities in the treatment of chronic musculoskeletal pain has been comprehensively reviewed. It was found that the duration or extent of therapy was more important than the kind of therapy performed, that the benefit did not outlast the therapy, and that long-term improvement was not the norm; in the two studies that showed long-term benefit, exercise was part of the therapeutic program.[41] As the move toward evidence-based medicine becomes more widespread, treatment modalities will be increasingly scrutinized to see if they are effective.

Treatment can be classified as (1) physical modalities, including both traditional physical ther-apy and manual or manipulative medicine as practiced in the United States by osteopathic physicians and by chiropractors; (2) pharmacologic management; (3) invasive nonsurgical treatment (e.g., trigger point injections, acupuncture, and epidural blocks); and (4) cognitive management (psychological). Any one patient often receives a combination of therapeutic approaches. Treatment principles in LBP overlap with those for myofascial pain syndrome, as that is the cause of pain for many patients with LBP.

Physical therapy and manipulative medicine address several issues. One is the immediate relief of pain, which may be accomplished by the application of heat or cold, the use of electrical stimulation, the use of soft tissue manipulation by local compression or pressure, massage of various sorts (local massage over the tender zone, friction massage, shiatsu, trigger point massage), muscle stretching and ultrasound, or articular manipulation. The other is the long-term control of pain by the correction of those factors that promote musculoskeletal pain, including myofascial pain syndromes. The long-term goal is accomplished by identifying mechanical stresses and correcting or alleviating them. This includes an assessment of body biomechanics that literally ranges from head to foot. Head and neck posture, such as forward head posture, influences spinal curvature and function. A round-shouldered, forward head posture with dorsal kyphosis is frequently accompanied by an increased lumbar lordosis and anterior pelvic tilt. Pelvic torsions (iliac rotations) cause pseudo–leg length inequalities that result in scoliosis. Postpartum pubic symphysis separation influences sacroiliac joint function and causes chronic pelvic region pain and LBP. Shortening of the iliopsoas muscle alters upright stance and tilts the pelvis anteriorly. Excessive foot pronation alters loading of the ankles, knees, and hips and can cause lower extremity pain and LBP. Ergonomic factors also fall under the heading of mechanical perpetuating factors. Sitting, lifting, and bending postures and load-handling affect the function of the low back and can promote chronic LBP when the mechanical loads exceed the tolerance of low back musculoskeletal structures. In addition, the long-term control of pain often requires lifestyle changes on the part of the patient in terms of strengthening of the low back, as weakness of low back musculature is a risk factor for chronic LBP.[42]

Common treatment practices have been called into question by the results of studies that showed that McKenzie exercises, chiropractic manipulation, use of lumbar supports, and back care education were all equally poor in their effectiveness in treating LBP.[20,21]

A 37-year-old woman with chronic LBP caused by an unstable spondylolisthesis is so obese that surgery is not considered an option, and in fact she does not want surgery. She also does not want to be reminded that her weight of more than 300 lb has an adverse effect on her back pain. She said that in the clinic she was enthused about exercise and treatment options, but when at home she had no desire to do anything to help herself. She bought an exercise video and tried to do floor exercises but came to the clinic subsequently saying that she could not do the exercises because she injured herself trying them, and moreover, she could not get off the floor when she finished. She said that she wanted to do other exercises such as Tai Chi but could not tolerate standing for even 5 minutes (a complaint not confirmed by observation in the clinic). Her idea for weight loss and pain control is that someone should do something to her (acupuncture, narcotics in increasing doses) rather than her deciding what she wants for herself and devising a plan to achieve her goals. She has had several years with no improvement and is still at the stage of needing to set a goal and deciding that she will take charge of her pain and of her life. These issues are the focus of the office visits.

In contrast, a 48-year-old lawyer with postlaminectomy pain and no option for further surgery tried to return to work but could not because he was unable to tolerate sitting and standing long enough either to get to the office or to accomplish work. He had been through a long process of therapeutic interventions before coming to our facility. These included epidural and selective nerve blocks, trials of antidepressant drugs, nonsteroidal anti-inflammatory drugs, and anticonvulsant drugs. He told us that his doctor did not think that the use of narcotic drugs was appropriate for what looked to be a lifelong pain problem. Therefore, he had not been treated with opiates. Physical exercise was not tolerated because of pain, although he had been physically active before his lumbar radiculopathy developed. He had been told to learn to live with his pain. Attempts at behavioral modification with a clinical social worker failed to increase useful activity, because his level of pain remained intolerable.

He was depressed and desperate because of financial pressures and lack of medical insurance and because he saw no hope of a pain-free life. He had found a job that he could take if he were able to travel to work, sit at a desk throughout an 8-hour workday, and concentrate well enough to abstract records and to produce analytical reports. Our initial discussions reviewed his previous treatments. He was not willing to invest more time in physical therapy, because it had previously failed and because he felt the need to be able to return to work in the immediate future. He thought that if his pain were controlled, he could return to work, his financial position would improve, he would again have health insurance, and his depression, which he thought was the result of his inability to function, would lift. He was uncertain about the chronic use of opiates but was somewhat reassured about the low addiction potential of slow-release, long-acting narcotics. He agreed to try them and found that their use controlled his pain well enough, although not completely, that he could return to full-time work and once again begin a physical therapy program. Because his pain has been adequately controlled, he feels less depressed. He is successful at work, and is progressing in physical therapy. His physical capabilities have improved, although he is not able to play tennis, as he desired.

This patient's case is distinguished by the fact that he had a clearly defined goal and a strong desire to regain control of his pain and his life. He became depressed when he saw no viable options. His previous treating physicians offered therapies that are effective for many people but that gave him no relief. The attempt to "learn to live with pain" and be a wage-earning individual able to provide financially and spiritually for his family was not achieved while his pain level was intolerably high. His depression lifted when his pain was controlled. In fact, he directed the treatment process himself. He was able to communicate his goals in terms that were measurable. Pain relief alone was not the issue. His goals were very practical: to ride the subway repeatedly, to sit in a chair for an hour, to attend to a written report well enough to analyze it. These were all measurable in the terms that were relevant to his perceived need of returning to work as an attorney.

These two individuals illustrate the importance of goal setting by the patient. The latter patient needed no help from the physician in setting goals but required assistance in achieving them. The former patient has been unable to even set achievable goals and represents a challenge to the physician, because the first steps of rehabilitation have not been achieved, as she has been resistant to making changes in her life. In fact, she told her physician that she was content to stay at home, largely on bed rest, while other family members shopped, cleaned, and cooked.

Myofascial Pain Syndrome

The elements of treating myofascial pain syndrome first involve an assessment of the pain complaint and of functional impairment. The cause of the pain must be determined. Muscles that contain trigger points that reproduce the individual's pain are identified. Muscles that do not actually contain trigger points that reproduce pain but that restrict movement or lead to weakness contribute to functional impairment and may need direct treatment to restore pain-free function. Myofascial trigger points can be the direct cause of all of the pain or be a direct cause of only a part of the pain but can be a major contributory factor. A single muscle can cause part of a person's overall pain but may not reproduce all of the pain. As one pianist told the author, "Each muscle alone plays just one note, but when they all hurt together, they play a symphony of pain."

Associated factors that are either primary, as arthritis, or secondary, such as trigger points that are related to scoliosis or leg length inequality caused by arthritis, must be identified for successful treatment. Arthritis can be treated symptomatically, but the underlying arthritis will not be altered. Trigger points associated with arthritis must be treated with this in mind. This applies, for example, to degenerative arthritis of the hip, where trigger points form as a direct result of the articular dysfunction and pain. Improvement in postural dysfunction caused by arthritis, scoliosis, or limited pelvic mobility can reduce myofascial trigger points related to these secondary manifestations of arthritis. Lumbar mobilization and stabilization can improve low back muscular pain syndromes in arthritis, and use of a heel lift can reduce stress on low back muscles and relieve pain in leg length inequality syndromes

caused by arthritis. Trigger points are also considered secondary when they occur as a result of the dysfunction caused by other trigger points. For example, trigger points in the trapezius muscle can alter the mechanics of shoulder function, and secondary trigger points will develop in other muscles that control shoulder movement, such as the infraspinatus or subscapularis muscles.

Treatment directed to the myofascial component of pain requires the inactivation of the myofascial trigger point either by manual means or by trigger point injection combined with manual therapy.[13,22] Manual therapy takes many forms, as the muscle responds to local compression (ischemic or trigger point compression), local stretch of the muscle using short strokes along the direction of the muscle fibers, and therapeutic stretching across the joint(s) acted on by the muscle being treated. Stretching the muscle to its full length is essential to eliminate the trigger point and restore normal function to the muscle and its functional muscle unit, the muscles that share its activity in moving or stabilizing a joint or part of the body. Stretching can be facilitated by contraction-relaxation techniques, which are incorporated into manual treatment techniques by the therapist and can be taught to the patient. Self-stretching is a therapeutic activity in which the patient can truly participate as a partner in therapy. Muscle can also be relaxed by passive shortening in a pain-free position, the principle behind strain-counterstrain.

Psychological stress can activate muscle trigger points and increase trigger point EMG activity.[43] Relaxation training can reduce psychologically induced muscle tension and results in the lowering of myofascial trigger point electrical activity.[44] Bringing patients into the therapeutic process is empowering to them, restores an element of control on their part, and shares responsibility for managing the pain between the patient and physician. Success is also shared, with patients taking credit for improvement that they achieved as well as the therapist.

The pharmacologic management of muscle pain, whether myofascial or fibromyalgia, uses the usual sequence of drugs for the relief of pain, starting with the nonopiate analgesics discussed previously. Muscle relaxants have been shown to be helpful in common musculoskeletal pain, but their use has not been examined specifically in myofascial pain or in fibromyalgia. Their long-term use has also not been well evaluated, either for effectiveness or for side effects. The use of opiates must be carefully considered because of the dependency issues and the problem of long-term reinforcement of pain behaviors. This is particularly true if significant improvement is possible through the use of effective physical therapy and manual treatment techniques. Biomechanical factors that affect muscular function and aggravate the myofascial component should be identified and corrected. These can be as simple as a pelvic torsion that causes functional leg length discrepancy and pseudoscoliosis that is correctable by manually rotating the ilium or as difficult as sacroiliac dysfunction after a lumbosacral fusion. In all instances, the patient must become a partner in therapy, learning and doing the stretches that keep the muscle at full length to minimize the recurrence of the trigger point.

Cognitive rehabilitation is an essential part of the recovery process in chronic myofascial pain as well as in fibromyalgia syndrome, which is discussed in the following section. As the diagnosis is being made, the patient's goals must be defined. The goals for the outcome of treatment may be refined and redefined during the diagnostic and treatment phase but must be kept in focus. The physician and the patient must be in agreement in developing the goal(s) of treatment. One patient may simply want to sleep through the night, whereas another may want to return to work, and a third patient may want to resume playing tennis, swimming, or skiing.

Patients with chronic myofascial pain and with fibromyalgia have learned to reduce their activity and to rely on others for daily needs, including household chores and even wage-earning activities. They often need help just to take the first steps (literally) in an exercise program. They need to learn that any pain produced by activity is transient and can be treated. They need to know that the physician or therapist is available to help relieve pain. Most of all, they need to find out that they have the resources within themselves to recover and take control of their lives again. Pacing activity helps them achieve specific goals without encountering disabling pain. The fear of suffering further pain is addressed. Patients learn that pain does not necessarily have to prevent them from performing many functions in their lives, as they learn ways to reduce and control pain.

A 55-year-old psychologist experienced an injury to the shoulder that resulted in chronic myofascial and neuropathic pain. After a long search for a drug that would reduce her pain without sedation, she found that a tricyclic antidepressant decreased both the burning and aching components of her pain, but she still had such severe pain that she could not concentrate well. She also had impairment of memory because of the distracting intrusion of pain so that she could no longer work as a clinical psychologist. She decided that instead of letting life pass her by, she would take control herself. She avoided talking about her pain, because focusing on it made it worse. Instead, she found new outlets in her life and has produced prize-winning works of art that can be created in her own time, allowing her to pace herself and take breaks as she finds them necessary. This redirection of a defeatist attitude and depressive reaction to the impairment caused by pain was accomplished with the help of a psychologist in the pain clinic in which she was treated.

Finally, attention must be directed to identifying and correcting physical and medical stresses that can be characterized broadly as ergonomic dysfunctions and metabolic abnormalities.[22] Ergonomic stress factors include poor workstation design, for example, a computer workstation with the keyboard and monitor positioned too high or too low or reference material placed so that the head must be turned too far to the side for long periods. Another common mechanical stressor for head and shoulder pain is the placement of the telephone tucked in the angle of the neck between the shoulder and the ear. The workplace must be made to fit the individual and allow the job to be done without undue musculoskeletal fatigue and injury. An example of a medical stressor is low tissue iron. Iron is obligatory for energy-creating cytochrome oxidase reactions and for the conversion of inactive thyroid hormone (T4) to active thyroid hormone (T3). When iron is depleted from muscle, at a serum ferritin level of approximately 15–20 ng/ml, the individual experiences fatigue and muscle cramps. Tissue iron deficiency produces a metabolic stress that is associated with chronic myofascial pain.[45]

The following case illustrates the value of working with the patient over time to uncover what was not obvious at the start. A 44-year-old physician and skier had constant left hip pain and restricted abduction of the hip. He came to the physician's office specifically because he thought that he had myofascial pain syndrome as the primary cause of the painful hip. Inactivation of the adductor muscle trigger points eliminated his pain temporarily but did not restore full abduction of the leg. It was necessary to explore other causes of hip pain. He was found to have degenerative arthritis of the hip that required a hip replacement. His pain was myofascial in part, but the myofascial pain syndrome was a secondary complication of arthritis.

The patient's previous physicians, including orthopedists, had not worked with him to find a cause but merely treated the condition symptomatically. He then had to consider among different treatment options, including analgesic drug therapy and nonsteroidal anti-inflammatory drugs, curtailment of skiing and seeking alternative exercise activities, and hip replacement. The distinction of secondary or associated myofascial pain syndrome from primary myofascial pain was important in this case, as it is in every case. The correct diagnosis of the underlying condition may not have been apparent at the start.

Fibromyalgia

Fibromyalgia is the other common chronic muscle pain syndrome.[4] It is characterized by widespread muscular pain and pain at tendon insertions and over bone, with no other identifiable cause. It is often associated with a sense that sleep does not restore a normal feeling of being rested and with an unusual degree of fatigability that can be disabling. It is a syndrome rather than a disease and is most likely heterogeneous or the end result of a number of different causes.[46] The common factor that seems to predispose to the unusual degree of muscle pain is hypersensitivity to many different kinds of stimuli.[28,47,48] It is, in fact, a syndrome of mechanical allodynia, or abnormally increased sensitivity to normally nonpainful stimulation. The hypersensitivity is not limited to mechanical stimuli, however, but is seen with both thermal and aural stimulation as well. Hypersensitivity may be the clinical manifestation of the elevation of substance P seen in fibromyalgia and some other chronic pain syndromes.[31] The finding of generalized hypersensitivity to non-noxious stimuli in patients diagnosed as having fibromyalgia

may be a most important result of diagnostic criteria that have at times been criticized for being the product of circular reasoning.[49]

The diagnosis of fibromyalgia syndrome is made by the identification of diffuse tenderness primarily, but not exclusively, in muscle. The criteria established by the American College of Rheumatology[50] require 11 of 18 specified sites to be tender in order to qualify for the diagnosis of fibromyalgia. The criteria were meant to be used for research studies to bring uniformity to the studies that were being done in increasingly greater numbers. They have come into general use for the clinical diagnosis of fibromyalgia, with the frequent caution that the number of tender points can vary from time to time. Thus, it is recognized that individuals can have greater or fewer than 11 tender spots at any given time, but it is the long-term involvement of muscle pain in at least three quadrants of the body that is diagnostic of fibromyalgia. No other criteria are required for diagnosis,[51] although the associated sleep disorder and fatigue are supportive, and a host of associated problems, including irritable bowel syndrome, dyspareunia, headaches, and interstitial cystitis, are said to be suggestive and also indicative of a more widespread "dysregulation syndrome."

Fibromyalgia is a clinical pain syndrome that affects a large number of persons. It presents a number of problems. The commonly used diagnostic criteria do not exclude myofascial pain syndrome unless the muscles are palpated for myofascial trigger points, an examination that is seldom performed. The diagnosis of fibromyalgia itself is daunting, because the condition is well known to be a chronic, lifelong disorder with no cure. No objective laboratory test is available to confirm the diagnosis. Therefore, a patient must convince the physician that she hurts (the overwhelming majority of fibromyalgia patients are women). If she is successful, she is then consigned to an unending treatment program that usually includes a tricyclic antidepressant and an attempt at an exercise program.

The protocol proposed here for management of fibromyalgia first evaluates the patient for identifiable causes of chronic muscle pain. This means a careful examination for myofascial trigger points and for biomechanical dysfunction. Medical causes of diffuse myalgia should be assessed, including hypothyroidism, Lyme disease, protozoan infection (especially amebiasis), drug-induced myalgias such as those associated with the "statin" drugs used to lower cholesterol, and inherited biochemical disorders such as myoadenylate deaminase deficiency. Psychological stressors should also be assessed, as they can induce generalized muscle pain as a manifestation of stress or as a form of somatization. Once medical and mechanical causes are excluded, the treatment of fibromyalgia can become the focus of attention.

Far from maintaining an active role in the home or in the workplace, so many persons with fibromyalgia find work difficult that disability retirement because of this condition has become epidemic.[52] The clear danger of the present approach is that the physician, and society through its disability programs, encourages the development of "sick behavior" and the need to demonstrate ongoing muscle tenderness (for which no reliable objective measure is available) to continue to qualify for disability. The goal of care therefore becomes the maintenance of sickness rather than the return to fitness and productivity.

The difference in approach can be striking. One 46-year-old man had allegedly contracted Lyme disease 20 years before his first visit. He reported that he had been diagnosed as having fibromyalgia 15–20 years before being seen. He was treated with amitriptyline, with continued pain, depression, and fatigue. He had stopped working as an accountant when he contracted Lyme disease but was not receiving disability payments. He had myofascial trigger points in the neck and shoulders. Attention was focused on relieving these specific sources of pain and improving sleep. A gradual, progressive exercise program was instituted. Through many discussions over the course of more than 1 year, he developed a plan of returning to school and trying to regain work as an accountant. The specific goal was to attend one class. He was successful and ultimately completed a 2-year program in accounting, earning straight As and taking the certified public accountant examination. He takes very little medication now and considers himself a success. The change in his attitude and addressing the issue of depression in this individual were critical. Without a focus and a specific, motivating goal, he had drifted for years in the sea of fibromyalgia.

The treatment begins when the patient steps into the room and the physician begins to listen to the patient's story. Often treatment is not directed toward any goal except pain relief, and no end to the treatment is anticipated. Redirection of goals and the development of a realistic plan to achieve them can restore the patient to a productive life, as the case of the psychologist described in the previous section illustrates. Pain may remain an impairment but does not necessarily have to lead to disability.

The medical model for treatment of fibromyalgia is less than satisfactory. Evidence for the effectiveness of pharmacologic management is poor. Only exercise has been proven to be of benefit, and then only for 4 years, after which no difference is seen between those who exercised and those who did not. As in any chronic illness that has no cure, a proliferation of treatments of unknown benefit are used, including dehydroepiandrosterone, guaifenesin, magnesium and malic acid, oxytocin, and other supplements. The physician has an important role in guiding individuals through the maze of unproven remedies.

The patient's pain alters the ability to perform activities and reduces enjoyment or pleasure in participating in activities. It makes tasks or recreational activities difficult. The inability to participate fully in life's activities, as well as chronic discomfort, leads to suffering. Treatment must deal with the suffering as well as the physical pain. As emphasized throughout this chapter, the impact of pain as an impairment is as important as weakness in musculoskeletal pain and sensory loss and weakness in neuropathic pain. Addressing the issue of pain directly as a cause of limited activity allows patients to find ways to limit its intrusion into their lives and enables them to regain control and responsibility for themselves. This element of cognitive rehabilitation is practiced by the clinician in all phases of patient contact, from the prescribing of medication to the prescribing of activity and the encouragement to the patient to try one step at a time in resuming activities that had been dropped. A 10-minute walk or eating one meal a day out of bed and at the table can be a triumph for a patient.

The need for continuity and the establishment of trust are illustrated by the following case of a 40-year-old woman diagnosed as having fibromyalgia. She had retreated to being solely in her home, in particular in her bed, for several years. She literally lived in bed, going out in a wheelchair only for groceries and to therapy.

Her first visit was a reluctant one, made at the insistence of her psychotherapist. She said she was willing to be worked on but had no desire to do anything herself or to change her way of life. She was told that we would work with her and provide her with the tools she needed to decrease her pain if she used them at home. She was also told that we would not work with her unless she made a "contract" with us to be an active part in the process. She left in an angry, defiant mood. Much to our surprise, she returned 2 weeks later, saying that she was willing to work but only if we promised to work with her. We struck a bargain: We would stick with her, even if she had a "down time," and she would do as we asked. Our first request was that she eat one meal every day sitting at the table. She tested us at first, saying that she could not do this activity. When she found that we were still willing to work with her, she began to trust us. She said that she was willing to try to do what we had requested because we had shown faith in her ability to succeed. Because we gained her trust and were not judgmental ("you are a good/bad person because you do/do not do _____") she trusted us and was willing to chance failure, and she became a more active participant in her recovery program. She soon gave up the wheelchair in the office and in therapy, has been eating all meals at the table, and is out of bed for several hours every day, playing with the cat that she bought to help her in her therapy. She now sees that she can perform activities that she had not done in years and that she is capable of success; she is now pushing us to help her do more. She still suffers from social isolation, a problem that remains to be solved.

In this case, a very small increase in activity was proposed to the patient after she had promised that she would try to meet our requests for reaching a mutually agreed-on goal. Meeting a small goal successfully translated into a strongly positive psychological reinforcement for further activity without any physical setback. Part of a therapeutic program is to address this problem directly by showing the patient that increasing activity produces only short-term and treatable consequences. In difficult situations, it may be possible to enlist the cooperation of the patient only in very small or seemingly trivial increases in activity. One has to be ready to address the pain in these situations, however, and to be supportive when the patient makes a positive effort, translated into a strongly positive psychological reinforcement for further activity without suffering any physical setback.

As Harding et al.[40] state, "Activity, activity-related goal setting, and pacing of activity play key roles in the rehabilitation of patients with chronic pain." As illustrated by this patient, and emphasized by these authors, setting an appropriate and achievable goal is essential, because it leads to increased self-efficacy, which is the key to a successful outcome.

In another instance, a young woman was referred by her physical therapist. She had a complex pain problem that involved the thoracic outlet, an ulnar entrapment syndrome, and a median nerve entrapment at the carpal tunnel. She required multiple surgical procedures to treat the nerve compressions and had undergone 13 corrective surgical procedures. The end point of treatment was initially determined by the surgeon to be the elimination of numbness, tingling, and pain. This was never achieved. She continues to have strange sensory complaints such as compression of a trigger point in the shoulder producing numbness in the leg. Goal setting was general (to be able to cook and shop again, but in a vague way), not specific. Her physical therapist characterized her as being very dependent and not likely to take over her own therapy. In fact, as some success was achieved in one area, she developed symptoms in other areas.

The patient had originally complained of numbness and tingling in the arms, especially when she lifted them to put blankets and sheets into the closet and when she did tasks that required prolonged arm use, such as ironing or cooking. She liked to sew and to make quilts but could no longer do either. Her arms became so painful that she could no longer perform even simple household chores.

Electrodiagnostic testing showed slowing of distal motor and sensory latencies compatible with carpal tunnel syndrome, which was then treated surgically. Her pain continued, and she developed numbness in the ulnar side of the hand and forearm up to the elbow, positive Tinel's sign at the ulnar nerve at the elbow, and pain on compression of the brachial plexus at the level of the medial scalene muscle. Electrodiagnostic testing showed slowing of nerve conduction across the cubital tunnel. The surgeons diagnosed cubital tunnel syndrome with ulnar nerve entrapment and thoracic tunnel syndrome. She underwent removal of the first ribs and decompression of the ulnar nerves at the elbow. However, she continued to have pain and tingling in the arms. She had a further complication in that her arms became flexed and restricted to the point that she could not extend them even to 90 degrees at the elbow. She became very disabled and had to rely on others for even simple household tasks and cooking.

The patient's physical therapist worked to stretch the upper arm and pectoral muscles to restore range of movement and function. An extension arm brace was used to maintain the improvement in arm extension, but it had to be worn day and night. She was referred to the pain clinic to facilitate restoration of arm function. The upper arm flexors were very tight, shortened, and tender. Myofascial trigger point injections into the biceps and brachialis muscles and into the pectoralis major and minor muscles allowed more complete extension of the arms, eventually to 175 degrees, and increased range of motion at the shoulder. The physical therapist and the author both taught her home exercises, which she did consistently. We worked with her to find activities that she could accomplish within the movement that she had, because increased activity and increased range of motion at the shoulder produced subjective tingling and objective duskiness of the arms and hands. We reviewed her activities and her wish list of things that she hoped to do. One of them was sewing. One day she brought in a decorative cloth that she had made, saying that she had not been able to sew since she had developed pain, but she was now trying and had succeeded in making a cloth bread cover.

The treatment of this woman raises issues of diagnosis and treatment of a complex chronic pain and neurologic impairment syndrome, for which no firm diagnostic guidelines have been formulated and for which the symptoms seem to lead the patient and physician onward in an endless round of treatment. Thoracic outlet syndrome was diagnosed clinically. No diagnostic test is available that has an acceptable degree of reliability for thoracic outlet syndrome. The diagnosis is based on a high degree of suspicion on the part of the physician, the finding of appropriate neurologic impairment, and the absence of other credible causes of pain and impairment. The electrodiagnostic tests for carpal and cubital tunnel syndromes are reliable insofar as they show abnormalities of nerve conduction and motor function, but the relation of the findings to the complaints of pain, clumsiness, and weakness remain matters of clinical judgment.

When the case selection is good, surgery for carpal tunnel syndrome has an excellent outcome for pain relief. Surgical decompression of the cubital tunnel is performed to relieve pain and to prevent progression of neurologic impairment. Both decompression of the carpal tunnel and of the cubital tunnel carry the small, but real, risk of producing severe postoperative pain that may take months to resolve. The decision to intervene surgically at the thoracic outlet (whether by first rib resection or scalenotomy), the cubital tunnel, or the carpal tunnel is most difficult when indications of nerve entrapment are present at all three sites. Selection of nonsurgical treatment options is also difficult because of lack of adequate guidelines that favor one over another. The treatment of postoperative complications is difficult because options are again limited, and outcomes are not well known or predictable. The patient and the doctor must both be aware of these limitations yet make decisions to proceed in spite of them.

Treatment goals must be selected and agreed on by both the patient and the doctor or therapist. In the case of the young woman just discussed, the initial goal of treatment to relieve pain through a series of surgical procedures was not realized. Short-term goals were established during her treatment with us, which took her from having a painful flexed arm through stretching and trigger point injection therapy and an uncomfortable mechanical splint to strengthening an arm that could be maintained with nearly full extension at the elbow. A therapeutic goal was once to extend the arm at the elbow to 45 degrees. A later goal was to use the arm when dressing, and still later it was to use the arm in simple household tasks, including cooking. A measurable outcome was the completion of a simple sewing project. A long-term goal not yet realized is to regain the ability to quilt. This case illustrates the problems of decision making when diagnostic studies are not conclusive, clinical judgment is uncertain, and treatment outcomes are not well predicted. It further exemplifies the goal-setting principles discussed by Harding et al.,[40] in which activity goals should not only be physical but also functional, involving daily tasks or activities, whether related to work, personal care, or recreation. The final activity goal is to reintegrate the individual into the social setting.

Chronic Neuropathies

The treatment of diabetic neuropathy is usually symptomatic and directed to diminution of pain. A goal that may or may not be stated, but one that may be primary to the patient, is to decrease the disruption of sleep and other daily activities caused by the pain.

A 48-year-old psychologist had well-controlled diabetes without known complications for 20 years. Once neuropathy developed, despite continued good diabetic control, pain increased over 18 months to the point at which it was not possible to control it with drugs. His pain was intense, and he was so distracted by the burning sensation that he could no longer work, and he could not sleep through the night. An immediate goal was to reduce his pain enough to let him sleep, and a long-range goal was to return to work.

The most effective approach to symptomatic treatment of painful diabetic neuropathy is to use drugs to block pain impulse transmission peripherally or alter transmission of pain impulses through the dorsal column of the spinal cord to the thalamus and the cerebral cortex. Pharmacologic therapy is designed to reduce the severity of pain and to promote sleep, goals that are intended to allow patients to resume more normal activities and regain control over their lives. The first level of drug therapy uses nonspecific nonopioid analgesics such as nonsteroidal anti-inflammatory drugs and acetaminophen. Adjuvant analgesics include the tricyclic antidepressant drugs[53] and the newer antidepressant drugs that similarly increase both serotonin and norepinephrine. The drugs of choice have been the tricyclic antidepressant drugs, notably amitriptyline, which have been subjected to careful clinical trials and have been demonstrated to be effective.[53,54] Selective serotonin reuptake inhibitors have not been shown to be as effective in neuropathic pain; indeed fluoxetine is not clinically effective at all, but citalopram and paroxetine have been shown to be useful in diabetic neuropathy.[55,56] These drugs have been shown to reduce the burning pain of neuropathy but are effective in virtually all of the chronic or recurring types of pain except the lancinating type, which is better treated with anticonvulsant drugs. The newer drugs, such as venlafaxine, have not yet been tested as the tricyclic drugs have. Steroids, either systemic or epidural, have not been proven to be effective. Anticonvulsant drugs are most useful in treating lancinating or paroxysmal pain and have been shown to be effective in different painful neuropathies including diabetes.[57] Gabapentin is one of the most recent of the anticonvulsant drugs to be studied by randomized controlled trial for the treatment of painful neuropathy in patients with diabetic mellitus. It has been shown to be effective compared with placebo both in the reduction of pain and in the improvement of QOL.[58] The γ-aminobutyric acid antagonist baclofen is also useful in treating these kinds of neuropathic pain. Capsaicin eliminates substance P from peripheral nerve endings in the skin and is effective in relieving pain in peripheral neuropathy, including diabetic neuropathy, postherpetic neuropathy, and even the pain of articular origin, but is often not well tolerated because it burns to a sometimes intolerable degree during the first week of application.

At times, however, drugs fail to relieve pain. Pain itself is the impairment that leads to the inability to sit, stand, or walk comfortably and also prevents thinking and concentrating, interfering with the ability to read or write or to interact reliably with others. Thus, pain can be the cause of the inability to perform the functions necessary to do work or to hold a job, as in the example of the person with diabetes recounted above.

Pain may be an associated cause of impaired function. An 84-year-old retiree with severe diabetes lost feeling in his hands to the extent that he could not hold items unless he was looking at them. However, the bitter complaint that led him to consider suicide was the unrelenting constant pain that never left him, that never let him sleep, and that prevented him from participating in the usual daily activities that he and his wife used to enjoy. Similarly, an 85-year-old woman had a 15-year history of sensory neuropathy of unknown etiology. During the first several years of the illness her major problem was numbness in the legs. However, over the years a burning, tingling pain developed that became more severe in the afternoon and evening, interfering with her sleep. Eventually, the symptoms spread to the hands and face and even caused burning in the tongue. Drug therapy failed to relieve the symptoms, clonazepam being the only drug that made the symptoms bearable, but at an unacceptable cost of memory loss and ataxia. Every day became a search for relief, and her life became bound up with doctors and ineffective treatment.

Pain is the dominant factor in both of these patients' lives. In the case of the man, he has reached a suicidal state of despair. In each case, the search for relief has become all consuming. Drug therapy has failed, and family support and behavioral modifications or cognitive therapy have been unsuccessful in relieving pain. The physician's role in treatment is to find the opening to a single achievable goal that will give some measure of success and re-establish the sense in patients that at least at times they can control their life even if they cannot eliminate the pain. This can be as simple as designating an hour of the day to a different activity that can be accomplished despite the pain. This was what was eventually done in these cases, so that even though the two individuals still have pain, they have learned that they can participate in other activities, and they have found that when they do so, their perception of pain is reduced. They have found a way, in other words, of using cognitive principles of pain management to engage in "well behavior" and lessen the impact of pain on their lives.

The response of a woman in her 50s is instructive as an example of a partially effective way of dealing with intractable chronic pain. Mary O. has a progressive painful neuropathy that has responded only slightly to anticonvulsant drug therapy. Doses of medication have been limited by side effects. She has both burning and electriclike pain and mechanical aching pain, as if she is standing on marbles or has steel bars pressing on her feet and hands. Her hands are so sensitive that she has to wear gloves to hold objects for everyday tasks. She has taken two part-time jobs, however, because she found that working "takes my mind off the pain."

Cognitive therapy or behavioral modification to reduce the impact of pain is well known.[59] Focusing on something other than the pain inhibits the transmission of painful input through the spinal cord to the brain. This is a goal of therapeutic intervention that uses imagery or other mind-absorbing activities to reduce pain and to help encourage resumption of normal behavior or activity. By working two part-time jobs, Mary O. has also taken control over part of her life rather than letting pain be the focus of all of her activities.

Measuring Effectiveness

Many treatments have been used for years and only recently have been subjected to careful assessment. An example of such time-honored treatments that were found to be of no benefit were bed rest and back-mobilizing exercises for acute LBP.[19] These treatments were once mainstays of nonsurgical treatment of back pain. Bed rest is now prescribed much less frequently and for shorter periods of time than the 5 or more days that were previously common. Back-mobilizing exercises are still in general use. Prolonged bed rest in the acute phase does no better than routine activity, deconditions the individual, and produces a financial hardship for the patient and employer alike. Thus, the ability to accurately assess the outcome of treatment becomes extremely important when prescribing therapy for persons with acute and chronic pain; the issue in chronic pain being even more important because treatment may be continued for long periods.

The practitioner must be aware of the general efficacy of the treatment proposed and, in addition, assess its usefulness in a particular patient. This issue is not only of practical importance to the patient being treated but is also of importance to government health regulation agencies, to insurance companies, to all who must finance health care, and to those who determine health care policy.[60] Treatment should be cost effective as well as therapeutically effective. Treatments without benefit must be identified and avoided. At the same time, lack of data about a particular therapy does not mean that it lacks efficacy but that it should be evaluated. Therefore, the treating physician must be capable of assessing the medical and personal needs of the patient and should have already assessed the effectiveness of available therapies and be able to present them to the patient.

A treatment program can then be developed by the patient and physician or therapist, with the patient a critical partner in determining the short- and long-term goals of treatment and deciding among different treatment options. The outcome must be relevant to the patient's perceived needs. Treating physicians and therapists may see reduction in the level of pain and a decrease in the use of analgesics as an acceptable and measurable goal. The patient may be more concerned with being able to sit in class for 1 hour, to work a full day, to play tennis or just walk for 15 minutes, or to engage once again in sexual activity. Treatment outcome is rarely measured in these terms of patient satisfaction.

Measurement tools have been developed to assess patient satisfaction, functional activities, and reduction in symptom severity to relate the effect of treatment to the needs of individual patients.[60] For example, whereas walking a mile, or 30 minutes, might represent an accomplishment for one patient, it might be an inappropriate goal for a marathoner. On the other hand, it might be an unthinkable goal for the person who spends 90% of his or her waking day in bed. Hence, the patient's goal(s) and the physician's goal(s) should be concordant rather than discordant.[61] It is the physician's role to make this happen.

Measurement of Impairments

Measurements of pain and suffering address the issue of impairment, in that pain and suffering are the elements of impairment that lead to disability. These tests do not relate pathologic changes of pain-producing conditions with pain, as the pathophysiologic basis of pain and the intensity of pain are not directly related. Instead, the tests measure the patient's perceived level of pain or functional or psychological impairment that occurs as a result of pain. Because many of these measurements are subjective, attempts have also been made to measure pain levels more objectively by assessing pain behaviors, including facial expression, postures, motor activity, and speech characteristics. Attempts to validate pain complaints with objective measurements of pathologic changes on imaging studies or laboratory tests as a condition of considering a complaint of pain to be "real" inappropriately eliminate from consideration those patients with chronic NSLBP, myofascial pain syndrome, fibromyalgia, and other causes of pain that do not have an established pathophysiologic or anatomic basis.

Instruments of Pain Measurement

Measurements of the degree of pain allow one to assess the effectiveness of treatment on an ongoing basis. The assessment of the psychosocial context of the pain experience and measures of pain intensity are reviewed in detail by Turk and Melzack.[62]

The Visual Analog Scale has been used as a subjective measurement of pain. Its advantage is that it is simple and easily understood, quick, and inexpensive and can be administered repeatedly during the course of care. The individual simply marks the perceived level of pain on a 10-cm line that is labeled as "no pain" at one end and "worst pain ever experienced" at the other. The distance in millimeters from the "no pain" end is measured and becomes the score. The test has content validity for intensity of pain, has test-retest reliability, and compares favorably with other measures of pain.

Pain drawing is a useful means for the patient to communicate to the doctor the location of pain. It can be used to indicate different intensities of pain in different areas. It was designed to identify nonphysiologic distributions of pain, thereby indicating when further psychological assessment was needed. Its drawback is that conditions such as LBP, myofascial pain syndrome, and fibromyalgia all have nonphysiologic pain patterns.

The Functional Capacity Evaluation (FCE)[63] is an attempt to assess what a patient can do at a specific time. It is a measure both of impairment, because its measurements depend on strength and range of motion, and of disability, as it measures ability to sit, stand, bend, lift, and so forth. It is not a measurement of what a person should do but rather what a person can do at the time of assessment. It is often used to predict whether a person can work at a job that entails elements of the activities studied, such as sitting for 2 hours at one time or repeated lifting and bending. The drawback of the FCE is that no standard set of activities is used that can be said to set a standard. Disability in certain tasks or activities does not necessarily mean that the patient has disability in other tasks. The individual may still be able to perform occupationally relevant tasks even if disabled in certain other activities. The reliability, relevance, validity, and reproducibility of the FCE have been questioned, in part because of lack of standardization.

The Minnesota Multiphasic Personality Inventory 2 (MMPI-2) has been used to assess patients with chronic pain. However, the standardization samples used for profile interpretation are not appropriate for these individuals. Hypochondriasis, depression, and hysteria scores tend to be high in patients with chronic pain and reflect disease activity rather than psychological status.[64] The test cannot distinguish organic from functional disease. It has three validity scales to evaluate how willing the subject is to answer honestly and 10 clinical scales, which include depression, hypochondriasis, hysteria, schizophrenia, psychasthenia, and paranoia. The overall pattern of responses is interpreted by the trained evaluator. The test has been used to predict how rewarding a person may find chronic pain. It has found its widest application in patients with chronic pain by its evaluation of psychosocial factors, which affect many people with chronic pain. Statistical associations have been made with MMPI-2 profiles and certain patient characteristics. However, computer-generated reports and applications to single individuals are more hypotheses about functioning than they are specific descriptions.

The McGill Pain Questionnaire[65] is a major tool in the assessment of pain, using words to describe the sensory, affective quality, and intensity of the experience of pain. This questionnaire has been shown to be valid, reliable, and consistent; to be reproducible; and to be very useful, even to the point of having discriminatory value to distinguish different pain syndromes from one another.

Measurement of Disabilities

The West Haven–Yale Multidimensional Pain Inventory[66] is a self-report measurement that assesses a broad domain of psychosocial variables associated with the chronic pain experience. It emphasizes the patients' own perceptions of their pain problems, their impact on their lives, and the responses of others to their pain. It addresses the experience of pain in the workplace, in social and recreational settings, and in the home. It is useful to measure the response to treatment, as it is sensitive to improvement in pain and functioning. It gives insight into pain-related disability as it examines the subjects' views of the impact of pain on their ability to carry out work, recreational, and home related activities.

Another measure of the chronic pain patients' capacity to cope and to function, and therefore their pain-related disability, is the Chronic Illness Problem Inventory.[67] This measures the ability of the subject to function within the restrictions of

physical limitations and looks at psychosocial function, health care behaviors, and marital adjustment. It focuses on the patient's competency in the face of chronic illness. It has been tested for validity in the pain patient population. These individuals reported more severe problems and greater restrictions in activity than other patients with chronic illness. The test is designed as both a screening test and a measure of treatment outcome.

The illness behavior inventory is a useful measure of improvement in pain with treatment. This questionnaire attempts to measure hypochondriasis and abnormal illness behavior. Patients with pain characteristically score high on the questions that indicate somatic preoccupation and that emphasize the physical rather than psychological basis of their pain. The questionnaire has utility in identifying patients who use illness behaviors to cope. It is limited in usefulness in developing treatment plans but has been shown to be sensitive to treatment effects.[68]

The Sickness Impact Profile[69] is a well-validated measure of perceived health status. The test was designed to be useful across cultural, medical, and demographic boundaries. It deals with the areas of rest and sleep, eating, work, home management, recreation, mobility, physical self-care, social interactions, alertness behavior, emotional behavior, and communication. It is a wide-ranging assessment of function that evaluates both disabilities (restriction or inability to perform an activity such as walking) and handicaps (the inability to perform functions, such as holding specific jobs, appropriate to age and gender). A modified version specific to the problem of LBP has been developed. A Spanish version has been tested for reliability and validity. It has been used both as a measure of outcome of treatment and as a research tool.

The Pain Disability Index (PDI)[70] is a brief and easily completed measure of the impact of pain on daily activities, such as recreational activity, social activity, occupational functioning, sexual behavior, self-care, and basic life support activities such as eating and sleeping. The PDI has been found to be sensitive and to have a high internal consistency in the assessment of functional disability. It is a measure of function, and as such, it measures handicap as well as disability.

An activity diary has been used to assess the subject's activity level, medication use, and pain. Questions have been raised regarding its validity, but findings are generally stable over 1 week. The diary can reveal how much time a patient spends reclining or in bed, an activity that leads to deconditioning.

Measurement of Handicap and Quality of Life

Attempts have been made to measure QOL using function and mood scales and assessments of the effect of illness and disability on life activities, such as work, home responsibilities, social activities, sexual function, and the like. The problem has been addressed very specifically in relation to cancer patients. The medical outcome studies short form[71] has been used for this purpose, looking at the areas mentioned previously and including mental health and health perception. A combination of tests may be needed to adequately assess QOL, however. Tests of depression and the previously described Sickness Impact Profile have been used to assess mood and function. The assessment of QOL looks at physical function and psychological status and the impact of symptoms on physical and social functioning. Many tests are general and do not specifically address the effect of pain on function but, in combination with tests of mood and assessment of social functioning, give a useful picture of the impact of pain on QOL. The PDI described above directly assesses QOL issues in addressing social and sexual functioning but omits assessment of mood, for example.

For those who deal with persons suffering from chronic pain and who attempt to evaluate the effect of the pain on their lives, the quality of the measurement is a significant issue. Tests are usually evaluated in terms of their reliability and their validity. Validity refers to the test measuring what it purports to measure. Is the test relevant to the function or activity that is under consideration? For example, are the items measured in an FCE relevant to the kind of tasks required in the subject's job? Reliability speaks to the consistency of the measurement. Does the test give the same result over time and between examiners (single rater reproducibility on repeat tests and inter-rater reliability among different examiners)? The issues of validity and reliability should be understood for each of the tests used in assessment of function and of psychosocial impact of pain on the individual by the person who is using the results to plan and monitor treatment.

The outcome of different therapies must be well understood, so that the physician can choose those treatment options that address the perceived needs of both the patient and the physician. Objective and subjective measures of the impact of chronic pain on function as well as assessment of perceived pain are useful in measuring the effect of an intervention on the patient's major problem. The goal in treating myofascial pain is not simply the elimination of the myofascial trigger point or even necessarily the reduction of pain; rather it is the restoration of desired function by the patient. The patient must have a realistic, achievable goal in this regard that is understood by both the patient and the doctor.

This chapter has attempted to illustrate that physical impairment is not necessarily the most disabling factor associated with chronic pain but that pain itself is an important impairment that leads to disability and hence results in handicaps that are expressed in truncated lives. Addressing the suffering from pain itself as an impairment is best done by enlisting the patient as a responsible partner in therapy. The physician should be mindful of the benefits to be obtained from encouraging the patient to become a partner in the treatment process.

References

1. Magni G. The Epidemiology of Musculoskeletal Pain. In H Voeroy, H Merskey (eds), Progress in Fibromyalgia and Myofascial Pain. Amsterdam: Elsevier, 1993;3–21.
2. Raspe H. Back Pain. In AJ Silman, MC Hochberg (eds), Epidemiology of the Rheumatic Diseases. Oxford: Oxford University Press, 1993.
3. Frymoyer JW, Cats-Baril W. An overview of the incidence and costs of low back pain. Orthop Clin North Am 1991; 22:263.
4. de Girolamo G. Epidemiology and social costs of low back pain and fibromyalgia. Clin J Pain 1991;7(suppl 1):S1.
5. Linton S. The socioeconomic impact of chronic back pain: is anyone benefitting? Pain 1998;75:163.
6. Verhaak PFM, Kerssens JJ, Dekker J, et al. Prevalence of chronic benign pain disorder among adults: a review of the literature. Pain 1998;77:231.
7. Becker N, Thomsen AB, Olsen AK, et al. Pain epidemiology and health related quality of life in chronic non-malignant pain patients referred to a Danish multidisciplinary pain center. Pain 1997;73:393.
8. Engel CC, Von Korff M, Katon WJ. Back pain in primary care: predictors of high health costs. Pain 1996;65:197.

9. Scudds RJ, Robertson JM. Empirical evidence of the association between the presence of musculoskeletal pain and physical disability in community-dwelling senior citizens. Pain 1998;75:229.

10. Solomon P, Tunks E. The role of litigation in predicting disability outcome in chronic pain patients. Clin J Pain 1991;7:300.

11. Becker N, Hojsted J, Sjogren P, Erickson J. Sociodemographic predictors of treatment in chronic non-malignant pain patients. Do patients receiving or applying for disability pension benefit from multidisciplinary pain treatment? Pain 1998;77:279.

12. Kost RG, Straus SE. Post-herpetic neuralgia–pathogenesis, treatment and prevention. N Engl J Med 1996; 335:32.

13. Gerwin RD, Dommerholt J. Treatment of Myofascial Pain Syndromes. In R Weiner (ed), Pain Management; a Practical Guide for Clinicians. Boca Raton, FL: St. Lucie Press (in press).

14. Fordyce WE (ed). Back Pain in the Workplace. Seattle: International Association for the Study of Pain, 1995.

15. Teasell RW, Merskey H. Chronic pain disability in the workplace. Pain Forum 1997;6:228.

16. Wallis BJ, Lord SM, Bogduk N. Resolution of psychological distress of whiplash patients following treatment by radiofrequency neurotomy: a randomized, double-blind, placebo-controlled trial. Pain 1997;73:15.

17. Turk DC. Efficacy of Multidisciplinary Pain Centers in the Treatment of Chronic Pain. In Pain Treatment Centers at a Crossroads: A Practical and Conceptual Reappraisal. Seattle: International Association for the Study of Pain, 1996;257–273.

18. Pal B, Mangion P, Hossain MA, Diffey BL. A controlled trial of continuous lumbar traction in the treatment of back pain and sciatica. Br J Rheumatol 1986;25:181.

19. Malmivaara A, Hakkien U, Aro T, et al. The treatment of acute low back pain—bed rest, exercises, or ordinary activity. N Engl J Med 1995;332:351.

20. Cherkin DC, Deyo RA, Battie M, et al. A comparison of physical therapy, chiropractic manipulation, and provision of an educational booklet for the treatment of patients with low back pain. N Engl J Med 1998;339:1021–1029.

21. van Poppel MNM, Koes BW, van der Ploeg T, et al. Lumbar supports and education for the prevention of low back pain in industry. JAMA 1998;279:1789.

22. Simons DG, Travell JG, Simons LS. Myofascial Pain and Dysfunction: The Trigger Point Manual (2nd ed), vol 1. Baltimore: Williams & Wilkins, 1999.

23. Hubbard DR, Berkoff GM. Myofascial trigger points show spontaneous needle EMG activity. Spine 1993;18:1803.

24. Chen JT, Chen SM, Kuan TS, et al. Phentolamine effect on the spontaneous electrical activity of active loci in a myofascial trigger spot of rabbit skeletal muscle. Arch Phys Med Rehabil 1998;79:790.

25. Hong C-Z, Torigoe Y, Yu J. The localized twitch responses in responsive taut bands of rabbit skeletal muscle are related to the reflexes at spinal cord level. J Musculoskel Pain 1995;3:15.

26. Gerwin RD, Shannon S, Hong C-Z, et al. Interrater reliability in myofascial trigger point examination. Pain 1997;69:65.

27. Granges G, Littlejohn G. Pressure pain thresholds in pain-free subjects, in patients with chronic regional pain syndromes, and in patients with fibromyalgia syndrome. Arthritis Rheum 1993;36:642.

28. McDermid AJ, Rollman GB, McCain GA. Generalized hypervigilance in fibromyalgia: evidence of perceptual amplification. Pain 1996;66:133.

29. Kosek E, Hansson P. Modulatory influence on somatosensory perception from vibration and heterotopic conditioning stimulation (HNCS) in fibromyalgia and healthy subjects. Pain 1997;70:41.

30. Lautenbacher S, Rollman GB, McCain GA. Multi-method assessment of experimental and clinical pain in patients with fibromyalgia. Pain 1994;59:45.

31. Russell IJ. Neurochemical pathogenesis of fibromyalgia syndrome. J Musculoskel Pain 1996;4:61.

32. WHO. World Health Organization International Classification of Impairments, Disabilities, and Handicaps: a Manual of Classification Relating to the Consequences of Disease. Geneva: World Health Organization, 1980.

33. Cassell E. The Nature of Suffering and the Goals of Medicine. New York: Oxford University Press, 1991;36.

34. Roy R. The Social Context of the Chronic Pain Sufferer. Toronto: University of Toronto Press, 1992.

35. Good M-JD, Brodwin PE, Good BJ, Kleinman A (eds). Pain as Human Experience. Berkeley: University of California Press, 1992.

36. Rudy TE, Kerns RD, Turk DC. Chronic pain and depression: toward a cognitive-behavioral model. Pain 1988;35:129.

37. Aronoff GM. Chronic pain and the disability epidemic. Clin J Pain 1991;7:330.

38. Brena SF, Turk DC. Vocational Disability: a Challenge to Pain Rehabilitation Programs. In GM Aronoff (ed), Pain Centers: a Revolution in Health Care. New York: Raven, 1988;167–180.

39. Morley S, Eccleston C, Williams A. Systematic review and meta-analysis of randomized controlled trials of cognitive behavior therapy and behavior therapy for chronic pain in adults, excluding headache. Pain 1999;80:1.

40. Harding VR, Simmonds MJ, Watson PJ. Physical therapy for chronic pain. Pain: Clinical Updates, 1999;VI:1.

41. Feine JS. An assessment of the efficacy of physical therapy and physical modalities for the control of chronic musculoskeletal pain. Pain 1997;71:5.

42. Leino P, Aro S, Hasan J. Trunk muscle function and low back disorders: a ten year follow-up study. J Chronic Dis 1987;40:289.

43. McNulty W, Gevirtz R, Berkoff G, Hubbard D. Needle electromyographic evaluation of trigger point response to a psychological stressor. Psychophysiology 1994; 31:313.

44. Banks SL, Jacobs DW, Gevirtz R, Hubbard DR. Effects of autogenic relaxation training in active myofascial trigger points. J Musculoskel Pain 1998;6:23.

45. Gerwin R. A study of 96 subjects examined both for fibromyalgia and myofascial pain. J Musculoskel Pain 1995; 3(suppl 1):121.

46. Turk DC, Okifuji A, Sinclair JD, Starz TW. Pain, disability, and physical functioning in subgroups of patients with fibromyalgia. J Rheumatol 1996;23:1255.

47. Bradley LA. Fibromyalgia: a model for chronic pain. J Musculoskel Pain 1998;6:19.

48. Norregaard J, Bendtsen L, Lykkegard J, Jensen R. Pressure and heat pain thresholds and tolerances in patients with fibromyalgia. J Musculoskel Pain 1997;5:43.

49. Quintner JL, Cohen ML. Fibromyalgia falls foul of a fallacy. Lancet 1999;353:1092.

50. Wolfe F, Smythe HA, Yunus MB, et al. The American College of Rheumatology criteria for the classification of fibromyalgia. Arthritis Rheum 1990;33:160.

51. Bennett RM. Fibomyalgia: the commonest cause of widespread pain. Compr Ther 1995;21:269.

52. Wolfe F. The fibromyalgia problem. J Rheumatol 1997; 24:1247.

53. Max MB, Lynch SA, Muir J, et al. Effects of desipramine, amitriptyline, and fluoxetine on pain in diabetic neuropathy. N Engl J Med 1992;326:1250.

54. Ollat H, Cesaaro P. Pharmacology of neuropathic pain. Clin Neuropharmacol 1995;18:391.

55. Sindrup SH, Gram LF, Brosen K, et al. The selective serotonin reuptake inhibitor paroxetine is effective in the treatment of diabetic neuropathy symptoms. Pain 1990;42:135.

56. Sindrup SH, Bjerre U, Dejgaard A, et al. The selective serotonin reuptake inhibitor citalopram relieves the symptoms of diabetic neuropathy. Clin Pharmacol Ther 1992; 52:547.

57. Swerdlow M., Anticonvulsant drugs and chronic pain. Clin Neuropharmacol 1984;7:51.

58. Backonja M, Beydoun A, Edwards KR, et al. Gabapentin for the symptomatic treatment of painful neuropathy in patients with diabetes mellitus. JAMA 1998;280:1831.

59. Fordyce WE. Behavioral Methods for Chronic Pain and Illness. St. Louis: Mosby, 1976.

60. Clancy CM, Eisenberg JM. Outcomes research: measuring the end results of health care. Science 1998;282:245.

61. Sledge WH, Feinstein AR. A clinimetric approach to the components of the patient-physician relationship. JAMA 1997;278:2043.

62. Turk DC, Melzack R (eds). Handbook of Pain Assessment. New York: Guilford Press, 1992.

63. Mayer TG, Gatchel RJ. Functional Restoration for Spinal Disorders: the Sports Medicine Approach. Philadelphia: Lea & Febiger, 1988.

64. Bradley LA, Haile JM, Jaworski TM. Assessment of Psychological Status Using Interviews and Self-Report Instruments. In DC Turk, R Melzack (eds), Handbook of Pain Assessment. New York: Guilford Press, 1992; 193–213.

65. Melzack R. The McGill pain questionnaire: major properties and scoring methods. Pain 1975;1:277.

66. Kerns RD, Turk DC, Rudy TE. The West Haven–Yale Multidimensional Pain Inventory (WHYMPI). Pain 1985;23:345.

67. Kames LD, Nabiloff BD, Heinrich RL, Schag CC. The chronic illness problem inventory: problem-oriented psychosocial assessment of patients with chronic illness. Int J Psychiatry Med 1984;14:65.

68. Waddell, G, Pilowsky I, Bond MR. Clinical assessment and interpretation of abnormal illness behavior in low back pain. Pain 1989;39:41.

69. Follick MJ, Smith TW, Ahern DK. The sickness impact profile: a global measure of disability in chronic low back pain. Pain 1985;21:67.

70. Tait RC, Pollard CA, Margolis RB, et al. The pain disability index: psychometric properties and validity data. Arch Phys Med Rehabil 1987;68:438.

71. Stewart AL, Hays RD, Ware JE. The MOS short-form general health survey: reliability and validity in a patient population. Med Care 1988;26:724.

Chapter 12
Management of Persons with Headache

Allan L. Bernstein

Nature of the Problem

Extent of the Problem

Incidence and Prevalence

Headache is one of the most common disorders, occurring in up to 90% of individuals in any given year. The most common forms are migraine and tension headaches, which account for the vast majority. Other headaches may be caused by trauma, infection, anemia, concurrent metabolic illness, and side effects of medications, or they may be secondary to disorders of the cervical spine. The condition is more common in women and most prevalent between the ages of 18 and 50 years, prime working years for most people.

Migraine, a well-defined primary headache disorder,[1] is a recurrent event, associated with headache, nausea, vomiting, photophobia, sonophobia, and visual disturbances. It is also associated with hypersensitivity to smells, motion, and many foods, including alcohol. In the United States, an estimated 17% of adult women and 8% of adult men are thought to have migraine.[2] In addition, up to 10% of all children have migraine, with an equal distribution between the sexes before puberty. Migraine is a hereditary disorder.[3] Families with migraine share their treatment strategies, prevention strategies, and fear of migraine.

Tension headaches occur equally between males and females. They are present in 40–60% of the adult population and may be equally prevalent in children, although the data are inconclusive at this time. They tend to be less severe but are more chronic than migraine headaches. They typically occur toward the end of the day, although they can be triggered by physical or emotional stress at any time. These headaches may be difficult to separate from pain that originates at the upper cervical vertebrae, joints, or disks. The characteristics of the pain include a bilateral location, a pressurelike feeling ("a band around my head"), and a distribution of pain, including the occipital region or the retro-orbital region, or both. The description of "pain behind my eyes" usually refers to a tension headache with an upper cervical component. The pain of tension headaches can extend to the periorbital region (often mistakenly called a "sinus" headache), the shoulders, or even into the teeth, triggering unnecessary dental treatments.

Burden of Care

When one family member has headaches, others are often required to take over for the disabled member.[4] Household chores, such as laundry and shopping, still need to be done. Meals must be prepared and cleaned up. Children need to be driven to school and after-school activities. A spouse may need to take time off from work to provide child care or to take the affected individual to the doctor or emergency department. Social events are canceled or not planned at all. Children may be resentful of a parent who is unpredictably unavailable or who needs assistance when they have other things planned.

The cost of headache can be measured in a variety of ways.[5-8] A dollar amount can be calculated by adding up the number of days lost from work and the salary per day. Other figures are available to calculate the cost of housework per day. Less reliable are the self-estimates of the degree of productivity while actually at work, although this amount of decreased work is significant. Loss of work by family members caring for the patient or the children or providing transportation for medical care needs to be included in the cost analysis.

The cost of medication can be substantial for many people who are not covered by comprehensive health insurance. Even those with health insurance may have a dollar limit on the total cost of medication, which is often exceeded for patients with difficult-to-control headaches. Typical headache medication can cost up to $40 per dose and may be needed up to three times a week. Other medications, specific to migraine, may cost $10–15 per pill, with medication bills of $100–300 per month not uncommon. Most medications are less expensive, but the potential exists for significant economic impact from headache, taking into account the combination of missed work, canceled travel plans, and cost of treatment.

The cost of headache needs to be measured in terms of direct financial cost, disability from work with potential loss of occupational advancement, emotional factors regarding "fear of headache," disability from the side effects of currently available treatments, and overall QOL.

Nature of the Disease

Headache is not a specific disease. It has been useful throughout this book to carry out the analysis of persons with chronic illness using the WHO classification, wherein analysis begins at the cellular level in terms of the underlying anatomic or physiologic basis. The level of "disease" has moreover been the primary focus of medical care leading to diagnosis. One can further identify the etiology (to the extent known), the biochemistry, or the genetics of the disorder. Prognosis can also be addressed at this level of analysis.

The natural history of the problem is the fundamental background on which the management of the person must proceed. In the case of chronic tension and migraine headaches, the natural history is that of intermittent illness, generally nonprogressive with periods of greater or lesser frequency and severity.

Pathogenesis

Chronic headache, the subject of this chapter, is a symptom of a multitude of conditions that involve pain-producing structures in the head. Patients often describe their headaches by location rather than etiologies. Hence, "sinus headaches" may have nothing to do with diseases of the sinus cavities but instead reflect pain localized to the region over the frontal, maxillary, or ethmoid sinuses. Similarly, "eye pain" or temporomandibular joint pain more accurately describes a location of pain than an etiology. The headaches associated with cerebral vasodilatation, such as from migraine, alcohol, or hypoxia, may be diffuse or localized but do not reflect focal disease.

Acute conditions within the head tend to give nonlocalizing pain such as increased intracranial pressure or infections of the meninges. Ruptured blood vessels may initially present as a localized painful process, but the symptoms rapidly become generalized. Ischemic strokes may be painful at the onset as one area of the brain becomes ischemic and the collateral vessels dilate to compensate for the lost flow. This localized pain generally subsides and is not useful in identifying the underlying etiology of the ischemic event.

Because headache is a symptom of diverse conditions, it has no specific anatomic or biochemical marker. Some specific headache disorders, such as migraine, are associated with changes in serotonin levels during acute attacks. Others, such as chronic tension headaches, are associated with low serotonin in the spinal fluid on a chronic basis. Chronic pain of any origin may show the same decrease in CSF serotonin. Headaches of cervicogenic origin have no demonstrable pathology. Cluster headache, although probably related to migraine, has chemical abnormalities (histamine) that can only be detected during acute attacks. Cluster headache also appears to be related to sleep disorders.

The role of serotonin in migraine headaches has been controversial. Although low serum serotonin is seen during acute attacks, and serotonergic drugs such as the triptan group seem to relieve acute migraine, selective serotonin reuptake inhibitors have not proved useful in the prevention or treatment of migraine. In addition, tricyclic antidepressants with primarily serotonergic properties have been less effective than antidepressants with mixed serotonergic and adrenergic properties in preventing migraine. Evidence has shown that dopamine may be a significant factor in migraine.[9] Dopamine-blocking drugs (phenothiazines, meclopropamide) have been used for acute treatment for many years without a full understanding of the mechanism. The newer theories help clear up some of the confusion.

Depression and migraine seem intimately related. They both are associated with low serotonin levels. Both are seen primarily in women, and both have strong familial associations. Frequent migraine attacks may produce situational depression and exacerbate an endogenous depression. Acute and chronic depression are associated with an increasing number of headaches.

Hormones are a factor in most headaches in women. Headaches often begin at menarche and occur in a cyclical pattern for most of a woman's life. The headache pattern changes with pregnancy and returns to baseline after delivery. Secondary headaches may develop in women with young children in the house (related to sleep deprivation), added marital stress, and concern over finances. The onset of menopause, although a time of decreasing headaches for some women, is associated with increased headaches in others. Some women consider having a hysterectomy as a means of controlling their headaches, although this has not proved to be effective. Women who had hysterectomies for medical reasons reported no change in their headache pattern. One study on hormone-related headaches suggested that the rate of decline in estrogen was the key factor in producing perimenstrual headaches.[10] Supplemental estrogen was only partially effective in preventing these headaches. Oral contraceptives and hormone replacement therapy have been inconsistent in their effect on headaches.

Many headaches are secondary to medications. These can be analgesics, which give rebound headaches, or medications taken for other conditions, with headache as a side effect. Typical examples include vasodilators such as nitrate drugs, antibiotics such as tetracyclines, histamine H_2 blockers such as cimetidine, and vitamins, including vitamin A, vitamin D, and niacin.

Diagnosis

Headache is one of the few disorders in which the diagnosis is made almost exclusively by the history and physical examination. The primary headache disorders, notably migraine, tension headache, and cluster headache, have no commonly available diagnostic tool other than the history and a physical examination. A history of repeated, similar attacks with periods of return to baseline health is the hallmark of a primary headache disorder.[1] Imaging studies are not indicated in patients with typical headaches and nonfocal neurologic examinations. Similarly, laboratory testing is not indicated for these disorders.

If the history and physical examination are not consistent with a primary headache disorder, further evaluation is indicated. Focal neurologic abnormalities on examination require a more detailed workup, often including imaging and laboratory studies. The more ominous neurologic conditions, such as tumors, AVMs, and aneurysms, rarely present as episodic headaches. They also would have atypical histories and, usually, abnormal neurologic examinations.

Medical conditions may give secondary headaches. These are often chronic rather than episodic. Conditions associated with low cardiac output give headaches, presumed to be related to relative hypoxia of the brain with a compensatory vasodilatation of cerebral vessels. Chronic lung disease may also give headaches, presumably by the same mechanism. Anemia is associated with chronic headaches. Ironically, the anemia may be secondary to chronic analgesic use, taken initially to treat episodic headaches. Hepatic and renal disorders are associated with headaches, but the mechanism is less clear. Chronic infections, especially in the head, neck, and sinuses, are associated with headaches. Dental infections may present as chronic headaches. Myofascial pain syndromes often include the facial muscles. When chronic bruxing is part of the condition, headaches may be the presenting complaint. Waking up with headaches and tender face muscles are the clues in the history taking that help make the proper diagnosis.

Emotional disorders may present as headaches. The most common condition to present as chronic headaches is depression. This is an important diagnosis to make, because these headaches are resistant to treatment unless the depression is also addressed. Anxiety disorders are associated with headaches. Patients with bipolar disorders appear to have a high incidence of headaches as well, although more seem to occur during the depressive phase than the manic phase.

Mechanical factors may be significant causes of headaches. The headache of eye strain usually is related to either squinting the facial muscles to compensate for poor focus or leaning the neck forward for the same reason. Staring into computer screens may cause these headaches. Trying to read written material at a distance (driving, classrooms) may also cause activity-specific headaches. The cervical spine is a source of headaches to many people. Often, these patients describe the onset of the headaches by putting their hands on their necks. Others may describe headaches after reading in bed, talking on the telephone, or bird watching.

Cervicogenic headaches often give referred pain to the retro-orbital region. The "pain in my eyes" is most frequently referred pain from the neck. Detailed histories from these patients, focusing on the mechanical aspects of their daily activities, may give a clearer picture of the etiology of the headache.

Headache is a symptom that is usually intermittent and often unpredictable. It occurs at all ages. In children it can lead to impaired school performance as well as a fear of participating in socializing activities. It may limit an entire family's plans for travel or other recreational activities. In young adults, headache may be a factor that limits occupational opportunities as well as impacting family life. In older adults, headaches may be more predictable but more chronic, limiting one's total QOL.

Nature of the Impairments

It is useful once again to use the WHO formulation and the distinction made between impairment and disability.[11] (WHO, 1980) Impairment is defined as "any loss or abnormality of psychological, physiological or anatomic structure or function." Impairment thus can be considered to be at the "organ" level. Normal medical practice uses impairments to deduce the underlying pathology or disease process. The aim is to reduce the degree of impairment with the use of medication or other techniques.

A migraine attack can be a severe event, occurring unpredictably and causing complete disability to carry out any sort of functions. Alternatively, it can be a minor inconvenience, occurring infrequently and responding to mild nonprescription medications or just minimal rest. Migraine can occur without the inclusion of headache, although these events with nausea, vomiting, visual distortions, speech dysfunction, weakness, and numbness may be as severe as a more typical migraine attack with headache.

Whatever the disease process, one major disturbance is the existence of pain in these syndromes. Pain is considered to be an impairment. One objective of management can be to reduce the degree of impairment. One can seek to try to reduce the various components of pain. One can also attempt to reduce the intensity, frequency, and duration of the headaches. In the absence of abolition of pain or its extensive alleviation, and given the costs in terms of the side effects of medication and so forth, the objective can also become the reduction of the disabilities, that is, the degree of disruption of one's life despite the continued existence of the recurrent pain. Particularly helpful in the case of migraine is relief from the unexpected nature of the episodes.

Nature of the Disabilities and Handicaps

Disability refers to the functional (behavioral) consequences of any pathology or impairments, or both. The WHO definition of disability is "any restriction or lack (resulting from an impairment) of ability to perform an activity within the range considered normal for a human being." *Disabilities* refer to the effects that the impairments have in the life of the person. They are a result of the interaction of the impairment, in this case chronic intermittent headache, and the person who is experiencing them. As such, they cannot be deduced merely from the medical-neurologic examination. Input from the patient is necessary for their proper identification. The specific disabilities to be ameliorated vary with the goals and the characteristics of the person. Normal rehabilitation practice deals with this level of analysis. The aim is to reduce the degree to which the person with headache is disabled by it.

The term *suffering* in the context of the existence of pain relates to the overwhelming impact it can sometimes have on the person and his or her family.

Cassell[12] is eloquent in describing this feeling. This phenomenon addresses the degree to which the pain is perceived to be a threat to the integrity of the person who is experiencing it. It can be seen as a result of one's sense of loss of control. Suffering can relate more specifically to the degree to which one is prevented from carrying out one's roles. Pain and suffering are not the same, although they are often closely identified. Suffering can occur in the absence of pain. Conversely, pain can be present without the subjective feeling of a sense of suffering. It is thus possible that one can help alleviate suffering without necessarily doing away with the pain.

In the context of chronic headache such as is described in this chapter, suffering can be felt when the pain is recurrent and without apparent end. Moreover, in the case of intermittent pain such as in migraine, patients with recurrent pain even suffer in the absence of their pain, merely anticipating its return. They may constantly worry whether it will reappear to ruin another important occasion.

Headache can cause disability by a number of mechanisms. The obvious one is that people with headaches are not able to function at their normal level. This may imply that they do not go to work or school because of headaches, do not partake in normal recreational or family activities, or function at a very reduced level of effectiveness. Various studies have been carried out to document these points, including a Canadian,[13] an English,[14] and an American study.[15] Headache results in loss of work days. In addition, it causes people to go to work but not accomplish very much. The employers are paying for a full day's work but getting only a fraction of it. The person with the headache has to make up the lost productivity on subsequent days, increasing emotional and physical job stress and the risk of triggering another headache.

Certain occupations are more difficult for people with headaches. Occupations that require rotating shifts tend to produce increased headaches in people with migraine. Emergency medicine and nursing, fire fighting, police work, and flying on commercial airplanes are good examples of industries to which people with migraine have a difficult time adapting. They either avoid these positions or go into them with the realization that they are likely to have increased sick time due to increased frequency of headaches. Exposure to strong smells increases headache risk. Working in cosmetic sales or in refin-

eries may be off limits for people with recurrent headaches. Agricultural chemicals, exhaust fumes, and tobacco smoke, to name a few, all can produce headaches and may limit job choices for people who experience them.

Case 1

A 46-year-old nurse-anesthetist had a history of migraine since age 12 years. The migraines generally occurred five or six times a year, producing 1 or 2 days of disability each year. With the onset of perimenopausal symptoms, her migraine attacks increased in frequency and intensity. She noted that doing on-call work and overtime work usually triggered a disabling event the next day. Her request to be taken off the on-call schedule and to limit her work to daytime only was initially denied by her supervisors. Eventually a compromise was reached in which she was able to work only the day shift, but at a significant reduction in her base pay and with no chance to increase her income by filling in, even on days, for people on leave or on vacation.

This is an example of some of the economic impact of headache that is not appreciated when describing it as "just a headache." It is still difficult to qualify for disability in most states because of headaches. The lack of a positive imaging study, laboratory test, or physical finding makes many physicians and most disability evaluators uncomfortable in acknowledging headache as a chronic illness that can limit one's ability to work.

A migraine attack in any member of the family affects the lives of the whole group. People with a history of severe headaches will not plan family activities due to the risk of having to call everything off. The entire family either limits their plans or proceeds without the one family member who may "slow things down." Various activities are minimized due to the possibility of inducing a headache. Because altitude changes and long car trips can lead to headaches, trips to the mountains, the beach, or an outdoor concert may all be limited because of the fear of triggering an event. Even such simple activities as going to a baseball or a soccer game are risky for people with headache, because sunlight and hot weather can set off an attack. Indoor events are often limited due to the risk of a headache-inducing exposure to perfume or other strongly scented products. Children who complain of getting headaches in church every Sunday are often (unknowingly) making the observation that the use of perfume, scented hair sprays, and deodorants by the people around them is making them sick.

Exercise can induce migraine in some people. This limits other recreational options and social activities even further. This limitation may in turn influence the entire family and its recreational planning. Going to national parks, where hiking to specific sights is often required, may be avoided because of the risk of inducing a headache. Camping, with the need to carry supplies, is also avoided in the interest of preventing a headache.

Most people try to treat their headaches rather than ignore them. The single most common treatment, aspirin, has proved its effectiveness and relative safety. It does not impair cognitive function, and excessive use is usually marked by gastrointestinal upset or tinnitus, or both, causing people to reduce their intake or change to a different medication. The second most common treatment is acetaminophen. This medication has also proved to be effective, but, because of a lack of rapid feedback, when it is used to excess, liver and kidney problems can occur before the patient is aware that the medication is being overused. Other common nonprescription treatments include caffeine, ibuprofen, and naproxen. All of the nonsteroidal anti-inflammatory drugs can cause gastrointestinal upsets as well as hepatic and renal damage. Caffeine, a component of many headache remedies, causes sleep disturbances as a side effect as well as increased muscle tension.

A recently recognized complication of many of these nonprescription medications is the phenomenon of rebound headaches.[16] Daily headaches of increasing severity gradually begin to develop in patients who have had intermittent headaches. These typically occur on awakening in the morning and can be alleviated by taking one of the offending medications. The headache returns in a few hours, and the process is repeated. Significant amounts of medication (10–30 pills per day) may be consumed before the patient seeks professional help. A gradual and often uncomfortable drug withdrawal program is usually needed to treat the rebound headache before treatment of the original headache can start.

Case 2

Bilateral occipital headaches developed in a 44-year-old male physician 1 year before he was seen in the neurology department. Because he was frequently on call, he treated himself with a nonprescription medication that contained aspirin, acetaminophen, and caffeine. He felt that this was a safe treatment and would not impair his judgment if he had to return to the hospital at night. The headaches gradually increased, and his medication usage gradually increased as well. Within 6 months of the onset of this treatment, he was taking two pills every 4 hours around the clock. If he did not take them, his headache would become "unbearable." He began waking with headache at 4:00 AM and found that two or three pills would alleviate his symptoms and allow him to return to sleep and wake up in the morning headache free.

By the time this patient was seen in the neurology department, he was taking 18 pills per day and still having headaches, of varying severity, every day. His neurologic examination was normal. No other etiology for his headaches could be found. A gradual drug withdrawal program was instituted, and his headaches diminished to their baseline level (one to two per week) within 6 weeks of his withdrawal from analgesic and caffeine. A biofeedback program and relaxation training were started, with significant reduction in his headaches. No new medications were prescribed.

This is not an uncommon problem in patients with headaches that start as intermittent events and become chronic daily headaches. The diagnosis is made by the normal examination and the history. A review of nonprescription analgesics and vitamin intake is essential, because it is not usually included in the medical history and may be omitted as "unimportant" by the patient.

Headache is clearly a significant cause of disability. It is extremely common and affects patients throughout their life. The disability can be from the pain, nausea, vomiting, photophobia, sonophobia, motion sensitivity, food intolerance, or medications used for treatment. A significant factor is fear of headache, which causes depression, emotional stress, medication overuse, and a very poor sense of overall well-being, even when the patient is not having a headache. Headache affects the entire family unit, with decreased ability to plan activities and the need to curtail activities when they may be only partially completed.

Headache is expensive. Major costs accrue from their effects. These include cost of medical visits, medications, imaging studies, laboratory studies, time off work, reduced efficiency while at work,[17] time the spouse is off work to care for the patient, and costs of canceled plans.

Character of the Solution

Overall Plan

The goal is to reduce the burden of illness. Recognizing that headache is a generally benign condition, the treatment plan has to focus on self-management and avoidance of treatment-induced complications. Reduction of pain is the goal of most individuals with headache. A more realistic goal might be reduction of the functional and emotional disability associated with chronic headaches. How to achieve these goals is a multifaceted task.

Diagnosis is critical to the overall plan. Although no specific tests are available for most headaches, the ability to define the headache with some degree of certainty is essential for patients to become active participants in the treatment plan. As long they still think that they have a brain tumor, they can never accept that the next headache is anything other than the sign of impending disaster. Headaches secondary to other medical conditions may be amenable to actual cure, and headaches secondary to medications may be totally avoidable. Headaches from toxic chemicals can be identified and prevented. When mechanical factors aggravate existing headaches, these can often be modified. Making a diagnosis of an emotional disorder such as depression is likely to lead to more appropriate treatment and understanding of the headache than is treating the headache alone.

Fear of medical personnel is another issue that must be addressed. Most patients with chronic or recurrent headaches have had experiences with the medical system that have been unproductive in addressing the patients' concerns. They have been brushed off as not being ill or being told that "it's all in your head." They are often accused of drug-seeking behavior. This fear may lead patients with long-standing, disabling headaches to fail to get appropriate treatment even when new treatments are available. It is necessary to establish an ongoing relationship with the health professional that is based on trust. Continuity of care is a basic principle.

Often the headache is a composite of a primary headache disorder such as migraine, complicated by analgesic rebound, sleep disorders, emotional upset over the headache, family and job stress (often related to the headache), and a sense of being out of control. Good care requires the practitioner to identify each of these issues and set up a plan with the patient to address them. One principle of adequate management must be a comprehensive approach.

"Fear of headache" is an extremely important issue to address with the patient. Every little twinge of a headache induces fear of a major headache with associated buildup of muscle tension, anxiety, and depression. It also leads to consumption of large amounts of medication in an attempt to prevent the progression of the headache. It causes people to cancel plans or not to make plans for that day or that weekend because of a possible headache. The fear factor often makes a small headache into a large one. Drug addiction may occur secondary to the fear of headache. It also creates a disability where one need not exist.

Medications used in the treatment of headache have potential side effects that are often overlooked in this generally healthy population. Sedation, depression, impaired judgment, decreased exercise tolerance, drug addiction, hair loss, weight gain, loss of libido, behavioral changes, hypotension, and hypertension are all seen as potential complications from headache medications. Headaches may be annoying and potentially disabling on an intermittent basis. What the medications often do is to create a chronic problem out of an intermittent one and change an annoying, benign process into a potentially lethal one as a result of drug complications.

Medication side effects can be a significant factor in the cost of headache. Somnolence may be significant with many of the drugs used for acute care or prevention. Gastrointestinal upset is another common problem. Constipation is seen with all narcotic analgesics. Depression and exercise intolerance are a problem with beta blockers. Ataxia, slurred speech, weight gain, and poor sleep are seen with many of these medications. In the treatment of a "benign" condition, many patients may become disabled or significantly impaired due to the side effects of the treatments. One principle in the management of persons with chronic headache is to make such care effective with minimal use of medication.

The cost of medical care needs to be considered in people with headaches. Costs are distributed among the insurers, the medical providers, and the patient. The cost of phone calls to the doctor's office, office visits, emergency visits, laboratory tests, imaging studies, and even hospitalization may be substantial in this group of patients. The cost of a phone call can be calculated in terms of the staff time, chart review, and call-back time. A visit to the office is another cost that can be substantial if done frequently. Simply walking in the door to an emergency department is costly. Even for patients with insurance, the copayment factors for visits can add up to a substantial amount of money over a year (or yearly over many years). Many patients who come to a new provider have imaging studies performed or repeated. Routine laboratory tests are also ordered and repeated as patients return to the medical setting, often seeing new providers on each visit, especially if the visits are during off hours.

Another principle relating to the cost-effectiveness of management must be concern with continuity of care. This enables the patient not only to reduce the frequency with which he or she needs to seek medical advice but provides the ability to deal with problems so that emergency care, which is more costly and less effective, is needed less often.

A working partnership must be established, with realistic goals regarding the nature of the problem and planned improvements. Most headaches do not go away. They can be managed in such a way that they no longer induce panic at the onset and no longer are running, and ruining, a person's life. The starting point for all treatment plans must involve patients taking an active rather than passive role in their care. The principles of cost-effective management of persons with chronic headache are those of continuity of care over time, comprehensive care dealing with the whole patient, and treatment in a fashion that is collaborative, enlisting the patient or family, or both.

Individual Treatment Plan

Ongoing comprehensive care can be considered to be a recurrent planning and evaluation process in which patients become better able to plan and evaluate themselves. The details of the collaborative planning and treatment process are described in Chapter 2. Its application in dealing with the management of persons with chronic headache is illustrated.

Several ground rules are useful to establish at the start but need to be reinforced again and again. One is, *Nothing we do will work all of the time.* One should be realistic in expectations. It is not always someone's fault that a headache occurred and interfered with some planned activity. Sometimes a headache is a way of telling patients that they need a break from the daily grind.

Another ground rule is, *Everything we do will have some impact on the headache, no matter how small.* Small changes add up. The total impact of headache on one's life will be reduced, but slowly.

Basic is acceptance of the principle that the overall goal is to reduce disability: *Headache is a lifelong condition that we "manage" rather than cure.* Again, realistic expectations can avoid the frustration that most patients with chronic recurrent headaches have felt. It is also important for the doctor to realize that a cure for headache is rarely available. We would not expect ourselves to cure diabetes, but we assume that a benign condition such as headache should be curable.

What Is the Problem?

The process of planning with the patient starts with the definition of the problem. Patients need to think about the question, "What gives you a headache?" They need time to consider a vast variety of possibilities. Often, off-the-cuff remarks such as "it's my kids" or "it's my spouse" need to be taken seriously. They often are the first open admission of stress factors at home. "It's my job" or "it's my boss" are equally telling statements that provide a point at which to begin further evaluations. Many patients are able to identify foods that give them headaches but may not be aware of combinations or amounts of certain items needed to induce headaches. Alcohol is an important issue in a headache interview. Some patients report that alcohol helps their headache, whereas others report it as a trigger factor. Many people state that they do not use it at all. When questioned further, some say that they have never liked alcohol or that it makes them sick. That answer is suggestive of a migraine diagnosis, with alcohol intolerance as one of the major factors. Every subsequent visit needs to include the question, "What is giving you headaches now?"

This question should also address the ways in which headaches are affecting the patients' lives. In addition to defining the causes of the headaches and, it is hoped, reducing their frequency and intensity, one is also trying to reduce the disability. One needs to help the patient make the transition to deal with goals that reflect the functional aspects, even if the headaches continue.

What Is the Goal?

The number of "good days" in a month might be a starting point. Each month with an increasing number of good days would be considered a successful month. Alternative goals might relate to the ability to carry out certain activities that are of high priority for that particular person. The definition of a good day can vary and become reflective of a higher level of performance, and it can also become more specific. It is important for the goal to be clear enough that it can be measured by the patient. This can enable the person to see progress. Another goal could relate to simultaneously reducing the amount of medication. Still another goal could be the ability to identify some of the precipitating factors of headaches to increase the predictability of the episodes, thus limiting the amount of disturbance in the life of the patient.

What Are the Outcomes?

A detailed headache diary is an essential starting point in an overall headache care plan. The first step is to identify the days and the times during the day that headaches occur, and the relationship to stress factors, foods, weather, travel, medications, and sleep and hormone cycles. Part of the diary would include self-assessments as to severity, how long the headache lasted, and what degree of disability was associated with the particular headache event. In general, the headache diary should monitor the goals that were established.

Case 3

A 45-year-old woman was seen for new-onset headaches. They were diffuse and throbbing and occurred daily. No aura and no obvious trigger factors were present. The headaches became progressively severe to the extent that they would interfere with sleep. The lack of sleep and the headache eventually caused her to go on disability from her work (clerical). Medical history included hepatitis 20 years ago with chronically elevated liver function tests. She denied the use of any medications or alcohol or tobacco products. A complete neurologic examination and imaging studies were normal. Her headaches disappeared for one month, only to recur with increased intensity. During the remission, she denied any change in her lifestyle, emotional status, or occupational state. Her husband was concerned about the progressive illness and eventually brought in some tubes of tretinoin (Retin-A) that she had been using for the past 6 months for her new-onset acne. The medication was not prescribed by a physician but was given to her by a friend who had found it helpful. Because it was a skin cream and not a "drug," she never mentioned it during the review of her history. During the 1 month that the headaches had disappeared, she had stopped the medication, only to restart when her acne got worse again. When the amended history was known, the Retin-A was stopped. The headaches disappeared in 2 weeks and have not recurred. Because retinols may be poorly detoxified in patients with pre-existing hepatic abnormalities, and retinol toxicity is known to give throbbing, diffuse headaches, in retrospect, this should have been an easy diagnosis to make. In reality, it took many months because of the lack of a complete medication review.

What Works?

By keeping this type of diary, patterns appear. One is interested in establishing a relationship between the outcomes and the actions taken (or not taken) by the patient. Addressing this question begins to change the perception of the patient as to his or her sense of control over the outcomes. With the headache diary, one can begin to help the patient address this crucial question.

One can begin to recognize patterns regarding headache trigger factors. They may be subtle: For example, one's tolerance for alcohol may be reduced 1 week before menses, whereas it is unaffected during other times of the month. The pattern may be very obvious, such as Monday morning headaches before going back to school or work. Saturday or Sunday headaches may occur after sleeping late or not drinking coffee at the usual hour. Headaches may follow long car trips or occur most often when one skips meals. Food triggers, such as chocolate, pork, monosodium glutamate, beans, or artificial sweeteners, may be identified. Headaches in the workplace can be difficult to sort out because of emotional factors; the ergonomic factors of the work site; not eating on a regular schedule; and strong smells from cosmetics used by coworkers, visitors, or customers. The type of lighting may influence headaches, and toxic chemicals may be a factor. All of these would need to be evaluated by gradual elimination, as much as that is possible.

A headache diary also allows one to recognize mood swings as contributors to the problem. Emotional reactions to situations ("my mother-in-law gives me headaches") are important to identify in helping to establish control over the headaches. New medications may be a factor in aggravating existing headaches or triggering new ones. Nitrates, cimetidine, and tetracyclines are typical examples of medications that are associated with headaches. Sometimes it takes serious detective work on the part of the patient and the doctor to identify the culprit.

Another important question needs to be what the patients feel will make their headaches better. Their expectations are essential to establishing a working plan for better headache control. Patients who only want medications are not likely to be receptive to a first suggestion that they need relaxation training. Similarly, patients who are asking about alternative therapies do not want to hear about daily prophylactic medications. Many people are willing to listen to alternative treatments if the physician can acknowledge their first concerns and make them part of an overall plan. One can start treatment using one modality of care and gradually add in others to achieve an acceptable balance. Most people are willing to change their lifestyles and eating patterns as part of a headache treatment plan, but they need to know that the physician is willing to expand to other modalities "if this isn't working." The working relationship between provider and patient must allow for realistic expectations by both.

Most patients with headaches either are using medications or have used them in the past. The goal is to design a plan that the patient and the practitioner are comfortable with as to how to use medication effectively, if at all. Some patients only feel comfortable if they have "something" to take when they feel that a headache is starting. Others prefer not to use medications at all. The general concept is that daily analgesics are not advisable, as they are likely to lead to analgesic rebound headaches. Simple, over-the-counter analgesics are preferable to prescription medications for treating acute headaches because they are likely to be less expensive, have fewer side effects, and have less addiction potential.[18] Depending on the type of headache being treated, specific analgesics, antianxiety medications, muscle relaxants, and antimigraine medications may be appropriate.[19] Again, the goal is to use the least amount of medication possible, with a plan to eventually eliminate the need for any drugs.

One concept in headache care is stepwise use of medication with specific guidelines as to when to move from one level to the next. At the onset of a mild headache, some sort of relaxation technique can be applied and, if needed, followed by a nonprescription analgesic. If the headache progresses after 2 hours, a stronger analgesic is used. If the headache can be defined as a migraine by the patient, a migraine-specific medication can be used. In this system, taking large amounts of ineffective medication would be reduced, with reduced frustration and anxiety as well as reduced medication side effects. The risk of rebound headaches is also decreased using this system.

If the headaches are chronic, occurring almost daily or causing significant disability, prophylactic therapy is indicated.[20] In general, daily headaches from analgesic rebound respond poorly to this form of treatment, but for most other headaches, prophylaxis is the appropriate therapeutic approach. Various categories of drugs can be used, including beta blockers, calcium channel blockers, antidepressants, muscle relaxants, antiepileptics, ergotamine derivatives, and anti-inflammatory medications. New medications continue to be developed. Older medications are still used in treating chronic headaches. The problem with chronic daily medication is the occurrence of side effects. Although these are often an acceptable tradeoff in people with severe underlying illnesses, most patients with headaches are younger, basi-

Table 12-1. Common Side Effects
of Preventive Medications

Preventive Medications	Side Effects
Beta blockers	Asthma
	Fatigue
	Exercise intolerance
	Depression
Tricyclic antidepressants	Weight gain
	Drowsiness
	Urinary retention
	Dry mouth
	Blurred vision
Valproic acid	Tremor
	Weight gain
	Nausea
	Hair loss
Calcium channel blockers	Constipation
	Hypotension
Ergotamine derivatives	Tingling hands and feet
	Retroperitoneal fibrosis
	Nausea
Nonsteroidal anti-inflam-	Gastrointestinal irritation
matory drugs	Hepatic injury
Muscle relaxants	Drowsiness
	Incoordination
Gabapentin	Drowsiness

Table 12-2. Common Side Effects
of Abortive Medications

Abortive Medications	Side Effects
Aspirin	Gastrointestinal irritation
	Tinnitus
Acetaminophen	Hepatic injury
Caffeine	Insomnia
	Irritability
	Addiction
Barbiturates	Drowsiness
	Slowed thinking
	Addiction
Narcotic analgesics	Slowed thinking
	Short acting
	Addiction
Ergotamine derivatives	Nausea
	Peripheral vasoconstriction
	Addiction
Triptan medications	Chest tightness
	Peripheral vasoconstriction
Dopamine blockers	Movement disorders
	Drowsiness
	Restlessness

cally healthier, and less tolerant of side effects. Typical medications and their potential side effects are described in Tables 12-1 and 12-2.

A number of nonpharmacologic treatments for headache have been used over the years. They are now accepted as part of comprehensive care for patients with this chronic and potentially disabling condition. They should be considered a part of an approach that seeks to minimize the problems caused by medication. Nonpharmacologic treatment plans are essential for women who are pregnant, plan to be pregnant, or are nursing. They are also important for patients with other medical conditions that may preclude their use of typical headache medications.

Stress management has been used to reduce muscle tension, reduce chronic bruxism, and improve sleep patterns. All of these factors are important in preventing headaches as well as in treating them once they begin. Biofeedback has also been used for many years. It is most effective in treating migraine but has been successfully used to treat temporomandibular disorders, ten-

puncture and acupressure are ancient techniques that are being used increasingly to treat all varieties of headaches. Physical therapy and chiropractic treatments are being used in headache care, especially when mechanical factors in the neck and base of the skull are contributing to the painful condition. Exercise programs act to prevent headaches, perhaps by increasing circulating endorphins. Group meetings of people with headache may help relieve some of the anxiety and stress through understanding that others have similar problems and have learned coping skills that they are willing to share.

The most effective nonpharmacologic treatment is education. This involves the patient and the family. A clear understanding of the nature of the problem is important. Being able to recognize the dos and don'ts as well as the maybes is part of learning how to live with a chronic condition and not panic at every new event. Making ample reading material available lets patients know that they are not alone in this situation. As they become more familiar with the methods that work for themselves, the ideas become modified and their own.

Case 4

A 52-year-old woman reported increasing headache disability. She began getting headaches associated with menarche at age 14. They typically would be associated with her menstrual cycles, although they "disappeared" for approximately 10 years between ages 25 and 35. Over the last 10 years, they have been increasing in frequency and severity. She holds two jobs and feels she cannot take time out to deal with her headaches. Her use of nonsteroidal anti-inflammatory drugs increased until gastritis developed, at which time she was forced to use acetaminophen-containing combination analgesics. When these were no longer effective, she began using a triptan medication, gradually increasing her intake to 10 pills a week. The amount of time she was missing from work, the decrease in her job performance rating, and the increasing cost of her medications forced her to seek further care for her headaches. Her family was concerned about her being continuously ill and unable to take part in social events.

A detailed history and physical examination established the diagnoses of migraine, tension headache, and analgesic rebound headache.

Treatment plans included realistic work, sleep, and eating schedules. This required her to acknowledge the necessity of relaxation time and the need to say no to added activities. An exercise program was agreed on, starting at twice a week for half an hour with increments each month. A medication reduction plan was instituted with a goal of no daily medications and limiting analgesics or triptans to twice a week. Two weeks of medical disability was scheduled to allow the treatment plan to start without other conflicting issues. She was advised to join a headache support group in the community.

The improvements took place in a stepwise manner. She rapidly decreased her medication use because of economic necessity. She was able to reduce her overtime and extra projects at work. Starting a regular exercise program was met with resistance but eventually occurred. She enrolled in a biofeedback program, which reduced her need for medications below the original goal. She still has headaches but is more in control of her life.

Not all treatment plans are successful from a medical point of view. The patients define the degree of pain, suffering, disability, and when to ask for help. The patients also define what is an acceptable level of improvement. The physician's role is to agree on common goals and appropriate ways to attain them.

Treatment of headache has to involve realistic expectations from the patients, their families, and the physicians. Most headaches are managed rather than cured. This means that treatments need to be discussed frequently regarding potential benefits, side effects, and costs. Costs in this setting may be financial but may also be the cost of a change in lifestyle, change in diet, or other behavior modification. Medications are often a major aspect of headache treatment. The disability from the medications may outweigh the disability from the headaches. Medications often lose their effectiveness over time and need to be changed or rotated. New treatments for headache are always in the news but are not appropriate for every patient. The physician and the patient have to decide together about many of these issues.

Measuring Effectiveness

Outcome measurements are used to monitor effectiveness of various treatments. In accordance with the WHO classification we have been using, outcomes can be measured on several levels. Number and severity of headaches are measures of the degree of impairment. The degree of headache-related disability also needs to be monitored. Treatment-related problems such as medication side effects can be part of the overall equation as well. One of the most important and least used items is the QOL score. The goal of medical care has always been to improve the QOL of our patients. Effective headache care may be one of the most significant improvements that we can make in a patient's overall QOL.

The goals of headache management are to reduce suffering, reduce disability, reduce reliance on the medical care system, and improve QOL. The measurements may be as simple as a self-report of "I'm much better, thank you," to a complex formula involving cost of resource utilization, disability rating scales, emotional cost, out-of-pocket costs, and QOL and depression ratings.[21-23]

We are able to calculate the cost of resource utilization. Cost of care is of concern to many people but is probably not significant when measured against the true cost of headache disability. It includes the cost of office and emergency department visits, cost of prescription medication, and cost of imaging and laboratory studies as well as the cost of telephone contact with the medical offices regarding headache. Inpatient costs may be included in this calculation, although this modality is rarely used.

The cost of headache-related disability is slightly more subjective. It includes the cost of days lost from work, whether compensated (sick leave) or uncompensated, because the day's work is still lost. If the patient is employed in a management position in which other people's work is dependent on his or her decision making, a much larger amount of work is lost due to this one person's impaired functioning. These costs remain uncalculated. Other costs of disability may include a spouse taking time off from work to care for the patient or to care for the children.

The Migraine Disability Assessment[24] has been developed to try to quantify the burden of migraine. It is a seven-question instrument that asks how many days of work were missed and during how many days (at work) productivity was less than 50% due to headache in the previous 3 months. The same questions were asked regarding housework and missing family, social, or leisure activities. The questionnaire includes disability due to side effects of the medications. It gives the physician and the patient substantial information and realistic goals when trying to define treatment plans.

Emotional cost can be documented in depression rating and QOL scales.[25–28] QOL scores include issues of being out of control of one's life, fear of headache, and feelings of letting others down because of one's inability to participate in activities. Additional issues in QOL scores focus on fatigue related to headache or medication, poor concentration, needing to ask for help, and feelings of frustration. Family ratings should also be used when evaluating the outcome of headache treatment and QOL scores. The patient may report little or no change, but family members may notice a great difference in day-to-day functioning. The opposite may also occur.

Out-of-pocket expenses related to headache may include tickets to events that were not used or canceled trips with nonrefundable deposits or plane tickets. The costs of nontraditional treatments, such as acupuncture, biofeedback, massage, or chiropractic, are often not a covered benefit on people's health insurance. The cost of nonprescription medications and herbal remedies may become significant and is rarely covered by insurance. The

multiple trips to the medical offices or hospital are usually accompanied by copayments.

As noted above, headache is an expensive condition to the patients, their families, their employers, and the medical health care system.[29] A headache management program was established at the author's medical center to try to address as many of the concerns as possible in a cost-effective manner.

Identification of appropriate candidates was made through the primary care departments with a yes answer to the question, "Are headaches a problem for you?" Anyone who sought care in the emergency department for their headaches was also referred. Patients were then asked about their interest in a teaching program to give them skills to manage their headaches, in addition to whatever other treatments might be appropriate. They were also asked to fill out a more detailed questionnaire regarding their headaches, the impact of the headaches on work and family, and the extent of disability related to headaches. This questionnaire served to address concerns and provided the basis for the eventual development of goals by each patient.

The emphasis of the treatment, carried out by a nurse practitioner, was to provide the patients with opportunities for reducing the likelihood of headaches. Further, a goal was to reduce the sense of unpredictability to alleviate the need for emergency department treatment. The focus was on appropriate use of medications along with lifestyle changes and other techniques to reduce dependence on medication. An educational approach was taken, with an initial group meeting and then subsequent individual sessions that lasted approximately 15 minutes each.

At the initial group meeting, the patients had a chance to share concerns, some of the precipitating factors that seemed to be relevant to each as well as what may have helped to prevent headaches. At the end of the session each would also set goals. The goals were not necessarily in terms of reducing the incidence and severity of the headaches per se. Rather, the focus was on improving QOL and on greater control over one's life. The concept of keeping a diary to reflect the goals that had been met was also introduced. The group process was itself useful because commonality was found in the answers to many of the planning questions.

At an individual follow-up session approximately 1 month later, the diary would be reviewed as a measure of status in relation to the goals that were originally set. Particular attention would be paid to the relationship between the headache and any triggers. Eventually patients could critically review the diary on their own and recognize such relationships. A new goal would then be set, for example, to reduce the use of emergency treatment.

Medications were adjusted, often downward, due to prevalence of analgesic rebound headaches in this group. During the course of a year, cost of medication for headache used in the medical center decreased by one-third. This was true even though more individuals were being specifically treated for migraine. The reduction in total cost would reflect medications being used more effectively because the cost per patient was less. Prevention strategies may have also contributed to this result by reducing the number of headaches per person. Emergency visits for treatment of headache decreased by 27%. Apparently, many of the persons who had previously come for emergency treatment now had the skills both to prevent headaches and to properly medicate themselves when needed. They were also less likely to be fearful of their headaches because they had a regimen that they could follow. Furthermore, disability days decreased by 40%.

The use of this relatively inexpensive headache management program has been able to give patients the skills both to prevent headaches and to treat themselves appropriately when a headache occurs. The treatment process was based on the recurrent use of the basic planning questions. Assessment of effectiveness deals not only with the reduction in the number and severity of headaches but extends to the effects on the patient's QOL and degree of disability and the impact on the health care system. All these parameters must be measured if one is to develop plans for the management of persons with chronic neurologic illness due to headaches.

References

1. Headache Classification Committee of the International Headache Society. Classification and diagnostic criteria for headache disorders, cranial neuralgias and facial pain. Cephalalgia 1988;8:9–96.
2. Stewart WF, Lipton RB, Celentano DD, Reed ML. Prevalence of migraine headache in the United States. JAMA 1992;267:64–69.
3. Stewart WF, Staffa J, Lipton RB, Ottman R. Familial risk of migraine: a population-based study. Ann Neurol 1997;41:166–172.
4. Lipton RB, Stewart WF, Von Korff M. Migraine impact and functional disability. Cephalalgia 1995;15(suppl):4–9.
5. Osterhaus JT, Gutterman DL, Plachetka JR. Healthcare resource and lost labour costs of migraine headache in the US. Pharmacoeconomics 1992;2:67–76.

6. Stewart WF, Lipton RB, Simon D. Work-related disability: results from the American migraine study. Cephalalgia 1996;16:231–238.
7. Mounstephen AH, Harrison RK. A study of migraine and its effects in a working population. Occup Med 1995;45: 311–317.
8. Ziegler DK, Paolo AM. Self-reported disability due to headache: a comparison of clinic patients and controls. Headache 1996;36:476–480.
9. Peroutka SJ. Dopamine and migraine. Neurology 1997;49:650–656.
10. Somerville BW. Estrogen withdrawal migraine. Neurology 1975;25:239–244.
11. World Health Organization. The International Classification of Impairments, Disabilities and Handicaps. Geneva: WHO, 1980.
12. Cassell E. The Nature of Suffering and the Goals of Medicine. New York: Oxford University Press, 1991;36.
13. Edmeads J, Findlay H, Tugwell P, et al. Impact of migraine and tension-type headache on life style, consulting behaviour and medication use: a Canadian population study. Can J Neurol Sci 1993;20:131–137.
14. Clarke CE, MacMillan L, Sondhi S, Wells NEJ. Economic and social impact of migraine. QJM 1996;89:77–84.
15. Schwartz BS, Stewart WF, Lipton RB. Lost workdays and decreased work effectiveness associated with headache in the workplace. J Occup Environ Med 1997;39:320–327.
16. Rapoport A. Analgesic rebound headache. Headache 1988;28:662–665.
17. Lipton RB, Stewart WF, von Korff M. Burden of migraine: societal costs and therapeutic opportunities. Neurology 1997;48(suppl 3):S4–S9.
18. Capobianco DJ, Cheshire WP, Campbell JK. An overview of the diagnosis and pharmacologic treatment of migraine. Mayo Clin Proc 1996;71:1055–1066.
19. Moore KL, Noble SL. Drug treatment of migraine: part 1. Acute therapy and drug-rebound headache. Am Fam Physician 1997;56:2039–2054.
20. Noble SL, Moore KL. Drug treatment of migraine: part II. Preventive therapy. Am Fam Physician 1997;56:2279–2286.
21. Jacobson GP, Ramadan NM, Aggarwal SK, Newman CW. The Henry Ford Hospital headache disability inventory (HDI). Neurology 1994;44:837–842.
22. Solomon GD, Skobieranda FG, Gragg LA. Does quality of life differ among headache diagnoses? Analysis using the medical outcomes study instrument. Headache 1994;34:143–147.
23. Solomon GD. Evolution of the measurement of quality of life in migraine. Neurology 1997;48(suppl 3):S10–S15.
24. Sawyer J, Edmeads J, Lipton RB, et al. Clinical utility of a new instrument assessing migraine disability: the migraine disability instrument (MIDAS) questionnaire. Neurology 1999;53:988–994.
25. Santanello NC, Hartmaier SL, Epstein RS, Silberstein SD. Validation of a new quality of life questionnaire for acute migraine headache. Headache 1995;35:330–337.
26. Hartmaier SL, Santanello NC, Epstein RS, Silberstein SD. Development of a brief 24-hour migraine-specific quality of life questionnaire. Headache 1995;35:320–329.
27. Osterhaus JT, Townsend RJ, Gandek B, Ware JE. Measuring the functional status and well-being of patients with migraine headaches. Headache 1994;34:337–343.
28. Stewart WF, Shechter A, Lipton RB. Migraine heterogeneity: disability, pain intensity, and attack frequency and duration. Neurology 1994;44(suppl 4):S24–S39.
29. Fishman O, Black L. Indirect cost of migraine in a managed care population. Cephalalgia 1999;19:50–57.

Index